David W. Brook, MD
Henry I. Spitz, MD
Editors

The Group Therapy
of Substance Abuse

Pre-publication
REVIEWS,
COMMENTARIES,
EVALUATIONS . . .

"**D**avid Brook and Henry Spitz, two very highly respected clinicians, have brought us a resource that can be of great assistance to anyone treating patients with substance abuse problems. It has long been demonstrated that group approaches to addictions (including self-help groups such as AA) are powerful modalities. In this book, the editors have brought together a stellar cast of experts who show us how to thoughtfully use a variety of group treatments with a variety of substance-abusing populations.

The text, while covering a vast amount of material, is well organized and logical. The first section covers a variety of introductory topics and a summary of different types of group treatments. The second section focuses more on treatment settings, while the third portion focuses on differing treatment populations. The book then moves to a review of the use of groups with specific diagnostic categories, and it finishes with an examination of research and ethical issues as well as some attempts to predict future trends. This book is a marvelous buffet that offers more than any single provider will need, but certainly has something for everyone treating substance abusers."

J. Scott Rutan, PhD
Senior Faculty, Boston Institute
for Psychotherapy; Past President,
American Group Psychotherapy
Association

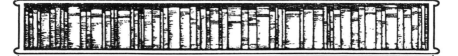

More pre-publication
REVIEWS, COMMENTARIES, EVALUATIONS . . .

"**B**rook and Spitz have edited what will become the standard text on the group therapy of substance abuse. They have assembled the leading experts on group therapy of addicted patients. Group therapy is an essential and effective method of treating patients with addictive disorders. Many of these patients have grown up with parents who are sometimes wonderful, sometimes terrible, and often addicted, and they tend to trust their siblings and peers more than authority figures. They can benefit from self-help and professionally led groups as much or more than individual counseling. These groups need to be tailored to patients with addictive disorders, comorbidity, and special populations. This book covers all of these issues and while it is evidence-based, it also takes advantage of the clinical wisdom of major leaders in the field.

A variety of group approaches from network therapy, cognitive behavioral approaches, interpersonal approaches, and self-help are expertly described. The book is scholarly yet readable and suitable for students and experienced practitioners, whether they are psychiatrists, psychologists, social workers, nurses, addiction counselors, school counselors, or based in law enforcement."

Richard J. Frances, MD, FACP, FAPA
President and Medical Director,
Silver Hill Hospital,
New Canaan, CT

"**G**roup therapy has been a mainstay of substance abuse treatment and the field has needed a comprehensive presentation of the varying approaches used to work with groups of substance abusers. This book provides just that. The chapters are well organized for the busy clinician to address a particular method of group therapy. They provide useful case material that specifically applies the principles of each therapy method within a group context. The chapters also have a coherence of themes as the authors use various 'stages of change' models in their groups to fit patients' attitudes and progress toward recovery from their addictions. Within these recurrent themes, the permutations of group treatments are illustrated for not just outpatient settings, but for therapeutic communities, inpatient programs, and a range of special populations such as women, adolescents, and schizophrenics. The group participants are also not limited to patients, but include family members and even employers when using network therapy. This book provides a wide variety of options for the work of relapse prevention in a chronic relapsing disorder."

Thomas Kosten, MD
Professor of Psychiatry,
Yale University

The Haworth Medical Press®
An Imprint of The Haworth Press, Inc.
New York • London • Oxford

The Group Therapy of Substance Abuse

HAWORTH Therapy for the Addictive Disorders
Barry Stimmel, MD
Senior Editor

The Facts About Drug Use: Coping with Drugs and Alcohol in Your Family, at Work, in Your Community by Barry Stimmel and the Editors of Consumer Reports Books

Drug Abuse and Social Policy in America: The War That Must Be Won by Barry Stimmel

Pain and Its Relief Without Addiction: Clinical Issues in the Use of Opioids and Other Analgesics by Barry Stimmel

Drugs, the Brain, and Behavior: The Pharmacology of Abuse and Dependence by John Brick and Carlton K. Erikson

The Love Drug: Marching to the Beat of Ecstasy by Richard S. Cohen

Alcoholism, Drug Addiction, and the Road to Recovery: Life on the Edge by Barry Stimmel

The Group Therapy of Substance Abuse edited by David W. Brook and Henry I. Spitz

The Group Therapy of Substance Abuse

David W. Brook, MD
Henry I. Spitz, MD
Editors

The Haworth Medical Press®
An Imprint of The Haworth Press, Inc.
New York • London • Oxford

Published by

The Haworth Medical Press ®, an imprint of The Haworth Press, Inc., 10 Alice Street, Binghamton, NY 13904-1580.

Medicine is an ever-changing science. As new research and clinical experience broaden our knowledge, changes in treatment and drug therapy are required. While many suggestions for drug usages are made herein, the book is intended for educational purposes only, and the author, editor, and publisher do not accept liability in the event of negative consequences incurred as a result of information presented in this book. We do not claim that this information is necessarily accurate by the rigid, scientific standard applied for medical proof, and therefore make no warranty, expressed or implied, with respect to the material herein contained. Therefore the patient is urged to check the product information sheet included in the package of each drug he or she plans to administer to be certain the protocol followed is not in conflict with the manufacturer's inserts. When a discrepancy arises between these inserts and information in this book, the physician is encouraged to use his or her best professional judgment.

The authors have exhaustively researched all available sources to ensure the accuracy and completeness of the information contained in this book. The publisher and authors assume no responsibility for errors, inaccuracies, omissions, or any inconsistency herein.

Cover design by Anastasia Litwak.

Library of Congress Cataloging-in-Publication Data

The group therapy of substance abuse / David W. Brook, Henry I. Spitz, editors.
    p. cm.
  Includes bibliographical references and index.
    ISBN 0-7890-1781-4 (hard : alk. paper) — ISBN 0-7890-1782-2 (soft : alk. paper)
    1. Substance abuse—Treatment. 2. Group psychotherapy. I. Brook, David W. II. Spitz, Henry I., 1941-

RC564 .G755 2002
616.86'0851—dc21

2002068656

To our wives and families—
Judith, Adam, Jon, and Nicole
and
Susan, Becky, and Jake—
for their love, good humor, and support

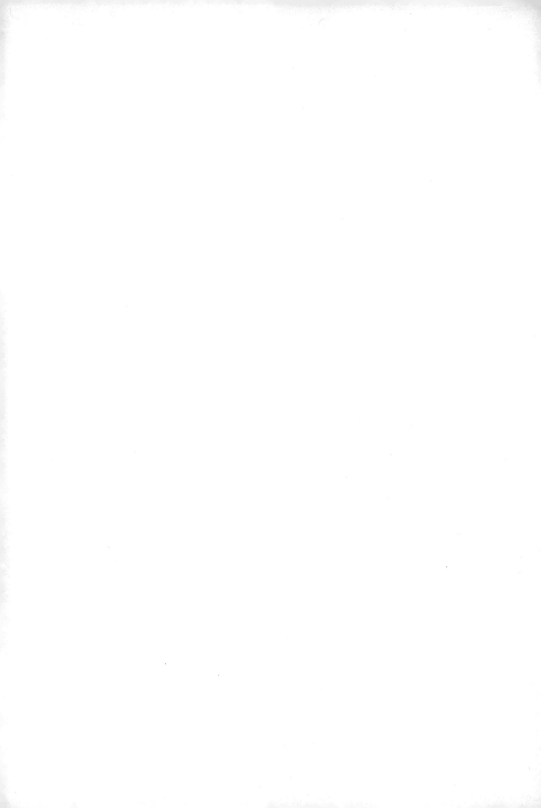

CONTENTS

SECTION II: SPECIFIC TREATMENT SETTINGS AND GOALS

SECTION III: SPECIFIC PATIENT POPULATIONS— DEMOGRAPHIC ISSUES

SECTION IV: SPECIFIC DIAGNOSTIC POPULATIONS

SECTION V: INTEGRATION AND IMPLICATIONS

ABOUT THE EDITORS

Dr. David W. Brook is Professor of Community and Preventive Medicine at the Mount Sinai School of Medicine in New York City. Previously, he was Professor of Clinical Psychiatry at New York Medical College, where he served as Director of the Division of Drug Abuse Research, Prevention, and Treatment. Dr. Brook is certified in general psychiatry and addiction psychiatry by the American Board of Psychiatry and Neurology and is a Fellow of the American Society of Addiction Medicine. He has served as a member of the Board of Directors of the American Group Psychotherapy Association, and is a past president of the Westchester Group Psychotherapy Society.

Dr. Brook is the author or co-author of more than 100 scientific publications. He has also co-edited or co-authored five books, and published in the areas of group psychotherapy, substance use and abuse, HIV, behavioral medicine, and medical education. He is a member of the editorial committee of the *International Journal of Group Psychotherapy* and the editorial board of the *Journal of Addictive Diseases*.

Dr. Henry I. Spitz is Clinical Professor of Psychiatry in the Department of Psychiatry at Columbia University, College of Physicians and Surgeons, in New York City, Director of the Group Psychotherapy and Couples Therapy programs at the Columbia-Presbyterian Medical Center and at the New York State Psychiatric Institute, and Attending Psychiatrist at New York Presbyterian Hospital.

Dr. Spitz is the author of more than 50 scientific publications in the fields of group and family therapy, and substance abuse, including *Cocaine Abuse: New Directions in Treatment and Research; Group Psychotherapy and Managed Mental Health Care, A Clinical Guide for Providers; Substance Abuse: From Principles to Practice;* and *A Pragmatic Approach to Group Psychotherapy*. He is a member of the editorial committee of the *International Journal of Group Psychotherapy* and a member of the editorial boards of *Group* and the *Amer-*

ican Journal of Family Therapy. He is a regular reviewer of manuscripts for the *American Journal of Psychiatry,* and he is a member of the Board of Directors of the National Registry of Certified Group Psychotherapists.

Both Dr. Brook and Dr. Spitz are Fellows of the American Psychiatric Association and the American Group Psychotherapy Association, and both are Certified Group Psychotherapists by the National Registry of Certified Group Psychotherapists. Both co-editors have presented extensively in workshops at national and international meetings.

CONTRIBUTORS

Mark J. Albanese, MD, is Associate Chief of Psychiatry, Tewksbury Hospital; and Assistant Clinical Professor of Psychiatry, Harvard Medical School, Hawthorne Mental Health Unit, Tewksbury, Massachusetts.

Peter Banys, MD, is Associate Clinical Professor of Psychiatry, Department of Psychiatry, UCSF School of Medicine, San Francisco, California.

Aaron T. Beck, MD, is University Professor, Department of Psychiatry, University of Pennsylvania; and President, The Beck Institute, Bala Cynwyd, Pennsylvania.

Sheila B. Blume, MD, is Clinical Professor of Psychiatry, State University of New York, Stony Brook, New York; Medical Director, Alcoholism, Chemical Dependency, and Compulsive Gambling Programs, South Oaks Hospital, Amityville, New York.

Thomas Edward Bratter, EdD, is President, The John Dewey Academy, Great Barrington, Massachusetts.

Timothy P. Carmody, PhD, is Clinical Professor of Psychiatry, UCSF School of Medicine, San Francisco, California.

George De Leon, PhD, is Director, Center for Therapeutic Community Research, National Development and Research Institutes, Inc.; and Research Professor, Department of Psychiatry, New York University Medical School, New York City.

Philip J. Flores, PhD, is Clinical Group Supervisor, Department of Psychiatry, Emory University; and Adjunct Faculty, Georgia State University and Argosy University.

Marc Galanter, MD, is Professor of Psychiatry; and Director of the Division of Alcoholism and Drug Abuse, New York University School of Medicine, New York City.

Valerie Gibbs, CSW, PhD, is in private practice, Marion, Massachusetts.

Les R. Greene, PhD, is a staff psychologist, Psychology Department, VA Connecticut Healthcare System, West Haven, Connecticut.

David J. Hellerstein, MD, is Associate Professor of Clinical Psychiatry, Columbia University College of Physicians and Surgeons; and Clinical Director, New York State Psychiatric Institute, New York City.

Keith Humphreys, PhD, is Assistant Professor, Department of Psychiatry, Stanford University Medical Center, Palo Alto, California.

Anthony S. Joyce, PhD, is Associate Professor of Psychiatry, Department of Psychiatry, University of Alberta, Edmonton, Alberta, Canada.

Edward J. Khantzian, MD, is Clinical Professor of Psychiatry, Harvard Medical School at the Cambridge Hospital, Cambridge, Massachusetts.

Howard A. Liddle, EdD, is Professor of Epidemiology, Public Health, and Psychology; and Director, Center for Treatment Research on Adolescent Drug Abuse, Department of Psychiatry and Behavioral Sciences, University of Miami School of Medicine, Miami, Florida.

Morton A. Lieberman, PhD, is Professor and Director, Memory Clinic and Alzheimer's Center, Department of Psychiatry and Langley Porter Psychiatric Institute, University of California, San Francisco, California.

Bruce S. Liese, PhD, is Professor of Family Medicine and Psychiatry and Associate Chair for Research, Department of Family Medicine, University of Kansas Medical Center; and Director, Kansas City Center for Cognitive Therapy, Kansas City, Kansas.

David M. McDowell, MD, is Assistant Clinical Professor of Psychiatry, Columbia University College of Physicians and Surgeons; and Medical Director, Substance Abuse Treatment, Research, and Service Unit, New York State Psychiatric Institute, New York City.

Roy Nelson, PhD, is Geropsychologist, Colmery-O'Neil VA Medical Center, Topeka, Kansas.

Jeanne L. Obert, MFT, MSM, is Executive Director, Matrix Institute on Addictions, Los Angeles, California.

William E. Piper, PhD, is Professor of Psychiatry, Department of Psychiatry, University of British Columbia, Vancouver, British Columbia, Canada.

Eloise Rathbone-McCuan, PhD, MSW, is Professor and Director, Graduate Social Work Education, University of Missouri–Kansas City, Kansas City, Missouri.

Richard A. Rawson, PhD, is Associate Director, UCLA Integrated Substance Abuse Programs, UCLA Department of Psychiatry and Biobehavioral Sciences, UCLA School of Medicine, Los Angeles, California.

Richard N. Rosenthal, MD, is Professor of Clinical Psychiatry, Columbia University College of Physicians and Surgeons; and Chairman, Department of Psychiatry, St. Luke's-Roosevelt Hospital Center, New York City.

Cynthia L. Rowe, PhD, is Assistant Professor of Psychology, University of Montana, Missoula, Montana; and Investigator, Center for Treatment Research on Adolescent Drug Abuse, Department of Psychiatry and Behavioral Sciences, University of Miami School of Medicine, Miami, Florida.

Kim Seaton, MA, is a graduate student in the Department of Psychology, University of Kansas, Lawrence, Kansas.

Lee Shomstein, CSW, is a social worker, Department of Psychiatry, Beth Israel Medical Center; and Group Therapist, Combined Psychiatric and Addictive Disorders Program, Beth Israel Medical Center, New York City.

Andrew Edmund Slaby, MD, PhD, MPH, is Clinical Professor of Psychiatry, New York University; and Adjunct Clinical Professor of Psychiatry, New York Medical College, New York City.

Arnold M. Washton, PhD, is Executive Director, Center for Addiction Psychology, New York City.

Foreword

As we continue to progress in our efforts to understand, prevent, and treat drug abuse and addiction, it is more imperative than ever that we rapidly disseminate these findings to the clinicians who can use this information to treat the 13.6 million Americans who are known to abuse drugs on a regular basis.

We have made tremendous progress over the past several decades that has revolutionized our understanding of drug abusers and addiction. We now know that drug abuse is a preventable behavior and that drug addiction is, fundamentally, a treatable, chronic, relapsing disease of the brain. Our research efforts have yielded practical applications for clinicians as well—providing them with a variety of behavioral and pharmacological treatments that can effectively reduce drug use, help manage drug cravings, prevent relapses, and restore people to productive functioning in society. Of the many approaches to the treatment of substance abusers, group methods have shown their broad utility, and are the focus of this text.

Although this text focuses particularly on group therapy, it is important to understand that no one treatment is appropriate for all patients. Moreover, drug treatment is not a unitary concept. As Avram Goldstein has suggested, the general approach to addiction treatment can best be described as breaking a big task into manageable bits; the combination of elements to be employed is tailored to the needs of the individual patient. Because of addictions' complexity and pervasive consequences, treatments typically involve many components. Effective treatments must attend to the multiple needs of individuals, not just their drug use.

Clinicians and researchers working with and/or researching group psychotherapy techniques have begun to explore the theoretical bases and pragmatic applications of group therapy in a variety of settings for the treatment of addiction. A judicious combination of group therapy, individual interventions, and pharmacological methods (when available) likely represents the best treatment currently available for most patients.

Group therapy has been found to be both clinically effective and cost-effective. Although both individual and group therapy have been gaining increased acceptance in the field over time, no book to date has brought together in one volume the work of a variety of expert contributors, the treatment of a range of patients representing the breadth of patients seen in the field, or the use of groups in such a wide and diverse variety of treatment settings.

Clinicians treating addicted patients can use this book to gain an increased understanding of the theories and techniques that have practical and immediate applications to clinical treatment. The organization of the book clearly delineates methods of thinking about patients in a systematized yet flexible way, and indicates techniques currently in use in a variety of settings. Clinical vignettes and the references to the literature help the clinician understand both particular treatment techniques as well as the research data on which these techniques are based.

The burgeoning interest in and use of the group setting in the treatment of substance abuse/addiction parallels our increasing understanding of the importance of groups in the development of these disorders. Group therapy is becoming more firmly embedded in the process of scientific inquiry, as the scientific method is now more widely applied both to our understanding of how groups work and to their effectiveness in the treatment of a greater range of disorders than ever before. Group therapy has been moving from a reliance on case reports and anecdotal evidence, to more complete descriptions of the group process, and into focused empirical studies designed to evaluate both the processes and outcomes of treatment. The group therapy of substance abuse is undergoing the same process, which will lead to our increased ability to use group experiences with more specificity to meet the unique needs of substance-abusing patients.

This book comes at a critical time for both patients and clinicians and represents "cutting edge" efforts to use group therapy to help substance abusers and addicts. This fine collection assembled by Drs. Brook and Spitz adds both depth and breadth to the clinician's understanding of how best to address the complex problem of addiction.

Alan I. Leshner, PhD
Director, National Institute on Drug Abuse
National Institutes of Health

Preface

The field of substance abuse has made great advances in the areas of etiology, diagnosis, epidemiology, and treatment using a multidisciplinary approach and a biopsychosocial model. There have been innovations in cognitive and behavioral therapies, relapse prevention, the use of self-help groups, psychopharmacology, family therapy, individual psychotherapy, and group psychotherapy.

Although this book focuses on group therapy, a particular kind of psychosocial intervention for the treatment of substance abuse, it is useful to briefly review our current understanding of the substance use disorders. They include substance abuse, substance dependence (addiction), and the organic brain syndromes resulting from substance abuse or dependence. Substance abuse and dependence are viewed as chronic and relapsing disorders of the brain, with acute episodes, and with psychosocial, behavioral, and cultural antecedents and effects. People take drugs to alter their feelings or thinking, and because they like the effects of drugs of abuse on their affective states and perceptions of their lives. The use of drugs of abuse in large amounts and over a long period of time results in a variety of changes in the brain.

It is likely that the interaction of a genetic diathesis for substance abuse (perhaps more than one type) with certain psychosocial and cultural risk factors results in the phenotypic expression of substance abuse and addiction. These psychosocial and cultural risk factors (and corresponding protective factors) include the parent-child mutual attachment relationship, peer interactions, personality and behavioral issues, and cultural factors such as ethnic identification. One model of the expression of such risk and protective factors in the etiology of the substance use disorders is known as "family interactional theory." The pharmacological effects of the drugs also play an important role in causation. This hypothesis is known as the "risk diathesis" or "stress diathesis" hypothesis of substance abuse. Substance abuse and addiction are indeed biopsychosocial disorders.

In their own right and because of the risk for HIV transmission that they pose, substance abuse and addiction are significant public health issues. Both disorders also play an important role in the occurrence of adolescent, domestic, and interpersonal violence, and place a heavy financial and medical burden upon our society. Since we think it is more effective and less costly to prevent these disorders and their sequelae, as opposed to later intervention, prevention efforts are of great importance in society's struggle against the ongoing epidemics of drug abuse and addiction. Research into cost-effective and well-structured prevention programs has been underway for some time, and a number of innovative programs have been developed and implemented. In addition, clinical efforts have been directed to more effective methods of rehabilitation and the prevention of disability in substance-abusing patient populations.

Fortunately for those who do suffer from the adverse effects of substance abuse, several kinds of treatments are available. Although a discussion of the full range of these treatments is beyond the scope of this book, progress is being made in the areas of pharmacological treatments and a variety of psychosocial therapies. Such research efforts are relatively recent, and much has been funded by the National Institute on Drug Abuse and the National Institute on Alcohol Abuse and Alcoholism.

As noted previously, this book focuses on one class of psychosocial interventions, group therapy, in its many forms and diverse uses. In the past, substance abuse treatment was split between two groups: those who believed in substance abuse recovery programs, typified by AA and other twelve-step self-help programs, therapeutic communities, rehabilitation programs, as well as groups espousing relapse prevention, and the medical/psychiatric community, which has used psychiatric treatment as the means to achieve often similar goals. The former believed that group treatment was effective, abstinence was the goal of treatment, and helping the abuser/addict to relearn more constructive and less self-destructive behavior relating to substances of abuse as well as to interpersonal relationships was the main process leading to recovery. The latter used a variety of forms of psychiatric treatment, including individual and group psychotherapies as well as psychopharmacologic intervention and were interested in treating comorbid disorders as well. In recent years, there has been a recognition that an integrated treatment program, combining features of both models, is more successful than either approach used alone. In both designs, the use of group treatment has been increasingly recognized as the most therapeutically and economically effective method of reaching out and helping these difficult-to-treat patients. Group therapy and integrated substance abuse treatment programs have grown rapidly, both as fields of knowledge and in their more widespread clinical applications.

Because of its therapeutic efficacy and cost-effectiveness, group therapy has come to play an increasingly important role as the psychosocial therapy of choice for ever-increasing numbers of patients with both psychiatric disorders and substance abuse disorders. Group experiences of varying types play a major role in treatment programs in inpatient, outpatient, and partial hospitalization settings. The mutual support and understanding that group members offer one another can have a major therapeutic impact on the lives of substance abusers in areas such as child and adolescent development, parent-child interactions, sibling and peer relationships, health maintenance and the prevention of disability, and, particularly important for substance abusers, the prevention of HIV transmission. Both time-limited and long-term groups can be effective for such purposes; the appeal of the reduced cost of group therapy lends itself to treatment in managed care environments. Group treatment approaches have been incorporated in the treatment guidelines adopted by the American Psychiatric Association, and group substance abuse treatment efforts have been increasingly included in the meetings of the American Group Psychotherapy Association and local affiliated group therapy societies.

The purpose of this book is to act as a bridge between the fields of substance abuse treatment and group psychotherapy. Although group therapy has been recognized by many researchers and clinicians as the primary psychosocial intervention in the treatment of substance abusers, there has been no previous attempt to address the many different perspectives and uses of the group treatments for these patients. The book will serve as an overall survey of the ideas and methods currently in use in the field. The chapter contributors are prominent in their areas of expertise, as scholars, clinicians, and teachers. The book is meant to serve as a resource for the burgeoning number of clinicians now using groups to treat substance abusers, and it can also be read as a survey of the work now being pursued in the field. Each section is grouped by a number of related themes. In addition, each chapter can also stand on its own as representing the current work of its author.

Each contributor will focus on the core topics in his or her area, presenting both theory and techniques, as well as clinical examples. Research advances as well as suggestions for future research are delineated in a form useful to clinicians. Owing to the diversity of approaches and the ever-changing nature of this field, each chapter will present group therapy in the context of the comprehensive treatment of substance abusers, and the place of that particular group approach in the broader area of psychosocial approaches to treatment in general. The goal of each chapter is to present material in a form that clinicians can readily translate into practice, and which other interested people can use to expand their knowledge of a rapidly growing field.

Section I consists of chapters that discuss the basic theoretical approach on which most group treatments of substance abusers are based, as well as an introductory chapter on the practice of group treatment in the age of managed care. The interpersonal approach, the psychodynamic approach, cognitive-behavioral methods, self-medication theory, and modified group psychotherapy are explored.

In Section II, the uses of group treatment approaches in specific treatment settings to achieve specific goals are discussed. Outpatient treatment groups, group relapse prevention approaches, inpatient group treatments, and partial hospitalization groups, including multifamily groups, the use of groups in therapeutic communities, time-limited groups, network therapy, in addition to self-help and twelve-step groups are included in this section.

Section III examines group treatment with certain specific patient populations. It begins with a discussion of ethnicity and culture in the group treatment of substance abusers and proceeds to include chapters on group treatments for female substance abusers, gay, lesbian, and bisexual substance abusers, two different perspectives on adolescent substance abusers, and elderly substance abusers.

Section IV focuses on group treatment approaches for specific diagnostic categories of patients and contains chapters about schizophrenic substance abusers, smoking cessation groups, and medically ill substance abusers.

The concluding chapters in Section V look at research issues in the group treatment of substance abusers, and the implications and future trends for public policy and the ethical treatment of this patient population.

We hope that this book can help clinicians employ groups more effectively, and specifically, to reach out to the large numbers of substance-abusing patients already in treatment and the even larger numbers of such patients not yet engaged in treatment.

Acknowledgments

The editors wish to acknowledge the contributions of many friends and colleagues in providing support and encouragement throughout the course of development of this book.

To begin with, we gratefully acknowledge one of the founding fathers in the field of group therapy in the postwar period, the late Dr. Aaron Stein, who taught and nurtured our growth through his own interest in both group therapy and substance abuse. He gave both personal and professional guidance and mentorship to our endeavors and contributed to our professional growth.

Our thanks go also to our chapter contributors, all of whom have expertise in their fields. We are grateful for their contributions, communications, patience, and collegiality. Without their great talents and wisdom, this book would not have come into being.

A number of colleagues were instrumental in their support, particularly in the early stages of the book, including Howard D. Kibel, K. Roy MacKenzie, and J. Scott Rutan.

We would like to thank Bruce Carruth, Barry Stimmel, and Bill Palmer of The Haworth Press for their encouragement, support, advice, and skills. We are also very grateful to Linda Capobianco, Rebecca Sugerman, and especially to Dorothy Marion for their prodigious efforts in organizing the manuscript in its many drafts and redrafts.

Most important, we would like to thank our wives for their rare blend of professional expertise, personal wisdom, and unwavering support. Judith S. Brook, Professor of Community and Preventive Medicine at the Mount Sinai School of Medicine, and Susan Spitz, Clinical Instructor of Psychiatry, Columbia College of Physicians and Surgeons, gave invaluable advice and encouragement throughout the book's progression with regard to both group therapy and substance abuse.

The work of David W. Brook, MD, is funded in part by grants from the National Institute on Drug Abuse of the National Institutes of Health.

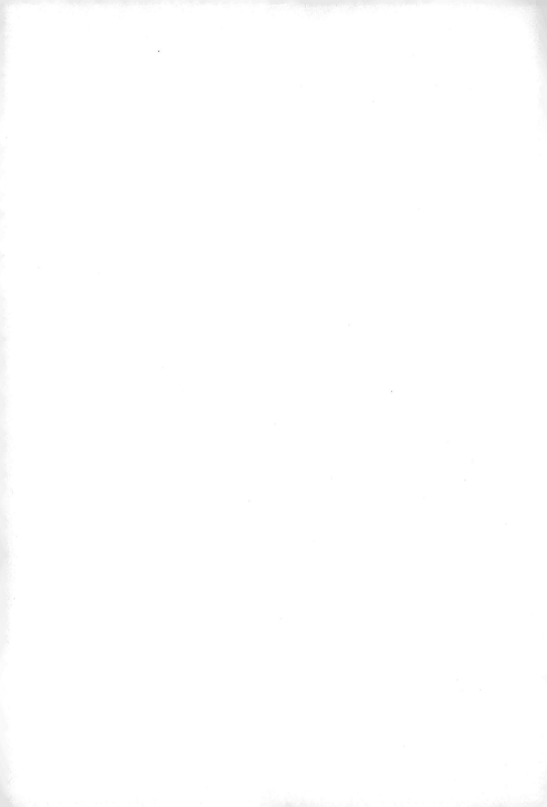

SECTION I:
INTRODUCTION AND GENERAL THEORETICAL ISSUES

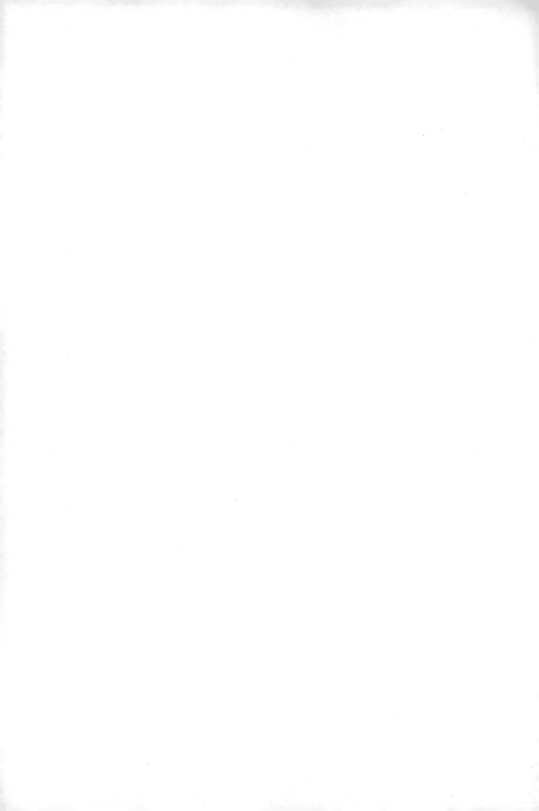

Chapter 1

The Impact of Managed Care on the Group Therapy of Substance Abuse

Henry I. Spitz

THE CHANGING CLIMATE OF HEALTH CARE: OVERVIEW OF THE PROBLEM

The past decade has been witness to a virtual revolution in the field of health care. Driven by concerns over costs of medical and mental health services, government, insurers, and others involved with the financing of health care have focused on creating ways to establish cost-containment while still providing high quality patient care. The implications of these changes are profound.

Optimists feel that radical change is inevitable in order to prevent the system from going out of control. To accomplish this goal, changes in conventional methods of health care delivery are inevitable. A wide range of alternatives have been proposed and instituted as experiments designed to stem the tide of runaway costs. These systems are broadly subsumed under the rubric of managed health care. Pessimists fear that we are seeing the "corporatization" of medicine and the end of psychiatric therapies as now practiced. The principles and language of business and economics threaten to shatter the cornerstones of practice, such as the doctor-patient alliance and patient confidentiality. With financial profit as the goal, many believe that quality care will inevitably suffer.

Although health care reform affects all segments of medicine, it does not affect them equally. Specifically, mental health services are treated as carve-outs in many managed care systems (Galanter et al., 2000). Furthermore, substance abuse and alcoholism treatment risk being adversely impacted by those programs that preferentially reimburse treatments which are brief, documentable, and able to be conducted by the least skilled practitioners whose fees are less than those of practitioners who characteristically provide these services.

This chapter will highlight some of the changes that have taken place under managed care, with a particular emphasis on the problems that face providers of group therapy for substance abuse treatment.

ETHICAL CONCERNS EMANATING FROM MANAGED CARE MODELS

Managed care has been in existence long enough for most clinicians to have experienced the potential intrusions into diverse aspects of psychiatric treatment. Concerns over patient confidentiality, the alteration of the psychotherapeutic relationship between therapist and patient, and decisions regarding what therapy is acceptable to managed care are but a few of the recognizable issues that have arisen as causes of concern.

Despite enlightened attitudes on the part of many, mental illness and substance abuse remain stigmatized. Information concerning people in treatment for these conditions needs to be handled sensitively. The clinician has a responsibility to patients to ensure that data about an individual will not be misused. Managed care, predicated on sharing information about patients in order to determine eligibility, medical necessity, and authorization for further treatment, is faced with the ethical challenge of procuring patient data from providers without violating traditional concepts of confidentiality and the patient's rights to privacy.

The expressed advantages of sharing relevant patient information have largely to do with streamlining care, reducing redundant, time-consuming administrative and clinical efforts, and coordinating treatment plans so that they can be truly integrated, well managed, monitored, and assessed for efficacy. Clinicians in managed care programs must inform patients about the nature of the information that will be shared about them. The clinician may need to inform the patient with whom it will be discussed, toward what purpose, and what will happen with that information in terms of where it will be stored, to which individuals and organizations it is accessible, and how long it will be retained.

IMPACT OF MANAGED CARE
ON CLINICAL SUBSTANCE ABUSE PRACTICE

The managed care model has infringed on the clinician's sense of independence in many ways.

- administrative conflicts
- denial of approval for services
- problems involving the selection of providers for inclusion on managed care panels
- delays in payment for service rendered
- errors in the review process
- problems with the pharmacological formulary restrictions
- low reimbursement scales
- contractual issues including "gag clauses" and requirements for disclosing patient information
- barriers to providing integrated treatment for patients

These changes have shifted the patterns of practice of many mental health and substance abuse practitioners. The increased value placed on brevity of treatment has resulted in an expansion of the use of short-term psychiatric interventions. The concern here is not with the broader use of brief therapies, since that has led to greater clinical and research understanding in the appropriate applicability of short-term methods. The view of brief therapy as a panacea is dangerous. This view may lead to misplacement of patients into treatments that make good economic sense but may be harmful to seriously impaired patients.

Despite the conflicts between the economic and therapeutic agendas involved in patient care, there are economically prudent ways to provide quality care for substance-abusing patients. The increased use of group psychotherapy is a prime case in point. When clinicians are skilled, many people, formerly relegated to expensive, long-term, inpatient or outpatient therapies, can be seen in a group setting. Short-term, symptom-focused groups emphasize specificity of treatment focus, teach skill acquisition, and disseminate accurate information about issues shared by group members. Moreover, with the increased enthusiasm for short-term therapies, a renewed appreciation for the effects of treatment over the course of a patient's life has emerged. Participants learn to identify when they are in need of psychological help and to seek treatment at the earliest possible stage in that process, thereby further reducing potential treatment costs by supplying a mechanism for relapse prevention and earlier intervention should symptoms recur.

Managed care's emphasis on standardization of treatment and determining what is commonly accepted practice for given psychiatric conditions has led to interest in the establishment of practice guidelines for treating specific psychological and substance abuse problems. Practice guidelines are just guides for effective and generally accepted protocols. They are not a substitute for individual clinical judgment. Guidelines are designed to be reviewed and updated periodically in order to include the latest research findings.

The two sets of American Psychiatric Association practice guidelines most relevant to this text are the treatment of patients with substance use disorders (1995), specifically cocaine, alcohol, and the opioids; and the treatment of nicotine dependence (1996). Both of these documents are clear at the outset that they are "not to be construed or . . . serve as a standard of care" (American Psychiatric Association 1995, p. 1; 1996, p. 1), but are guidelines only. Clinicians and managed care reviewers can utilize practice guidelines to help speak a common language of psychiatric treatment. Accountability to third-party payers demands ways of distinguishing treatments with documented efficacy.

EMERGING TRENDS IN RESPONSE TO MANAGED CARE

The proliferation of managed care models has raised a number of clinical, policy, and philosophical questions. The fundamental nature of the interaction between therapist and patient has been influenced if not directly altered by the presence of managed care. Starting with the first encounter, a person seeking help is aware of the presence of a third party in the treatment process. Patients must first learn of their rights as participants in therapy financed by managed care before they can agree to be involved, informed participants in their treatment. This policy awareness works against a cooperative therapist-patient relationship.

Termination of treatment is also directly determined by outside influences. No longer can patients and their therapists decide when a working relationship has served its purpose and plans to terminate therapy are in order. Abrupt, involuntary disruptions and terminations of treatment are much more common under managed care. Therapists who find themselves caught in this situation have an added responsibility to find ongoing professional support for patients whose treatment they regard as incomplete.

The shift from using conventional psychiatric diagnosis to reporting on the basis of functional impairment of patients is another offshoot of the managed care system. Symptom specificity is the hallmark of reporting case material. Global goals such as improvement of self-esteem are being discarded in favor of measures of performance in vocational, academic, and family settings. Similarly, interventions that are behaviorally oriented, aimed at specific functional difficulties, and are circumscribed in their duration of treatment are more likely to be approved for reimbursement.

Those in academic and research circles are greatly distressed by the reduction of funding directed toward professional education, training, and clinical investigation. Managed care is primarily interested in outcome research regarding the varied forms of psychiatric treatment, focusing on which interventions are the most cost-efficient. Although it is critical to account for costs, this is only one dimension of the spectrum of research avenues. The trend away from innovation, teaching, and exploration on a broad scale is troubling.

In sum, managed care has had a profound effect on the character of contemporary psychiatric services. Although the temptation to be critical of the profit motives of managed care at the expense of patient care is high, some serendipitous results are worthy of serious consideration (i.e., increased awareness of the appropriate applications of brief therapies; interest in patient therapist matching; incorporating functional assessments in diagnostic evaluations). Yet, an ongoing need remains for refinement and further study of creative ways to control cost without compromising the access to and quality of substance abuse care.

MANAGED CARE
AND SUBSTANCE ABUSE TREATMENT

The interplay between managed care and substance abuse treatment poses some issues unique to drug and alcohol treatment.

Conceptual Issues

The emphasis on brief and inexpensive treatment, which characterizes the spirit of managed care, runs counter to the experience of those who work with problems of substance abuse. Addiction stands as a model of a chronic, relapsing condition, which must be seen as time unlimited, a condition that calls for more than one element in its treatment plan. As Alan Leshner (1997), the Director of the National Institute of Drug Abuse, emphatically stated, "Addiction is and must be seen by all as the quintessential biobehavioral disorder, with clear biological, behavioral, and social aspects. Combined biological, behavioral, and social or whole person treatments are clearly the direction we must continue to go" (p. 105).

Scientific advances in brain research have shed light on the anatomy, physiology, and neurochemistry of the addictions. Functional magnetic resonance imaging (fMRI) and positron emission tomography (PET scan) have demonstrated which centers in the brain are activated by the use of various drugs of abuse and the presence of drug memories, which can be elicited and measured even in addicts with long periods of abstinence from active drug use. Investigation into medications that treat aspects of addiction including LAAM (levo-alpha-acetylmethadol), naltrexone, and methadone further substantiate the biological basis for substance abuse.

In addition to biological factors, psychological influences play a central role in the genesis and maintenance of addictions. The narrow definition of addiction as a mere dependence on any substance that has a physiological withdrawal state associated with its discontinuance is being revised. Studies demonstrate that other elements play pivotal roles in the process of addiction. Two factors, compulsive behavior and the mood-altering properties of drugs per se, are specifically broadening the definition of addiction, reflecting a shift to a broader concept of addiction.

In essence, the view of substance abuse as a multifactorial entity involving neurological, psychological, cultural, familial, socioeconomic, ethnic, and gender related factors appears to be much more consistent with empirical findings than were former definitions.

Programmatic Issues

The construction of effective alcohol and drug abuse treatment programs requires scientific and clinical understanding coupled with the concern for cost containment. An overview of some of this work will provide a sampling of issues to be taken into account in order to address both sets of needs.

The question of how best to evaluate a person with drug or alcohol problems is a subject of great importance given the complex nature of addiction. Comprehensive assessment is the cornerstone of any treatment plan. The initial assessment of a patient has to encompass biological, psychological, and social factors in order to be as precise as possible in designing both an individualized therapy plan and a therapy plan that meets the criteria for reimbursement under managed care. Lewis (1997) presents a comparison between adaptive and ineffective approaches for the evaluation and treatment of alcoholism in a managed care environment. Once a balanced diagnosis is made of the extent of the addiction, as well as other comorbid psychiatric and medical conditions, a logical progression toward individualized treatment goals, empirically based treatment planning, selection of appropriate cost-effective therapies, and methods for documenting outcome or provider accountability will flow more naturally.

Many methods and measures for assessment of substance abuse can be incorporated into a managed care context. With problems of substance abuse, it is always helpful to include an awareness of issues of gender, ethnicity, languages, illiteracy, homelessness, religion, pregnancy and child care responsibilities, culture, age-specific concerns, and other factors that have direct bearing on evaluation and treatment planning but may not be a part of standardized instruments used to measure addiction. Inclusion of these factors leads to patient-specific decisions about level of care needed, intensity of treatment, and inpatient or outpatient setting.

Once the initial evaluation has been completed, questions will arise concerning the proper placement of patients in treatment programs. Several aspects of this process are being addressed in current studies of alcoholism and drug abuse treatment. One example is the theme of matching. Two major examples of matching under managed care are therapist-patient matching and problem-service matching. Specificity and economy are reflected in these efforts.

One of the better known illustrations of an organized attempt to address the issue of matching patients to appropriate treatments is reflected in the U.S. Department of Health and Human Services' program conducted under the auspices of the Substance Abuse and Mental Health Services Administration (SAMHSA). Through the creation of uniform patient placement criteria (UPPC) a systematized effort has been made to bring consistency and stability to patient placement.

The treatment of addiction requires freedom of movement through a number of treatment settings as the patient's clinical course changes. The ability to conceptualize the process of addiction and its consequent need for enduring care at various levels is essential. Once the level of care is determined, then specific therapeutic interventions or modalities can be employed. On all levels of care, biological, psychological, and sociocultural treatment modalities can be tailored to the individual needs of the patient.

Psychological modalities can include options ranging from drug counseling and education to more ambitious forms of psychotherapy including cognitive, behavioral, group and family or couples therapy approaches. Once sobriety has been attained, the focus on relapse prevention strategies allows a number of social and community support options to be matched to the patient's current needs. At this juncture, attendance at twelve-step meetings, vocational rehabilitation, culturally specific experiences, and social skills training will be available as therapeutic choices. The reduction of program costs and increased efficiency helps reduce redundancy and avoidable cost overruns in well-designed programs.

General Treatment Issues

Although it is tempting to talk of managed care as a uniform entity, considerable variation exists among different managed care systems. This is particularly true when dealing with the treatment of substance abuse. Insurers and reviewers do not use standardized criteria for assessing aspects of addiction treatment. In fact, managed care rules seem arbitrary to many providers of addiction services. The only point of universal consensus under managed care is that the least expensive forms of treatment are the most preferred.

Substance-abusing patients have unique needs and these must be factored into any treatment plan if it is to be successful. Medical illnesses which regularly accompany addiction (e.g., HIV, hepatitis C, tuberculosis) broaden the concept of comorbidity and dual diagnosis beyond just the psychiatric syndromes ordinarily associated with the use of these terms. The simultaneous treatment of coexisting medical and psychological problems is a complex, time-consuming, and labor-intensive effort on the part of the professional treatment team. No shortcuts are possible without compromising the essential aspects of patient care. Despite these liabilities, managed care has placed restrictions on various dimensions of addiction treatment, including group treatment.

Evidence for this can be found at all stages of treatment. Reviewers and physicians treating the patient often disagree on what constitutes detoxification. Even though it is well established that the propensity for relapse is very high during the period immediately following detoxification, a reviewer may not judge this as sufficient grounds for approving continued inpatient treatment.

Outpatient care has its own associated administrative and managerial problems. Most managed care companies assume that outpatient treatment will include elements of twelve-step participation, regular urine screening, and community-based support and education programs. If the provider feels that a level of care greater than outpatient treatment is indicated or that continued outpatient treatment of longer than one year's duration is required, the rationale for this opinion must be presented. Whether this will be approved depends upon many variables, not just the patient's insurance coverage.

In many instances a distinction exists between the extent of coverage for psychiatric conditions (affective disorders, schizophrenia, or other psychoses, etc.) and substance abuse conditions. Coverage for the former is usually greater than for the latter. A familiar tug-of-war ensues between the clinician, who emphasizes the medical necessity for treating both entities, and the managed care reviewer, who supports the view that substance abuse is the primary problem and that reimbursement decisions should be based on treatment of the less expensive diagnosis.

In the rehabilitation phase of addiction treatment, still other problems arise. Presently, the trend among case reviewers is to authorize less time for rehabilitation. Three reasons for this tendency are: (1) it has traditionally been difficult to document the efficacy of rehabilitation with good scientific data; (2) the structure of insurance benefits for many patients is such that an extended rehabilitation phase would exhaust their benefits and leave them uninsured in the case of future relapse; (3) since much of what transpires during rehabilitation carries a strong, somewhat standardized, educational component, it is assumed that repeated exposure to the same material over time will have diminishing returns.

Assessing Substance Abuse Treatment Outcome

Accurately measuring outcome of substance abuse therapies has always been of prime concern to clinicians. The introduction of managed care to the equation has only made this process more complex. Treatment providers and managed care payers are faced with the generic problems inherent in trying to assess outcome in a substance-abusing patient population.

Even under the best circumstances, outcome research into substance abuse and alcoholism treatment still invites certain controversies. A representative sampling of questions that arise include whether patient satisfaction is really a measure of treatment quality, whether the same measures are appropriate for public and private sector patients, how adaptable medical patient satisfaction measures are for the addictions, and how reliable or truthful the responses of a substance-abusing patient population are when many of the drugs they use and the methods used to obtain them are illegal.

Regardless of one's position in the managed care versus traditional patient care debate, all concerned will be beneficiaries of the results of thoughtful investigation of what contributes to successful outcome in the treatment of addictions.

MANAGED CARE AND GROUP PSYCHOTHERAPY

Interface Issues

While the relationship between the group leader and group member is based upon therapeutically derived principles, managed care is economically driven and largely based on cost containment. Four general areas of vulnerability under managed care can potentially threaten establishment of a constructive working relationship between a group therapist and his or her patient, which can even preclude the formation of a meaningful therapeutic alliance. These areas are the therapist's fiduciary obligation to group members, the patient's participation in health care decision making, access to adequate treatment, and the quality of the care itself (Spitz, 1996; 1997). In a managed care system, the payer requires a great deal of information from the therapist in order to make determinations about diagnosis, medical necessity of the proposed treatment plan, and the duration of benefit approval. This is of great significance in group treatment. Although managed care organizations are familiar with individual psychotherapeutic models, they are not as yet as advanced in their understanding of the breadth and variety of group treatment options.

A narrow view of group therapy restricts treatment choices to those patient populations and/or psychological conditions that lend themselves to management in brief cognitive-behavioral or psychoeducational formats. There are people at every level of psychological functioning who appear to derive little benefit from these models of treatment. Patients in the neurotic range of the diagnostic spectrum run the risk of being relegated to symptom-oriented group therapy, while their less healthy counterparts are told that long-term treatment is not compatible with managed care. Consequently, many of the more seriously impaired psychiatric patients are assigned to psychotropic medication management and social support groups, leaving no place for more ambitious therapeutic work with these patients.

A similar problem exists for the treatment of patients who have DSM-IV Axis II diagnoses under managed care. No one from the managed care community has clearly espoused the benefits of group therapy in the comprehensive treatment of patients with personality disorders, though group therapists know this method of treatment to be empirically and scientifically valid. Other well-supported group treatment plans also appear to remain foreign to those who are responsible for treatment decision making in the managed care community. These include "maintenance group psychotherapy" for the severely ill psychiatric patient, time-limited group psychotherapy for borderline patients (Marziali and Munroe-Blum, 1994), and periodic serial group experiences as represented by the adult developmental model of Budman and Gurman (1988) and others still appear to be foreign to those in positions of treatment decision making in the managed care community.

If left unchecked, this trend of mismatching treatment and over-looking options has predictably deleterious effects. In essence, what will happen is a "downward drift" of the most seriously ill or "highest risk" patients into medication-only groups; issues of interpersonal function will be ignored or dealt with only superficially; and groups will become the dumping ground for patients who are regarded as difficult to treat. Undoubtedly, although it has a certain appeal, forming treatment decisions based solely on economics will cause clinical care to suffer.

When group therapists share their expertise with those in managed care circles who are receptive to group therapy, then the gap between a managed care perspective and therapeutic considerations can be narrowed. Managed care professionals need to be informed about the flexibility and diversity of group experiences. Group therapists strongly believe that there is hardly a psychiatric, medical, and/or social condition for which a constructive group experience cannot be created. The advances found in group therapy with substance abuse patients offer a prime example of the confluence of the psychological, physical, and social needs of patients addressed simultaneously in one form of treatment. This model is not merely cost-efficient, it makes for high quality treatment with high degrees of patient specificity.

Impact of Managed Care on Aspects of Group Therapy

Managed care has made its presence known in many ways. There are, however, a few issues that specifically affect group therapy treatment and are worthy of separate mention.

The demand by consumers to specify which clinicians are specially trained to perform particular psychological services has met with a favorable response among group therapists. This concern for setting standards and evaluating qualifications of group services providers is evident in the creation of The National Registry of Certified Group Psychotherapists. The registry represents a major outreach effort to assist the public and managed care organizations in determining which group treatment practitioners are the most qualified. The national registry demonstrates that group therapists are very interested in maintaining the highest ethical standards in clinical work and are willing to hold themselves accountable for the same levels of excellence that they expect from other managed care providers.

As managed care companies continue to profile providers, interest is growing among psychotherapists for performing a parallel evaluation process of the managed care company. Such information could help to distinguish organizations that are group knowledgeable from those that are not. In this way, group therapists will be able to target their education and training efforts toward those managed care organizations that are less informed about the value of contemporary group psychotherapy.

With the advent of managed care, issues of education and training have been profoundly influenced. Naturally, several questions emerge regarding changes in the current and future training needs of the group therapy practitioner in the managed care environment. What skills will the group therapist need to add to the existing therapeutic armamentarium in order to maximize the benefits of group therapy practiced in the arena of health care reform? How will these skills be best acquired? How will the current education and training of group therapists need to be updated in order to keep pace with emerging trends in managed care?

Training psychiatric residents in the managed care age will be different from the past. The settings in which training takes place are likely to expand from the traditional models of inpatient hospital and outpatient clinic and agency work to new venues that are by-products of managed care. Employee assistance programs (EAPs) in corporate settings, managed care clinics, primary care satellite locations, consultation-liaison services, and multispecialty interdisciplinary practitioner groups may all be new sites of learning for group therapists treating substance abusers.

Clearly a need exists for group therapists to collaborate with managed care in order to determine how to successfully incorporate group therapy into managed care systems. In-service training for members of managed care organizations can help teach effective collaborative skills between managed care representatives and members of the health care provider community, and heighten awareness group therapy as a primary modality or as the treatment of choice. In order to accomplish all of these goals, managed care must make efforts, such as ensuring that intake personnel and intake forms are geared to group as well as individual therapies. Similarly, computerized information systems and software programs need to be organized to incorporate data relevant to group placement and tracking of patients referred to group therapy. Toward these goals, group therapists who are used to dealing with these potential pitfalls can share their experiences with the managed care personnel in order to refine and make information systems user-friendly to therapists.

EFFECT OF MANAGED CARE ON THERAPIST MORALE

Changes in health care financing have had demoralizing effects on practitioners of psychotherapy. The positive aspects of the professional identity of the group therapist as caregiver, collaborator, and guide are rapidly being eroded by policymakers for whom managed care equals managed cost. Consequently, empathy, trust, the relief of suffering, and the constructive use of the power inherent to groups are assigned lesser value, if any at all. A climate of fear, mistrust, and paranoia has replaced the cooperative spirit that has for so long defined the group therapy field. Moreover, the potential for therapist "burnout" is much greater than in the past because practitioners are given less time to do more work, including extensive administrative requirements, for fees that are not commensurate with the effort put forth. This is especially true in the group treatment of substance abusers, where the therapist's dedication, morale, and resilience are constantly being tested. Independence in clinical decision making is being co-opted by administrators, case managers, and other representatives of the managed care industry. These factors are even more demoralizing to the average group therapist than the decline in income that accompanies participation in a managed care plan.

Intense negative reactions in providers of psychotherapy services are becoming commonplace. Group leaders have to be particularly aware of their personal reactions to spare the group from any rage, despair, powerlessness, and other negative feelings they may displace in reaction to managed care. Differentiating "garden variety" therapist countertransference responses to group process from the leader's idiosyncratic emotional agenda emanating from a personal issue with managed care is becoming a more difficult task.

Is there any hope for this gloomy situation? Group therapists must be willing to redefine themselves while maintaining professional standards. This redefinition process for group therapists is likely to result in a shift toward technical eclecticism in group practice. The inclusion of outcome research into group practice is likely to result in an updated brand of group psychotherapy for the new millennium, an amalgamation of the old with some of the new.

Psychodynamic constructs do not need to be abandoned or regarded as antiquated. As was the case with the evolution of family therapy, group therapists with a psychodynamic orientation will flourish if knowledge of individual and group dynamics are combined to form the basis for timely group interventions. The conventional use of interpretation of resistance, analysis of transference, and other classical psychoanalytically oriented techniques provide only some of the needed strategies. The inclusion of out-of-session tasks that tap the relevant group and individual dynamics will help expedite the therapeutic process without shortchanging patient care.

By transforming conventional psychodynamic principles into active contemporary clinical form, the group leader can blend the best of the old with the best of the new. This process is challenging but it promises to be stimulating rather than inhibiting for clinicians.

The modern history of group psychotherapy reflects the ability of group therapies to adapt to social change. Whether the stimulus was the increased need for psychiatric services following World War II or the community mental health movement (both of which dictated that mental health professionals see more patients in shorter time frames), the field of group therapy has expanded exponentially. With new and enlightened policies, it is very likely that managed care will be the current impetus for change, innovation, and creativity among practitioners of group psychotherapy.

Group treatment of alcohol and drug-related problems represents the "cutting edge" of contemporary biopsychosocial treatment in the era of health care reform. The chapters that follow are all illustrative of how thoughtfully the group milieu has been adjusted to meet the unique needs of patients, clinicians, and third-party payers without compromising the quality of care. Group psychotherapy with substance-abusing patients serves as the prototype of such efforts.

REFERENCES

American Psychiatric Association. *Diagnostic and Statistical Manual of Mental Disorders,* Fourth Edition. Washington, DC: American Psychiatric Association, 1994.

American Psychiatric Association. Practice guidelines for the treatment of patients with substance use disorders: Alcohol, cocaine, opioids. *American Journal of Psychiatry* Supplement 152:11, 1995.

American Psychiatric Association. Practice guidelines for the treatment of patients with nicotine dependence. *American Journal of Psychiatry* Supplement 153:10, 1996.

Budman SH, Gurman AS. *Theory and Practice of Brief Therapy.* New York: Basic Books, 1998.

Galanter M, Keller DS, Dermatis H, Egelko S. The impact of managed care on substance abuse treatment: A report of the American Society of Addiction Medicine. *Journal of Addictive Diseases* 19:13-25, 2000.

Leshner AI. Drug abuse and addiction treatment research: The next generation. *Archives of General Psychiatry* 54:105-107, 1997.

Lewis JA. Treating alcohol problems in a managed care environment. In *Managed Mental Health Care: Major Diagnostic and Treatment Approaches,* edited by Sauber RS. Bristol, PA: Brunner/Mazel, Inc., pp. 297-311, 1997.

Marziali E, Munroe-Blum H. *Interpersonal Psychotherapy for Borderline Personality Disorder.* New York: Basic Books, 1994.

Spitz HI. *Group Psychotherapy and Managed Mental Health Care: A Clinical Guide for Providers.* New York: Brunner/Mazel, Inc., 1996.

Spitz HI. The effect of managed mental health care on group psychotherapy: Treatment, training and therapist morale issues. *International Journal of Group Psychotherapy* 47:23-30, 1997.

Chapter 2

The Interpersonal Approach

Philip J. Flores

INTRODUCTION

Many experienced clinicians believe that the interpersonal model can be most easily modified to meet the specific needs, unique difficulties, and distinct challenges the typical substance abuser brings to treatment. Techniques and strategies for the general psychiatric population often fail with this population. Consequently, substance abusers have usually been viewed as poor treatment risks because they are unmotivated and resistant. The Interpersonal Group Psychotherapy (IGP) approach, which specifically takes into consideration the special circumstances of these patients and makes intelligent changes in applied technique, is likely to prove successful.

Pragmatism

IGP provides a practical, results-oriented approach for a population that desperately requires such a technique. During the early phase of treatment when the window of opportunity for effectively engaging these patients is limited and brief, IGP proves extremely effective. IGP furnishes the group leader with a set of strategic tools that can be freely accessed and effortlessly applied. Moreover, IGP can be organized to provide enough structure to prevent the emergence of unproductive regression, while at the same time allowing the group members to have a group experience that is not leader-dependent or leader-centered. Unsurprisingly, many substance abusers will become resistant to a leader who is domineering or authoritarian.

IGP and the treatment of addiction complement each other in the establishment of the components of effective treatment for the substance-abusing population. The specifics of the IGP process include, but are not limited to, transference, support, containment, identification, confrontation, attachment, shame reduction, and ultimately the alteration of character pathology. The specific ways in which IGP accomplishes these tasks will be elaborated upon in the latter half of this chapter.

The Interpersonal Model

Interpersonal theory, true to its theoretical grounding in psychodynamic theory and the work of Sullivan (1953), holds the position that all patterns of interpersonal relatedness are established as a consequence of our earliest interpersonal relationships. These patterns become habitual later in life, ingrained, often maladaptive, and ultimately self-defeating. Much in the same way that classical psychoanalysis believes that dreams and slips of the tongue are royal roads to the unconscious, interpersonal theorists believe that the habitual and characterological ways individuals interact with one another also act as windows to the unconscious. Through the force of the repetition compulsion and the reparative attempt, we are constantly re-creating our past in the present. Moreover, as implied in this model, emotional attachment plays a central role in our developmental lives as do peer relationships.

It is within the realm of group therapy that many of the most innovative and creative applications of interpersonal theory have been made. As Yalom and Vinogradov state, "All group psychotherapy, regardless of the orientation of its leader, is by its nature largely interpersonal" (1993, p. 185). Over the last few years IGP has been expanded and influenced by object relations theory, self-psychology, and modern psychoanalytic (Ormont 1992) approaches. Despite the extent of other influences, it is impossible to accurately describe the IGP model without acknowledging the tremendous impact of Yalom's work (1995).

YALOM'S INTERACTIONAL GROUP PSYCHOTHERAPY

Yalom's model of interactional group psychotherapy is one of the most widely applied approaches to group therapy (Dies 1992). Although there are many advantages for utilizing the principles of intervention inherent to this approach, the reasoning behind the application of these principles is not always articulated in a cogent and encompassing fashion. Consequently, some have criticized interpersonal group therapy and have labeled it as an assortment of techniques in search of a theory. Most of this criticism is because, during the last twenty years, IGP has been almost exclusively aligned with Yalom's Interactional Model of Group Psychotherapy (1995). Yet despite his popularity and influence, Irvin Yalom is not the only IGP theorist.

Over the last ten years, IGP has evolved into a more thorough and comprehensive theory due to the persuasive influence of a number of different psychodynamic group theorists within the American Group Psychotherapy Association (AGPA). After having been singularly aligned with Yalom's interactional model, IGP now has its own identity and has developed into a more sophisticated and comprehensive theory, incorporating important aspects of object relations theory, self-psychology, attachment theory, and modern analytic perspectives. Psychodynamic group therapy is a generic model of group therapy that recognizes three primary dynamic forces operating in group all the time. Correspondingly, three levels of intervention possible in group are directly related to the three levels of dynamics above. These three levels of intervention are (1) intrapsychic, (2) interpersonal, and (3) group as a whole (systems theory).

The task of the group leader is to integrate all three intervention levels into a balanced, coherent flow, keeping in mind that many variables (i.e., stage of group development, introduction of new members, ego strength of individual members, etc.) influence each level. Ignoring any aspect of these three levels limits the full range of therapeutic possibilities and, conversely, an overemphasis on one level limits the other two levels. The art of psychodynamically oriented interpersonal group therapy is determined by the group leader finding the optimal balance among these interrelated forces and taking full therapeutic advantage of all three levels.

Despite the immense latitude the group leaders have in which to apply IGP, among IGP theorists there is a consensus regarding the essential elements of approach. Foremost among these agreements are

1. the necessity of establishing proper group cohesion with therapeutic norms, which allow group members the opportunity to

assume responsibility for the group, eventually promoting equal participation by all its members;
2. the importance and significance of the here and now in the group;
3. the interaction between group members;
4. the proposed and required activity level of the group leader to ensure active participation of all group members; and
5. the lack of emphasis, and at times a total disregard, for group-as-a-whole interventions.

Cohesion

Yalom (1995) has repeatedly placed a particular emphasis on the value of cohesion in group. Other IGP therapists draw parallels between an alliance in individual therapy and cohesion in group therapy, which may not be the case. Ormont (1992) suggests that if a group leader orchestrates the right mixture of emotional involvement and communication between all members, an important source of therapeutic power will be harnessed.

Object relations theorists have recently contributed alternative ways for understanding the role which cohesion plays in group. Group members can become emotionally attached to the group, in ways inaccessible in individual therapy because of the intensity of transference, object hunger, and shame. A properly managed group can become a good holding environment and a transitional object for group members, which will eventually allow a transference relationship to be established with the group acting as an internal object (Ganzarain 1992). The group as a substitute good mother can serve as an idealized transferential object while it keeps its members protected from the intensity of hostility to or dependency on a single person (the therapist) and the shameful longings of object hunger related to this dependency. Aggressive and hostile aspects can be projected "out there," thereby preserving a sense of togetherness until the group is more cohesive and mature. An example may help to clarify this point:

Mary, an addict with nearly two years of abstinence, had been progressing nicely in her therapy group since her discharge from an inpatient treatment program. Along with a gradual feeling of trust that she had been able to establish in her group, Mary had developed an idealizing transference with her female group leader. Mary would revel in any show of attention given to her by her "idol." However, her admiration came to an abrupt end one evening when the group leader supported another group member's observation that Mary was intolerant of anyone disagreeing with her. Mary exploded with rage, screaming at the group leader that she was "sick and tired of people betraying her and blaming her for everything."

All attempts at containment and interpretation by the group leader proved futile and only enraged Mary more. Mary was able to gain some solace from many of the other group members who seemed to understand her expressed feelings for they too had had similar experiences in their lives. She was encouraged by the group members not to leave the group, as she had threatened, and to deal with the group leader. In the following weeks, Mary continued to show up for group and interact with the other group members, but she refused to speak or even look at the group leader.

Eventually, Mary was able to engage with the group leader and even respond favorably to some of her interventions. Nearly six months after the initial explosion, Mary told the group about an argument she had been able to resolve with her supervisor at work. Pausing at the end of her story, Mary looked directly at the group leader and openly confessed, "You know, I think I was distorting her comments and overreacting just like I did with you six months ago." No interpretation or comment was required. The group had provided her with a safe holding environment, which allowed her to work through the transference feelings of disappointment and object hunger directed toward her therapist.

Here-and-Now

Yalom has long described here-and-now as the power cell of group. He suggests that the group leader should ensure that the group members focus their attention on their immediate feelings and thoughts toward the other group members, the group leader, and the group as a whole: immediate here-and-now events in group must take precedence over the events of the past and those outside of group (there-and-then). The here-and-now interactions can avoid distortions that so often accompany a patient's report of an event (Leszcz 1992).

Under the right circumstances, the past then becomes the here-and-now as in the following example:

Jim, an alcoholic with over three years of sobriety, had been in an outpatient group for nearly ten months. Despite his involvement in AA and the group, Jim continued to live alone and showed little progress in being able to establish a relationship with anyone inside or outside the program. Jim's engagement to the group stayed limited to talking about himself.

During the course of one evening, Jim began to speak to the group about his isolation and history of being ignored by his parents as a child. After Jim stated bitterly, "I don't think anyone in my family ever gave a damn about me," the group leader asked Jim if he was feeling ignored in group right now and if he thought anybody in here "gave a damn" about him. Jim said he didn't expect anyone in the group to care about him more than anyone else did in his life. At this point, a number of group members responded to Jim saying that they had grown fond of him over the last few months and that they were touched by his story concerning his home life. Ignoring their reaction, Jim returned to the subject of his past isolation. The group leader stopped him and asked Sally, one of the group members who had tried to respond to Jim, if she thought Jim had noticed her efforts to relate to him. Sally replied, "No, I don't think he did." Another group member agreed with Sally and said that he felt the same way. "In fact," he added, "I'm feeling ignored by you right now, Jim. It's as if my efforts to relate to you don't matter to you."

The group leader tried to encourage Jim to take advantage of the opportunity not to be alone here in group right now and to look at the ways in which he might be contributing to his own isolation. The group leader also asked another group member, who had been quietly shaking her head in agreement, if she wanted to tell Jim what she was agreeing with. She quickly added, "I think I know exactly how you must feel, Jim. I have this huge empty cavern inside of me that feels like a bottomless pit. One show of warmth or compassion will just ricochet off the empty walls and does little to make the emptiness go away. Consequently, I can do exactly what I see you doing in here. I push people away who are trying to relate to me."

With some gentle prodding by the group leader, the group was soon engaged in a rich emotional exchange that could have remained sterile and distant if he had not guided its members to interact with one another in a way to bring the "there and then" into the "here and now."

Interaction Among Group Members

No theory places more emphasis on members actively interacting with one another than IGP. Yalom has repeatedly identified interpersonal input, output, and learning as curative factors in IGP. Similarly, Ormont (1992), theoretically grounded in a modern analytic perspective, and Rutan and Stone (1993), theoretically grounded in object-relations theory and self-psychology, stress active interaction in group. Object relations theory indicates that introjected self and object representations carry intense affect within them. These internalized introjections contribute to individuals' propensity for projecting their internal experiences onto the external world. Through the power of projective identification, individuals are likely to coerce, induce, or provoke others unwittingly to contribute to their internal struggles and expectations in a self-fulfilled prophecy so that the external world begins to conform or fit internal expectations and experiences.

Modern analytic perspectives provide an important understanding of the significance of altering maladaptive behavioral patterns in interpersonal relations within a therapy group. Ormont (1992) contends that preoedipal patients pose special problems because of developmental failures that occurred early in life before these patients were able to use words effectively to describe their experiences. Such individuals are more likely to act out or emote than talk. Moreover, these patients do not respond favorably to words or interpretations; they can only be influenced by feelings and actions. Although insight alone is not enough to change powerfully conditioned self and object representations, a powerful corrective emotional experience—one that is more likely to happen if the group leader keeps the group members interacting, attached, and emotionally involved with one another—will have such an effect. A subtle but very important interplay occurs among attachment, cohesion, and interaction.

To help facilitate the task of communicating their immediate thoughts and feelings when group members are reluctant to react spontaneously, Ormont suggests the use of a technique he calls "bridging." Bridging is described as "any technique geared to evoke meaningful talk between group members, to develop emotional connections where they did not exist before" (Ormont 1992, p. 15). Spontaneity and immediacy give the group and its members a profound sense of authenticity and of actual experience only if there is total emotional involvement by every member. Only through the realm of shared emotional experiences with peers can many patients be influenced.

Activity Level of the Group Leader

If IGP is to reach its full potential, active leadership of a special nature is required. As the individual therapist acts as a participant observer, a group leader functions as a model for group members by reinforcing therapeutic norms in the group. The norms that are valued above all others are those that (1) keep the group members interacting with one another on an emotional level, (2) keep the interaction in the immediacy of the here-and-now as much as possible, and (3) establish a sense of cohesion to help facilitate emotional attachment in the group. If these norms are established, the group leader's activity level will be greatly reduced, requiring activation only when the group becomes emotionally stale, intellectual, or stuck in destructive or meaningless chatter.

The art and skill of competent leadership requires knowing when to be silent and how to be active, as well as the establishment of an accepting and nonjudgmental environment. Such an effort must be done skillfully, because if it is applied clumsily, nonjudgmental acceptance can easily come across as noncaring and indifferent.

Group-As-a-Whole

IGP recognizes that there will be times when the group and its members are impacted by the regressive pull of the group climate. If group-as-a-whole interpretations are required to help the group move beyond this obstacle, the IGP-oriented leader should use them as necessary. Rather than harp on these occurrences, IGP places much more emphasis on maintaining authentic relationships in the group. Group-as-a-whole interventions are helpful only when the group becomes stuck or embroiled in Bion's basic assumptions (1961). Within Bion's perspective, there are always two groups operating in every group encounter—the overt or work group and the covert or basic assumption group. While the work group is always established to accomplish an overt task, the unconscious contagion of the regressive pull of the basic assumption group operates covertly to subvert the conscious aim of the group. Bion asserts that the primitive states of mind operating covertly in the basic assumption group tend to dominate the work group, interfering with the declared task of the work group. The emotional valences organized in these basic assumptions are unconscious processes that fall into three distinct categories. These categories possess an "as if" quality and are identified as dependency, fight-flight, and pairing. However, as DG Brown (1985) has convincingly demonstrated, basic assumptions can be iatrogenically introduced, or encouraged, by the presence of an emotionally unavailable, passive group leader who inhibits, or does not promote, genuine human emotional contact within the group. IGP suggests that an active leader who promotes authentic contact between group members will encounter fewer group-as-a-whole resistances.

HISTORY OF IGP AND ADDICTION

The use of Interpersonal Group Psychotherapy to treat substance abuse has a relatively short, but important, history. The evolution of this model parallels many other important developments and changes that have occurred in addiction treatment during the past twenty years. Brown and Yalom's (1977) classic article on the use of Inter-actional Group Psychotherapy as an approach to treating alcoholics not only laid an important theoretical foundation for treating addic-tion in groups, but also exposed the futility of trying to use psycho-therapy with a practicing alcoholic. Brown and Yalom's research not only helped legitimize group therapy as the treatment of choice for addiction, it also helped substantiate Alcoholics Anonymous' (AA) contention that abstinence is the first requirement for successful ad-diction treatment.

Historically, because of AA's influence, group therapy had always held wide acceptance as an essential ingredient for the treatment of substance abuse. In spite of its popularity, empirical research into the effectiveness of group therapy either had been limited or equivocal. What empirical research was available led a number of researchers (i.e., Kanas 1982; Pattison 1979) to recommend that more specific guidelines and suggestions be constructed for group treatment of this population.

To meet this challenge, an increasing body of research and clinical literature has emerged in the last few years. In general, a consensus has grown among clinicians. Khantzian, Halliday, and McAuliffe (1990), Vannicelli (1992), S Brown (1985), Flores and Mahon (1993), Matano and Yalom (1991), and Flores (1988; 1997) have all provided extensive suggestions concerning group therapy strategies for substance abusers. These authors agree that abstinence is a crucial, if not the most impor-tant, element in recovery from a substance abuse disorder. Each author supports and recommends complementary twelve-step programs and the use of a group therapy format that includes an interpersonal ap-proach and relies heavily on Yalom's (1995) theoretical model of interactional group therapy. However, most clinicians have modified, adapted, and integrated many of Yalom's principles and techniques with those of psychodynamic group therapy.

PSYCHODYNAMIC THEORIES
OF ADDICTION AND GROUP THERAPY

The principles that guide the application of IGP thoroughly match the deficits that fuel the addiction process. They both recognize that a person's capacity for healthy interpersonal relatedness contributes to the elimination of forces that drive the need for chemical use and its subsequent abuse.

One premise is the recognition of an inverse relationship between addiction and healthy interpersonal attachment. Such a deficiency in being able to establish healthy relationships is related to both genetic and biological substrates, which contribute to an inborn or induced decreased capacity for attachment. The less able individuals are to establish emotionally intimate contact with others, the more they will be prone to substitute drugs and alcohol for intimacy. Early developmental failures leave certain individuals with vulnerabilities that enhance addictive type behaviors, often occurring as attempts at self-repair. Because of the deprivation of appropriate developmental needs, the substance abuser is constantly attempting to use something "out there" to substitute for what is missing "in here."

CONTRIBUTIONS OF SELF-PSYCHOLOGY AND ATTACHMENT THEORY

Addiction can be viewed as an attachment disorder. The individual's relationship to chemicals serves both as an obstacle and as a substitute for interpersonal relationships. Because of the potent emotional euphoric "rush" that drugs and alcohol produce, they are powerfully reinforcing. Self-psychology holds that deficits in psychic structure contribute to impairment of attachment and that substance use is often an attempt to compensate for deficits in structure. Psychic structure represents a class of psychological functions pertaining to the maintenance, restoration, or consolidation of self-experience. It therefore represents the capacity, or ability, to integrate and organize fragmenting affect into meaningful experience. Structure formation—the acquisition of patterns and meaning—is developed out of the internalization of the functions previously provided by external objects or sources, without relying excessively on self-objects.

The deficits in psychic structure that require external augmentation are usually the result of developmental failures or unmet age-appropriate attachment needs. Conversely, the successful formation and establishment of self-structure is a developmental outcome that reflects a capacity for self-regulatory functioning. Thus the treatment of deficits in self or psychic structure becomes the eventual long-term goal of group psychotherapy. Kohut (1984) and other object relations theorists view addiction as a condition resulting from a person's misguided attempt at self-repair of deficits in psychic structure. Physical dependence leads to further deterioration of existing physiological and psychological structures. Prolonged stress on these existing structures will lead to exaggerated difficulty in the regulation of affect, behavior, self-care, dependency, alexithymia, anhedonia, and character pathology.

Self-Care

Substance abusers are notorious for their self-destructive and self-defeating behavior. Because they suffer from a deficient or underdeveloped capacity for identifying and modulating their feelings, they are often unable to detect when they are tired, sick, hungry, anxious, or depressed. Many also smoke incessantly, do not exercise or over-exercise, and have poor dietary regimens. Such lack of self-care also leads individuals to be less aware, less cautious, and not worried or frightened enough to resist injurious or damaging behavior. Because they often have had poor parenting as children, they are inadequately prepared to properly evaluate the consequences of risky or self-defeating behavior. Therefore, they constantly place themselves in potentially destructive and painful circumstances.

Affect Regulation

Substance abusers are usually unable to identify, verbalize, and use feelings as signals or guides for managing and protecting against instability and chaos in their internal emotional lives. They have a disturbance in the regulation of affect.

Dependency and the Self

Self-deficits lead to failures in ego-ideal formation. Following Kohut's work on self-objects, substance abusers can be seen as having been deprived of the opportunity to adequately internalize the admired and admiring, encouraging, valued, and idealized qualities of "good enough" parental figures. They often lack self-worth and suffer from chronic feelings of poor self-esteem and shame. It is within the matrix of environmental responsiveness and emotional attunement that a specific process of psychological structure formation develops, as the consequence of minor, nontraumatic failures in response to empathic self-objects. These failures, or *optimal frustrations,* lead to a gradual replacement of the self-object functions by the child's developing capacity to soothe and calm himself or herself. Kohut called this process *transmuting internalization.* Self-regulation and self-soothing become internalized, allowing less dependence on external sources for gratification. However, as the attachment theorists remind us, we are always in need of some emotional regulation from one another. Denial of the need for others leads individuals to seek support elsewhere (i.e., drugs, alcohol, food, sex, work, gambling, etc.).

Alexithymia and Anhedonia

Alexithymia and anhedonia have been identified respectively as the inability to name and be aware of one's emotions and the inability to experience pleasure. Substance abusers' inability to verbalize feelings leads to the somatization of affective responses. This somatization results in their being confronted with sensations rather than with identifiable feelings. Consequently, the physiological sensations are not useful as signals, but remain painful and overwhelming. Thinking becomes operative, mundane, and boring. The capacity for empathy and development of utilizable transference is seriously diminished. Moreover, many substance abusers lose the capacity, if they ever had it, to experience joy, pleasure, or happiness without the use of substances.

IMPLICATIONS FOR TREATMENT

Looking at addiction and substance abuse from the perspective of self-psychology and attachment theory implies adjustments in strategies and techniques when applying IGP during its different phases. Therapists need to differentiate early treatment strategies from later stage treatment strategies (Wallace 1978). More recently, Kaufman and Reoux (1988) recommended that treatment strategies be adapted to fit three distinct phases of treatment: (1) achieving sobriety, (2) early recovery or abstinence, and (3) advanced or late stage recovery. In a similar fashion, Washton (1992) suggested that substance abusers should move through different sequential groups, which focus on issues relevant to their particular stage in recovery: (1) early recovery, (2) relapse prevention or maintenance, and (3) long-term recovery.

Early Treatment Issues

IGP must be adapted to fit the many unique characteristics and circumstances of the typical substance abuser in early treatment. While simultaneously helping the patient become emotionally attached to the group and actively involved in the treatment process, early treatment addresses the need for working through initial resistances. Moreover, recent suggestions for early treatment goals include getting patients "acculturated" to the group and the "culture of recovery" (Kemker, Kibel, and Mahler 1993), helping them to accept identification as an addict or an alcoholic while integrating the twelve-step recovery principles into the therapy format (Matano and Yalom 1991), and providing group members with the opportunity to understand their own attitudes and denial of addiction by giving them the opportunity to confront similar attitudes and defenses in other substance abusers (Vannicelli 1992).

Early treatment requires more structure and direction than later stage treatment. Most substance abusers will not be able to tolerate the frustration and regression inherent to the more classically influenced psychodynamic group approaches as outlined by Bion (1961) and Ezriel (1973). Substance abusers will usually respond more favorably to a group leader who is spontaneous, alive, engaging, and responsive than to one who adopts the more reserved stance of technical neutrality. An active group leader can counter the characterological deficits of these patients, who constantly battle feelings of boredom, deadness, meaninglessness, and inner emptiness that threaten to overtake them. However, overly charismatic behavior can induce fears of engulfment, destructive idealization, and competitive distractions. A passive group leader is likely to be experienced by the substance abuser as withholding, timid, weak, and dead. Such an adverse relationship stirs up unconscious fears of annihilation and nothingness, feelings associated with primitive identifications; transference distortions are heightened which, in turn, intensifies resistances.

Walant (1995), examining substance abuse from the perspective of attachment theory, emphasizes the need for an "immersion experience"—moments of complete understanding between the patient and the therapist—as a means for dislodging the alienated, disconnected inner self from its hiding place, so that the group will develop into a secure base that enables all patients to shift their object of attachment from substances to one another.

The group leader should not gratify the group members in an infantile manner. This is unrealistic, antitherapeutic, and ultimately impossible, and also feeds the substance abuser's infantile narcissistic grandiosity and demands for immediate gratification. Establishing a climate of *optimal frustration* provides a delicate balance between meeting the patients' dependency needs and making patients internalize control over their own emotions.

Substance abusers require much help early in treatment to identify their feelings, communicate these feelings to others, and establish intimacy and interpersonal relationships.

To establish such early treatment strategies, the group leader must modify the IGP approach so that leadership functions take precedence over therapy functions. The group leader should establish a safe, cohesive environment where boundaries are strictly maintained and the release of emotions are carefully modulated. This provides the opportunity for a corrective emotional relationship, allowing members to reclaim disowned shameful parts of themselves.

Late-Stage Treatment

Once group leaders have used the power and the leverage of the group to help patients internalize responsibility for abstinence from alcohol and drugs, they must then help them come to terms with the internal deficits that have contributed to substance abuse. This "coming to terms" is usually not possible until the substance abusers have had enough time and distance from their use of substances to allow cognitive processes to stabilize and emotional lability to be contained. During this stage of treatment patients begin to develop the capacity to understand substance use as a source of affect regulation and gratification.

Eventually substance abusers must come to terms with their character pathology and their inability to establish and to maintain healthy intimate relationships; this is a major contributing factor for relapses and the return to substances (Khantzian, Halliday, and McAuliffe 1990).

In a mature group, one in which the members have had the opportunity to achieve some degree of sobriety and abstinence, here-and-now exchanges prove more profitable. Since increased abstinence frees group members from the preoccupations of withdrawal and craving, the whole group is able to tolerate an approach that is less gratifying and more demanding than the one used earlier in treatment. The ultimate aim is to help group members develop interpersonal skills within the group that can be generalized and applied outside, in the real world. This late stage treatment operates on the principle that internal structural change is necessary for external behavioral change to be long-lasting and something other than adaptive compliance.

The alleviation of shame is related to structural change. This relationship among addiction, character pathology, and shame is becoming increasingly recognized (Alonso and Rutan 1993). Shame involves exposure and feeling diminished. It leads to hiding, dishonesty, and isolation. Because the activation of intense feelings of shame related to object hunger, dependency, and hostility associated with a transference relationship are too profound for substance abusers to tolerate in individual therapy, group therapy is required. By virtue of its size, a group dilutes the intensity of feelings that would otherwise inundate a patient. Thus, substance abusers in a group can spread their attachments and feelings safely to several people and the group itself. The responsiveness of the group leader and his or her firm, yet nonhostile, ability to absorb anger can lay the foundation for later identification. Consequently, fears of closeness, rejection, attack, and dependence are not as severe, and members feel less threatened. The group can also provide an alternative to the substance abuser's lifestyle, acting as a transitional object until a more stable sense of self is internalized.

CONCLUSION

By viewing addiction and substance abuse as components of an attachment disorder, group therapy works for the substance-abusing population. Substance abuse is the result of disturbances in attachment and reactions to injury of the self. No one ever escapes the need for satisfying relationships. The inability to form healthy interpersonal intimacy determines the degree of vulnerability to substitute substances for human closeness. There is an inverse relationship between an early experience of positive self-object responsiveness and the propensity to turn to drugs, alcohol, and other sources of gratification for missing or damaged relationships. Conversely, to success-fully give up misguided attempts at self-repair, one must develop healthy relationships to gradually satisfy the need for self-object responsiveness. Since relationships can also be addicting, substance abusers must learn how to establish and maintain healthy relation-ships within the group before they are able to have relationships out-side of the group. The goal of substance abuse treatment is very simi-lar to that of analysis for individuals suffering from narcissistic disturbances. In therapy, cure is obtained when a person can establish healthy relationships outside of the therapeutic milieu (Kohut 1984).

IGP provides a predictable and consistent holding environment that allows attachment and self-object needs to be met in a non-exploitive, destructive, or shameful way. Through identification with others in group, members will have the opportunity to accept in them-selves what they could not previously accept because they felt so unique in their badness. Acceptance at this level of emotional vulner-ability (immersion experience) can be tolerated by substance abusers only if they feel understood at a very basic, empathic level by another as vulnerable as they. Someone who feels like a peer or a true equal can best provide such an understanding.

True mutuality is the necessary catalyst for shame reduction and attachment. IGP group therapy can provide this mutuality much more effectively than can any other form of therapy.

REFERENCES

Alonso A, Rutan JS. Character change in group therapy. *International Journal of Group Psychotherapy* 43:439-452, 1993.
Bion WR. *Experiences in Groups.* New York: Basic Books, 1961.
Brown DG. Bion and Foulkes: Basic assumptions and beyond. In *Bion and Group Psychotherapy,* edited by Pines M. London: Tavistock Routledge, 1985, pp. 192-219.
Brown S. *Treating the Alcoholic: A Developmental Model of Recovery.* New York: John Wiley & Sons, 1985.
Brown S, Yalom I. Interactional group psychotherapy with alcoholic patients. *Journal of Studies on Alcohol* 38:426-456, 1977.
Dies RR. Models of group psychotherapy: Shifting through confusion. *International Journal of Group Psychotherapy* 42:1-18, 1992.

Ezriel H. Psychoanalytic group psychotherapy. In *Group Therapy,* edited by Wolberg LR, Schwartz EK. New York: Straton Intercontinental Medical Books, 1973, pp. 183-210.

Flores P. *Group Psychotherapy with Addicted Populations.* Binghamton, NY: The Haworth Press, 1988.

Flores P. *Group Psychotherapy with Addicted Populations: An Integration of Twelve-Step and Psychodynamic Theory.* Binghamton, NY: The Haworth Press, 1997.

Flores P, Mahon L. The treatment of addiction in group psychotherapy. *International Journal of Group Psychotherapy* 43:143-156, 1993.

Ganzarain R. Introduction to object relations group psychotherapy. *International Journal of Group Psychotherapy* 42:205-224, 1992.

Kanas N. Alcoholism and group psychotherapy. In *Encyclopedic Handbook of Alcoholism,* edited by Pattison EM, Kaufman SE. New York: Gardner Press, 1982.

Kaufman E, Reoux J. Guidelines for the successful psychotherapy of substance abusers. *American Journal of Drug and Alcohol Abuse* 14:199-209, 1988.

Kemker SS, Kibel HD, Mahler JC. On becoming oriented to inpatient treatment: Inducing new patients and professionals to recovery movement. *International Journal of Group Psychotherapy* 43:285-302, 1993.

Khantzian EJ, Halliday KS, McAuliffe WE. *Addiction and the Vulnerable Self.* New York: Guilford Press, 1990.

Kohut H. *How Does Analysis Cure?* Chicago, IL: University of Chicago Press, 1984.

Leszcz M. The interpersonal approach to group psychotherapy. *International Journal of Group Psychotherapy* 42:37-62, 1992.

Matano RA, Yalom I. Approaches to chemical dependency: Chemical dependency and interactive group therapy—A synthesis. *International Journal of Group Psychotherapy* 41:269-294, 1991.

Ormont L. *The Group Therapy Experience.* New York: St. Martin's Press, 1992.

Pattison EM. The selection of treatment modalities for the alcoholic patient. In *The Diagnosis and Treatment of Alcoholism,* edited by Mandelson JH, Mello NK. New York: McGraw-Hill, 1979, pp. 229-255.

Rutan JS, Stone WN. *Psychodynamic Group Psychotherapy,* Second Edition. New York: Guilford Press, 1993.

Sullivan HS. *The Interpersonal Theory of Psychiatry.* New York: WW Norton, 1953.

Vannicelli M. *Removing the Roadblocks: Group Psychotherapy with Substance Abusers and Family Members.* New York: Guilford Press, 1992.

Walant KB. *Creating the Capacity for Attachment: Treating Addictions and the Alienated Self.* Northvale, NJ: Jason Aronson Inc, 1995.

Wallace J. Working with the preferred defense structure of the recovering alcoholic. In *Practical Approaches to Alcoholism Psychotherapy,* edited by Zimberg S, Wallace J, Blume S. New York: Plenum Press, 1978, pp. 19-29.

Washton AM. Structured outpatient group therapy with alcohol and substance abusers. In *Substance Abuse: A Comprehensive Textbook,* edited by Lowinson J, Ruiz P, Millman R. Baltimore, MD: Williams & Wilkins, 1992, pp. 440-448.

Yalom ID. *The Theory and Practice of Group Psychotherapy,* Fourth Edition. New York: Basic Books, 1995.

Yalom VJ, Vinogradov S. Interpersonal group psychotherapy. In *Comprehensive Group Psychotherapy,* Third Edition, edited by Kaplan HK, Sadock BJ. Baltimore, MD: Williams & Wilkins, 1993, pp. 185-194.

Chapter 3

The Cognitive Therapy Addictions Group

Bruce S. Liese
Aaron T. Beck
Kim Seaton

INTRODUCTION AND THEORY

For the past decade we have provided individual and group cognitive therapy (CT) to hundreds of people with addictions (Beck and Liese 1998; Beck et al. 1993; Liese 1994; Liese and Beck 1997; Liese and Franz 1996; Wright et al. 1992). In this chapter, we describe our theory of addictions and offer guidelines for facilitating cognitive therapy addiction groups (CTAGs). Case examples from actual CTAG sessions are provided to illustrate salient concepts, activities, and interventions.

We believe that addictions result from complex interactions among cognitive, behavioral, emotional, family, social, cultural, and biophysiological processes—although naturally, we focus primarily on cognitive processes. Our model has been substantially influenced by previous cognitive-behavioral theories of addiction and relapse (e.g., Marlatt 1985).

Cognitive Processes in Addictive Behaviors

Cognitive processes cover numerous mental activities: thoughts, beliefs, ideas, schemas, values, opinions, expectations, philosophies, assumptions, and so forth. Those most likely to lead to addictive behaviors include anticipatory beliefs, relief-oriented beliefs, automatic thoughts, facilitative beliefs, and instrumental beliefs. We hypothesize that these cognitive processes interact with emotional, environmental, physiological, and developmental processes in ways that determine whether a person will manifest addictive behaviors. Our model is presented in Figure 3.1.

A thorough working knowledge of the cognitive model is essential for clinicians who facilitate CTAGs. In each session, the cognitive model is reviewed by the facilitator who relates it to the lives and problems of group members. Group members enter the CTAG with idiosyncratic maladaptive beliefs that perpetuate their addictive behaviors (e.g., "I'll go crazy if I quit smoking" or "Life without drinking would suck"). Group members come to understand that they are addicted largely because of their maladaptive thinking. In CTAGs, addicted group members learn to control their thought processes and their addictive behaviors.

Most addictive behaviors (e.g., smoking, drinking, gambling, overeating, overspending) can be traced to various *activating stimuli* (see Figure 3.1). These stimuli, also known as "triggers" or "cues," are both internal and external. *Internal cues* are most commonly experienced as emotions (e.g., anxiety, depression, anger, boredom) or physiologic

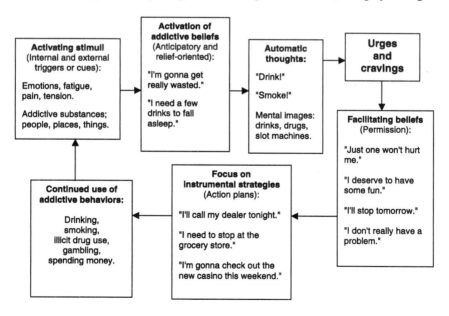

FIGURE 3.1. Cognitive Therapy Model of Addictive Behaviors (*Source:* Adapted from Liese and Franz [1996]. "Cognitive therapy of addictions: Lessons learned and implications for the future" [p. 477]. Copyright 1996 by Guilford Press. Reprinted by permission.)

sensations (fatigue, pain, tension). People use addictive behaviors as compensatory strategies to regulate and cope with feelings. They drink, smoke, and overeat to *relieve* boredom, anxiety, and depression. But they also use addictive behaviors to *make good feelings even better.* For example, Joe (a heavy drinker) feels *pretty good* on Friday afternoon. He stops at a bar, meets friends, and has ten to fifteen drinks in order to feel *even better.* Joe's *excitement* as he anticipates the weekend is an *internal cue* that activates his drinking. When he arrives at the bar where he meets his *friends,* he encounters numerous *external cues.*

External cues (e.g., exposure to addictive substances and various "people, places, and things") are synonymous with environmental triggers. Many addicted individuals feel helpless about the urges and cravings they associate with external cues.

According to our model, the *activation of addictive beliefs* kindles addictive behaviors. There are at least two types of addictive beliefs: anticipatory and relief-oriented. Anticipatory beliefs involve positive expectations about engaging in addictive behaviors. An example is, "I'm gonna get really wasted this weekend!" Relief-oriented beliefs involve a reduction in some aversive condition (e.g., depression, loneliness). An example of a relief-oriented belief is, "I need a few drinks before bedtime to fall asleep." *Automatic thoughts* (ATs) are brief, abbreviated ideas or mental images. Examples of addiction-related ATs are "Drink!" and "Smoke!" Mental images might include frosty mugs of ice cold beer, fat joints, or puffs on a cigarette. ATs precede urges and cravings, though they occur so quickly and automatically that they tend to go unnoticed.

Urges and *cravings* are experienced as physical sensations, such as hunger or thirst, for addictive behaviors. According to Marlatt (1985), an urge is a "relatively sudden impulse to engage in an act" while a craving is "the subjective desire to experience the effects or consequences of a given act" (p. 48). Urges and cravings do not necessarily lead to addictive behaviors. The process of detaching oneself from urges in order to abstain from addictive behaviors has been referred to as *urge surfing*. Marlatt explains, "the urge is similar to the swelling of a wave which the surfer hopes to 'ride' without getting 'wiped out' " (p. 64). CTAG members are advised to surf (rather than indulge) their urges. Group facilitators explain that urges eventually subside on their own. Group members often report that the image of urge surfing is helpful. Some seem to enjoy associating their recovery process with the courageous and exciting image of riding the crest of a wave.

Facilitating beliefs are quite common; they involve self-granted *permission* to engage in addictive behaviors despite wishes to stop such behaviors. An example of a facilitating belief is, "Just one won't hurt me." Those who indulge in addictive behaviors have given themselves permission to do so, while those who abstain from their addictive behaviors have developed such *prohibitive* beliefs as, "One hit will lead to two hits, which will lead to three hits, until I'm in big trouble." (These beliefs are called "prohibitive" because they prohibit subsequent addictive behaviors.)

Instrumental beliefs (or "action plans") are cognitive processes that lead to the acquisition of addictive substances or engagement in addictive behaviors (e.g., "I'll call my dealer tonight" and "I need to stop at the grocery store on the way home from work"). When instrumental beliefs are fully activated, individuals may become like "heat-seeking missiles" in pursuit of their addictive behaviors.

Addictive behaviors are characterized by certain overt actions (e.g., smoking, drinking, overeating, gambling, overspending), and more subtle rituals associated with addictive behaviors, such as cigarette breaks. An essential function of the CTAG is to help group members understand the rituals associated with their addictions.

In summary, CTAG facilitators teach group members that their thoughts and beliefs, not triggers per se, lead to addictive behaviors. As group members learn to attribute their addictive behaviors to internal cognitive processes, they can begin to take increasing responsibility for changing these behaviors.

The Development of Addictive Behaviors

Group members often ask, "How did this addiction happen to me?" To answer this common question, CTAG facilitators must be skilled at applying the cognitive model to the development of addictive behaviors (see Figure 3.2). As our model indicates, early life experiences lead to the development of certain schemas, basic beliefs, and conditional beliefs. These may be negative, positive, adaptive, maladaptive, or neutral, depending on the nature of early life experiences. They may also lead to certain dysfunctional conditional beliefs ("If I don't take advantage of others, they will take advantage of me"), which make people vulnerable to addictive behaviors follow-

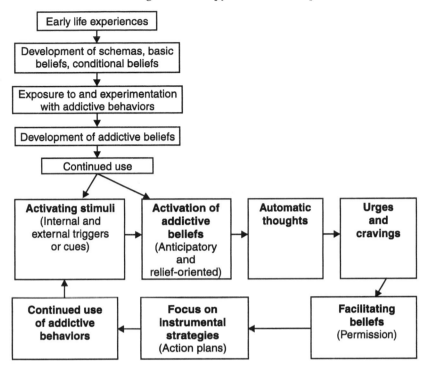

FIGURE 3.2. Cognitive-Developmental Model of Addictive Behaviors (*Source:* Adapted from Liese and Franz [1996]. "Cognitive therapy of addictions: Lessons learned and implications for the future" [p. 482]. Copyright 1996 by Guilford Press. Reprinted by permission.)

ing exposure. As a result of continued involvement in addictive behaviors, these beliefs become overlearned and predominant. It is important to note that this model does not deny the validity or importance of biological or genetic determinants of addictions. However, CTAG facilitators focus more on cognitive developmental processes than on genetic or biological processes.

OVERVIEW OF THE COGNITIVE THERAPY ADDICTIONS GROUP

Numerous cognitive-behavioral (C-B) therapies have been developed for treating addictions (Liese and Najavits 1997) and many addiction group interventions have been described and evaluated

(Stinchfield, Owen, and Winters 1994). Cognitive-behavioral addiction treatments mostly focus on modifying thoughts and behaviors and developing coping skills. Cognitive-behavioral programs are highly structured and psychoeducational, and easily adapted to both individual and group modalities. A well-designed, empirically validated cognitive-behavioral group for treating alcohol dependence (Monti et al. 1989) was modified for individual delivery in the MATCH study (Kadden et al. 1993). Likewise, our approach (Beck et al. 1993) was recently modified for delivery in a group setting (Maude-Griffin et al. 1998) and found to be superior to twelve-step facilitation. In the following sections we describe our CTAG in detail.

CTAGs are heterogeneous, composed of group members with a wide range of addictions and other psychosocial problems. Sessions provide a supportive, structured, educational environment where members are encouraged to develop effective cognitive and behavioral coping skills. Group size can range from small (two people) to large (ten people), with four to eight group members considered optimal. CTAGs meet at least once per week and sessions are ninety minutes in length. Group membership is "open" (i.e., members initiate and terminate involvement as they wish).

CTAG Facilitators

CTAG facilitators are mental health professionals of all kinds trained to conduct group cognitive therapy, with a working knowledge of cognitive theory and therapy. They should also have substantial knowledge of psychopathology and addictive behaviors.

CTAG facilitators should possess strong interpersonal and group facilitation skills (Flores 1997). The most effective CTAG facilitators strike a balance between being *task-oriented* (i.e., well-organized, focused, systematic) and *process-oriented* (i.e., adaptable, caring, empathetic, able to initiate and maintain productive group interaction).

CTAG Members

CTAGs serve a wide range of people with addictions and other problems. Individuals who enroll in CTAGs should

1. recognize that they have problems with addictive behaviors;
2. take some responsibility for their problems;

3. want this type of treatment;
4. understand cognitive therapy concepts and techniques; and
5. collaborate with other group members.

CTAG members vary in their addictive behaviors (e.g., smoking, drinking, gambling, shopping, etc.), patterns of use (e.g., chronic, episodic), and symptomatic behavior. In CTAGs, individual differences among group members are viewed as potentially beneficial. Effective CTAG facilitators can help group members learn important coping and recovery skills from one another's similarities and differences.

Goals of the CTAG

Although a high level of motivation is optimal, CTAG members vary in their readiness to change. Therefore CTAG facilitators should be familiar with the transtheoretical model of change (Prochaska and DiClemente 1992) and motivational interviewing (Miller and Rollnick 1991). Some group members may initially deny their problems and their need for treatment; some may be contemplating change; some may be prepared to change; some may be in the midst of change; and others may be maintaining long-term changes. Some may wish to reduce their addictive behaviors; others may wish to become fully abstinent; while others may already be abstinent but contemplating limited use. CTAG facilitators should give the clear message that the group is designed to help members *abstain from addictive behaviors and effectively cope with life's challenges.*

CTAG facilitators regularly encounter addicted group members who either recurrently relapse or choose to continue using rather than abstain. When this occurs, facilitators should be prepared to take a "harm reduction" (HR) approach (Marlatt et al. 1993; Marlatt and Tapert 1993). In HR, individuals are treated with respect and unconditional regard despite their persistent addictive behaviors.

Some group members are likely to interpret HR interventions as condoning addictive behaviors. The facilitator must explain that the long-term goal of the CTAG is *abstinence,* although HR may necessarily be a point along the way for some individuals. HR interventions are motivational strategies designed to move addicted individuals from one stage of change to the next.

Attrition is a major problem in the treatment of addictions (Liese and Beck 1997). A major goal of the CTAG is to retain group members even when they have difficulty abstaining. CTAG facilitators should encourage relapsing members to attend sessions unless they are disruptive to the group or they flaunt their substance use. Instead of giving group members the message, "Come to the group *only if you are abstinent,*" facilitators give the message, "Try to attend our group *no matter what.*"

STRUCTURE OF THE GROUP

The structure of the CTAG is among its assets. Each session consists of the following components:

1. *Facilitator introductions* (five minutes): Facilitators introduce themselves, the group, and the cognitive model.
2. *Group member introductions* (twenty to forty minutes): Group members introduce themselves, and the facilitator begins to relate their problems to the cognitive models in Figures 3.1 and 3.2.
3. *Challenging thoughts and beliefs that lead to addictive behaviors* (twenty to forty minutes): The *Cognitive Model Worksheet* (Figure 3.3) is used to elicit and challenge thoughts and beliefs that lead group members to engage in addictive behaviors.
4. *Coping Skills Training* (ten to twenty minutes): Group members are taught specific coping skills relevant to their current problems (e.g., mood regulation, relationship development and maintenance, crisis management).
5. *Goal setting and homework* (ten to twenty minutes): Each member is encouraged to set short-term and long-term goals and commit to homework assignments for achieving these goals;
6. *Closure* (five to ten minutes): Members reflect on what they have learned in the present group session.

In the following sections, these six components are more fully described.

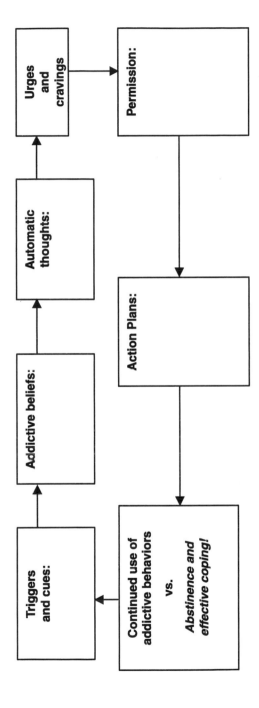

FIGURE 3.3. Cognitive Model Worksheet (*Source*: Adapted from Liese and Franz [1996]. "Cognitive therapy of addictions: Lessons learned and implications for the future" [p. 490]. Copyright 1996 by Guilford Press. Reprinted by permission.)

Facilitator Introductions

CTAG facilitators introduce themselves by telling who they are and why they facilitate the group. On occasion they will be asked about their own recovery status (i.e., "Have you ever been addicted?"). Self-disclosure may be appropriate at times to facilitate authenticity and group cohesiveness. CTAG facilitators with histories of addictive behaviors should be especially careful about self-disclosure. In general they are discouraged from *initiating* discussions about their addictions since group time is limited and member responses to self-disclosures are somewhat unpredictable. Facilitator self-disclosure, when it does occur, should be in response to group members' questions, and excessive detail should be avoided.

When making introductory remarks, the facilitator discusses the structure, content, and rules of the group. *Structure* includes the components listed above (i.e., introductions, challenging thoughts and beliefs that lead to addictive behaviors, coping skills training, goal setting, and closure). *Content* is partly determined by issues presented by group members, but the cognitive model of addictions is reviewed in every session. *Rules* of the group mostly involve confidentiality and respect for other group members. In addition, group members are asked to be as honest and immediate (i.e., in the here and now) as possible, rather than philosophizing or generalizing.

Group Member Introductions

After facilitator introductions are completed, group members introduce themselves. They state their names, past and present addictions, the status of their addictions, goals, and other issues. The facilitator limits each member's introduction to five minutes or less.

Introductions provide opportunities for group members to listen and learn vicariously from one another's successful and unsuccessful coping strategies. During introductions group cohesiveness begins to develop as members share their problems, fears, hopes, and plans for improving their lives. As group members introduce themselves, the facilitator completes the *CTAG Attendance and Summary Form*. This form helps organize information provided by group members during introductions, and it serves as a guide for discussions that follow. Later in the session the facilitator will need to choose a coping skills topic for discussion with the group. Notes taken on the *CTAG Attendance and Summary Form* can be very helpful for this purpose.

The following brief excerpt from an actual CTAG session provides a typical example of members' introductions. The facilitator has already introduced himself and asked group members to state their names, addictions, status, goals, and other problems. There are four members present and each has been attending this CTAG for at least several months. As group members talk, their responses are noted on the facilitator's *CTAG Attendance and Summary Form*.

FACILITATOR: Who wants to start?

BILL: I'll go first. My name is Bill and I'm an alcoholic. I haven't had anything to drink in seven years and I plan to keep it that way. I try to get to as many meetings as possible 'cause I always learn something. Maybe some day you guys will even convince me to quit smoking! Everything else seems to be going good in my life.

FACILITATOR: So, Bill, your addictions have been alcohol and cigarettes. You've been abstinent from alcohol for the past seven years, but you're still smoking cigarettes. How many packs a day are you smoking?

BILL: Two, but I've cut down from three.

FACILITATOR: Okay, two packs a day. But at least you're contemplating quitting.

BILL: I didn't say *that*. I just said '*Maybe* some day you guys will convince me to quit.' [Group members laugh.]

FACILITATOR: You can be sure we'll keep trying! [More laughter.]

FACILITATOR: Okay, who wants to go next?

KATHY: I'll go. I'm Kathy and I have been smoking marijuana for as long as I can remember. I'm not sure it's really a problem. I have lots of friends who smoke and they don't seem to have problems with it. I don't know. I guess that's why I'm here. I just don't know. I'll admit that my husband is really pissed at me for continuing to smoke. He says I ignore the kids.

FACILITATOR: So you're still considering the possibility that you are addicted to marijuana. How much did you smoke this week?

During group member introductions, the facilitator summarizes common themes, problems, and issues. The cognitive model is briefly introduced and applied to one or more group members.

FACILITATOR: Sue, do you mind if we discuss your situation?

SUE: I figured you would.

FACILITATOR: Is it okay if I use the cognitive model?

SUE: Yeah, actually I've been thinking about those boxes a lot. They've helped me understand why I'm having so much trouble.

FACILITATOR: Good, I'll draw them now. [Facilitator draws the cognitive model on the chalkboard.] According to the cognitive model of addictions, people are most likely to engage in addictive behaviors following certain triggers or cues. These triggers can be internal or external. Internal triggers include emotions such as depression, anxiety, boredom, anger, and loneliness, as well as physical sensations such as withdrawal symptoms, pain, hunger, and fatigue. External triggers can include people, places, and things associated in some way with your addiction. So, Sue, you shouldn't be surprised that you want to smoke more right now.

SUE: Yeah, this medical thing is about the biggest trigger I can imagine.

The facilitator explains the seven boxes of the cognitive model (Figure 3.1) and with each box he asks Sue to describe corresponding triggers, thoughts, feelings, or behaviors. In doing so he makes the model "come to life" for the group. After this review of the cognitive model the facilitator asks, "Any questions?" There are none and he moves on to the next phase of the group.

Challenging Thoughts and Beliefs That Lead to Addictive Behaviors

Following introductions and review of the cognitive model, the facilitator invites group members into the discussion by asking them to describe thoughts and beliefs that contribute to their own addictive behaviors. Each group member receives a blank copy of the *Cognitive Model Worksheet* (Figure 3.3), which is also drawn on the chalkboard. As they identify their maladaptive thoughts and beliefs they prepare to challenge (and hopefully modify) them. To encourage participation, the facilitator (starting with the "triggers" box) asks, "What are your triggers?" "Under what circumstances are you most likely to have strong urges?" and "When is it most difficult for you to keep from drinking, smoking, using, gambling, or overeating?" After group members describe their triggers the facilitator asks, "What can you do about these?" The facilitator helps the group discuss the management of both avoidable and unavoidable triggers.

Prior to challenging thoughts and beliefs that lead to addictive behaviors, the facilitator may first help group members understand the cognitive-behavioral change process.

As the facilitator discussed strategies for changing beliefs, group members are helped to generate thoughts and beliefs that counteract their addiction-related thoughts and beliefs. As group members respond, the facilitator notes their comments on the chalkboard and they are encouraged to write their idiosyncratic thoughts on their own copies of the *Cognitive Model Worksheet,* as well as challenges to these thoughts. Pointing toward the third box of the cognitive model of addictions, the facilitator defines automatic thoughts and permissive beliefs.

Group members are encouraged to identify and challenge their permissive (and other addiction-related) beliefs by means of the *Two-Column Technique.* To introduce this technique the facilitator draws two columns on the chalkboard. At the top of the left column the facilitator writes, *"Permissive Beliefs."* At the top of the right column *"Prohibitive Beliefs"* is written. Group members are asked by the facilitator to list their common permissive beliefs and one such belief is written in the left-hand column: "I deserve to have some fun." In the right-hand column the group generates a list of beliefs that prohibit addictive behaviors (e.g., " I deserve to have fun but I can have fun without drugs" and "Doing drugs now will lead to big trouble later"). At the end of this activity, the group is asked to reflect on what they have learned.

The facilitator next explains, "After people with addictions give themselves permission to use, many focus on action plans to prepare for indulging their addictive behaviors." The facilitator asks, "In order to indulge your addictive behaviors, what actions must you take?" Specific action plans, such as buying cigarettes or calling a dealer, are largely determined by each individual's unique addictive behaviors. The group facilitator points out that this may be the group member's final opportunity to stop the addiction cycle before it returns in full force. Some group members describe this process as "white knuckling" (i.e., where they use "brute force" to deny themselves their addictive behaviors in the face of strong urges and cravings). Group members are taught that white knuckling is perhaps the most fragile and uncomfortable approach to recovery since it occurs after urges and cravings have already taken hold. Alternatively, group members are encouraged to learn coping skills to reduce their vulnerability to addictive behaviors.

Coping Skills Training

The facilitator is next faced with an important, complex, and challenging task: choosing the coping skill to be discussed in the current session. Coping skills training is standard to most cognitive-behavioral addiction treatment programs (e.g., Glantz and McCourt 1983; Kadden et al. 1995; Monti et al. 1989; Najavits, Weiss, and Liese 1996). For some CTAG members, coping skills training provides specific strategies for addressing problems uncovered in "personal inventories." (For excellent discussions of AA and psychological change processes, see DiClemente 1993; McCrady and Miller 1993.)

The following is a list of five coping skills commonly taught to CTAG members, organized into modules:

1. *Developing and maintaining healthy relationships:* Healthy intimate relationships can greatly facilitate the recovery process. Conversely, unhealthy relationships can lead to emotional distress and the exacerbation of addictive behaviors.
2. *Mood control—coping with anger, depression, boredom, anxiety:* We assume that people use addictive behaviors to regulate emotions, moods, and feelings. Hence, many (if not most) people who quit addictive behaviors are likely to experience serious difficulties with moods. In this module, the cognitive models of anxiety, depression, and anger are taught to group members, as well as cognitive-behavioral techniques for mood management.
3. *Motivation, readiness to change, and self-discipline:* Motivation is a continuous (rather than static) process. People range at times from being highly *unmotivated* to being highly *motivated*. Some are motivated to engage in certain behavior changes but not others. In this module on motivation, group members learn about the processes and stages of change as well as strategies for making changes.

4. *Finding meaning:* As people become increasingly addicted, they are more likely to lose sight of values and activities that potentially make their lives fulfilling. Perhaps this is why so many addiction programs include a spiritual component. In this module, group members are helped to find meaning in their lives. It is emphasized that this process does not necessarily require a focus on God or religion—many people in recovery choose to search for meaning in their work, hobbies, and relationships.

5. *Crisis management:* Addictions and crises go hand in hand; crises trigger addictive behaviors and addictive behaviors trigger crises (Liese 1994). Many addicted people experience interpersonal, legal, medical, psychiatric, and financial crises. Although crises may involve threats, they may also offer opportunities for personal growth, and can become turning points where meaningful changes can begin to occur.

Most group members entering CTAGs admit that they lack essential coping skills that they wish to learn in the group. In fact, many continue to attend open group sessions long after achieving abstinence in order to continue learning coping skills. In a meeting of regular CTAG members who are successfully maintaining abstinence, at least half of the session may be spent discussing coping skills.

Cognitive therapy is well suited for the treatment of mood problems associated with addictions. In CTAGs, group members are taught that their thought processes profoundly affect their moods, and that each emotional problem has its own unique underlying cognitive pattern and process. Group members are taught to regulate their moods by learning to apply the cognitive models to themselves.

Many techniques for helping patients to regulate their emotions are taught to CTAG members as needed. For example, in some sessions group members may be taught to identify and label their own cognitive distortions, or to use *Daily Thought Records* (DTRs) to modify their thoughts and feelings.

DTRs are among the most basic of CT interventions. They provide a standardized method for evaluating and changing dysfunctional thoughts. A sample DTR is presented in Table 3.1. Group members complete DTRs by providing the information requested in each column. This practice enables them to recognize and evaluate their own thoughts and feelings. The following is a list of guidelines for using DTRs:

1. *Teach group members the rationale for using DTRs:* Explain that a major goal of cognitive therapy is to identify and change the beliefs that get people into trouble.
2. *Express confidence in the usefulness of DTRs:* Explain that many people have been helped by DTRs. Encourage group members to complete DTRs for an extended period.
3. *Provide specific instructions regarding the completion of DTRs:* Tell patients, "At least once a day identify a problem you have faced, as well as the time and date of the problem. Then write down the situation, how you felt, and what thoughts caused you to feel that way. Then imagine how you might feel if you had changed your thoughts."
4. *Explain that all sections of DTRs are important:* Tell patients that they need to provide all information asked for on the DTR.
5. *Emphasize the importance of completing at least one DTR each day:* Tell group members, "These forms are called *Daily* Thought Records because they really need to be done *every day* until you are able to monitor how you think and feel without them."
6. *Use real life situations from group members as examples:* Ask group members, "Who wants to help me with real examples for filling in a DTR?"
7. *Review DTRs assigned as homework:* Tell patients, "Please complete *at least one DTR per day* and we will review them in the next group session."
8. *Expect group members to make mistakes when first completing DTRs:* DTRs appear deceptively simple. In reviewing group members' DTRs, help them understand how to use them effectively.

Group facilitators who wish to have group members use DTRs should plan to spend at least twenty minutes demonstrating one with the group (see DTR in Table 3.1).

Instead of choosing "mood regulation" as a coping skill, the facilitator could have focused on "readiness to change." If this topic had been chosen, an *Advantages-Disadvantages (A-D) Analysis* (Table 3.2) might have been used to help group members understand how their perceptions of advantages and disadvantages affect their readiness for change. In completing an A-D analysis, facilitators help group members to complete the advantages and disadvantages of using or not using their addictive behavior.

TABLE 3.1. Daily Thought Record

Patient's name: _____ Sue _____   Date: _____ April 8

Date and time	Stimulus situation (trigger)	Feelings (Rate intensity 0-100)	Automatic thoughts or beliefs (Rate confidence 0-100%)	Alternative thoughts or beliefs (Rate confidence 0-100%)	Resulting feelings (Rate intensity 0-100)
4/6	My doctor says something is wrong with me.	Worried (100) Desperate (75)	"I probably have cancer." (60%) "I'm gonna die from this problem." (40%)	"Right now I don't have any way of knowing whether I have cancer or will die from it, so I'd better quit worrying myself sick over it." (85%)	Slightly less worried (80) Less desperate (50)

Directions: When you notice a mood shift, use this chart to identify the stimulus situation, your feelings, the thoughts that contribute to your feelings, alternate thoughts (to replace the original thoughts), and new feelings (resulting from the alternate thoughts). As you complete each of the last four columns, rate the intensity of your feelings and your confidence in the thoughts on a scale from 0 (none) to 100 (maximum). Complete these ratings *prior to moving to the next column.*

TABLE 3.2. Advantages-Disadvantages Analysis

	Using addictive behaviors (e.g., smoking marijuana)	Not using addictive behaviors (e.g., not smoking marijuana)
Advantages	Smoking relaxes me. Smoking is fun. Smoking is something to do with my friends.	I might have fewer problems with my husband. I'd save some money. I might feel better about myself.
Disadvantages	Smoking costs money. My husband doesn't like that I smoke. It's not that easy to quit.	My friends would think it was weird if I stopped smoking. I'd be losing an old friend. I love the feeling of getting high.

Goal Setting and Homework

Goal setting is common to most cognitive-behavioral approaches to addiction treatment. Early in each CTAG session group members receive *Personal Goal Sheets,* which are small slips of paper on which they write their names, the date, long-term goals, short-term goals, and homework. After discussing coping skills, all CTAG members are asked to use *Personal Goal Sheets* to list their goals and potential homework. An example of a long-term goal might be to "develop healthy intimate relationships." An example of a short-term goal might be to "spend more time with people who are clean and sober." An example of homework might be to "invite one person over for dinner."

Setting explicit goals can be difficult or intimidating for some group members, who believe that they may fail, or who find it difficult to envision goals for their lives. CTAG facilitators should take an active role in modeling or suggesting goal setting examples for the group. The following three steps can be helpful when teaching group members to identify goals:

1. Envision the future.
2. Establish goals that are specific and achievable.
3. Identify resources.

Brainstorming and sharing ideas may be helpful.

Homework may be self-assigned by group members, or facilitators may assign homework. *Personal Goal Sheets* provide a standardized method for self-assigning homework assignments, or group facilitators may recommend particular assignments. In all likelihood, the most appropriate assignment is an extension of what has been learned in the session. At the end of each session, group facilitators collect goal sheets for review during the next group session. Homework should be completed by the following week and discussed in the group (during introductions or goal setting). A number of self-help books focus on addictions and coping skills.

Closure

At the end of each session, at least five minutes should be set aside for *closure*. Closure provides an opportunity to review issues discussed or lessons learned in the present session. If there were any problems or crises unresolved, closure provides the facilitator with an opportunity to address these (or schedule individual follow-up as needed).

SUMMARY AND CONCLUSIONS

For approximately ten years we have been developing and refining our cognitive model of addictions. This model has been based on the assumption that addictive behaviors are strongly associated with certain maladaptive thoughts and beliefs. Corresponding with our theory, we have also been developing individual and group approaches for treating addictive behaviors.

CTAGs provide highly structured, supportive, educational environments where people with various addictions can learn to be more effective at managing their lives. In group sessions, members are taught to use the cognitive model to understand and resist their addictive behaviors. They also learn coping skills for adapting to life's many challenges. In CTAGs, group members are taught to develop and maintain healthy intimate relationships; they are encouraged to search for meaning; they learn about the processes and stages of change; they are taught strategies for regulating their moods; and they are helped with their crises. Ninety-minute group sessions are offered at least weekly, and some group members continue to attend sessions even after extended abstinence in order to continue learning coping skills.

Over the years we have discovered that CTAGs can be difficult to facilitate. At various times we have been challenged by hostile group members, relapsing group members, intoxicated group members, and group members who simply could not relate to the cognitive model. From these experiences, we have learned numerous lessons about addictive behaviors (Liese and Franz 1996). More important, we have learned that there is a vast need for services that collaboratively challenge addicted people to abstain from addictive behaviors and develop vital living skills. Each time this need is fulfilled, even for one CTAG member, the rewards are great.

REFERENCES

Beck AT, Wright FD, Newman CF, Liese BS. *Cognitive Therapy of Substance Abuse*. New York: Guilford Press, 1993.*

Beck JS, Liese BS. Cognitive therapy. In *Clinical Textbook of Addictive Disorders, Second Edition*, edited by Frances RJ, Miller SI. New York: Guilford Press, 1998, pp. 547-573.

DiClemente CC. Alcoholics Anonymous and the structure of change. In *Research on Alcoholics Anonymous: Opportunities and Alternatives,* edited by McCrady BS, Miller WR. New Brunswick, NJ: Rutgers Center of Alcohol Studies, 1993, pp. 79-97.

Flores PJ. *Group Therapy with Addicted Populations: An Integration of Twelve-Step and Psychodynamic Theory,* Second Edition. Binghamton, NY: The Haworth Press, 1997.

Glantz MD, McCourt W. Cognitive therapy in groups with alcoholics. In *Cognitive Therapy with Couples and Groups,* edited by Freeman A. New York: Plenum Press, 1983, pp. 157-182.

Kadden R, Carroll K, Donovan D, Cooney N, Monti P, Abrams D, Litt M, Hester R (eds.). *Cognitive-Behavioral Coping Skills Therapy Manual: A Clinical Research Guide for Therapists Treating Individuals with Alcohol Abuse and Dependence.* NIAAA Project MATCH Monograph Series, Volume 3. Washington, DC: U.S. Department of Health and Human Services, 1995.*

Liese BS. Brief therapy, crisis intervention, and the cognitive therapy of substance abuse. *Crisis Intervention and Time-Limited Treatment* 1:11-29, 1994.

Liese BS, Beck AT. Back to basics: Fundamental cognitive therapy skills for keeping drug-dependent individuals in treatment. In *Beyond the Therapeutic Alliance: Keeping Drug-Dependent Individuals in Treatment,* edited by Boren JJ,

---

*Recommended readings

Onken LS, Blaine JD. National Institute on Drug Abuse Monograph. Washington, DC: Government Printing Office, 165, 1997, pp. 207-229.

Liese BS, Franz RA. Treating substance use disorders with cognitive therapy: Lessons learned and implications for the future. In *Frontiers of Cognitive Therapy,* edited by Salkovskis P. New York: Guilford Press, 1996, pp. 470-508.*

Liese BS, Najavits LM. Cognitive and behavioral therapies of substance abuse. In *Substance Abuse: A Comprehensive Textbook,* Third Edition, edited by Lowinson JH, Ruiz P, Millman RB, Langrod JG. Philadelphia: Williams & Wilkins, 1997, pp. 467-478.

Marlatt GA. Relapse prevention: Theoretical rationale and overview of the model. In *Relapse Prevention: Maintenance Strategies in the Treatment of Addictive Behaviors,* edited by Marlatt GA, Gordon JR. New York: Guilford Press, 1985, pp. 3-70.*

Marlatt GA, Larimer ME, Baer JS, Quigley LA. Harm reduction for alcohol problems: Moving beyond the controlled drinking controversy. *Behavior Therapy* 24:461-504, 1993.

Marlatt GA, Tapert SF. Harm reduction: Reducing the risks of addictive behaviors. In *Addictive Behaviors Across the Lifespan,* edited by Baer J, Marlatt G, McMahon R. Newbury Park, CA: Sage Publications, 1993, pp. 243-273.

Maude-Griffin PM, Hohenstein JM, Humfleet GL, Reilly PM, Tusel DJ, Hall SM. Superior efficacy of cognitive-behavioral therapy for urban crack cocaine abusers: Main and matching effects. *Journal of Consulting and Clinical Psychology* 66:832-837, 1998.

McCrady BS, Miller WR (eds.). *Research on Alcoholics Anonymous: Opportunities and Alternatives.* New Brunswick, NJ: Rutgers Center of Alcohol Studies, 1993.

Miller WR, Rollnick S. *Motivational Interviewing: Preparing People to Change Addictive Behavior.* New York: Guilford Press, 1991.

Monti PM, Abrams DB, Kadden RM, Cooney NL. *Treating Alcohol Dependence: A Coping Skills Training Guide.* New York: Guilford Press, 1989.*

Najavits LM, Weiss RD, Liese BS. Group cognitive-behavioral therapy for women with PTSD and substance use disorder. *Journal of Substance Abuse Treatment* 13:13-22, 1996.

Prochaska JO, DiClemente CC. The transtheoretical approach. In *Handbook of Psychotherapy Integration,* edited by Norcross JC, Goldfried MR. New York: Basic Books, 1992, pp. 300-334.

Stinchfield R, Owen PL, Winters KC. Group therapy for substance abuse: A review of the empirical research. In *Handbook of Group Psychotherapy: An Empirical and Clinical Synthesis,* edited by Fuhriman A, Burlingame GM. New York: John Wiley and Sons, 1994, pp. 458-488.

Wright FD, Beck AT, Newman CF, Liese BS. Cognitive therapy of substance abuse: Theoretical rationale. In *Behavioral Treatments for Drug Abuse and Dependence,* edited by Onken LS, Blaine JD, Boren JJ. NIDA Research Monograph 137, DHHS Pub. No. 93-3684. Washington, DC: U.S. Government Printing Office 137, 1992, pp. 123-146.

50·b/s

Chapter 4

Group Therapy for Alcohol Dependence Within a Phase Model of Recovery

Peter Banys

INTRODUCTION

It has become a truism among substance abuse treatment professionals that groups are the treatment of choice for addictions, as groups are more effective than individuals at confrontation of denial. Self-help and psychotherapy groups also provide opportunities for change through the nonverbal process of identification for which emotional safety is essential. Groups provide safety, opportunities for identifications for patients who must find honor in the midst of being a "drunk," a holding environment in which lost or undeveloped capacities for human relations may be practiced, and, finally, groups help to restore capacities for love and altruism.

Whereas an individual relationship is potentially threatening and, for alcoholics, experienced as "out of control," a group meeting, such as Alcoholics Anonymous (AA), is highly predictable, safer, and, to some extent, ritualized. It is precisely the predictability of this social ritual that creates a safe holding environment within which a gradual shift occurs toward the painful identity, "I am an alcoholic." It may seem paradoxical that a group of unreliable alcoholics is experienced as more reliable than any individual relationship, but in early recovery any individual relationship is fraught with unpredictable dangers. A group avoids dangers that arise in individual relationships such as the other person's contempt or condescension, or the alcoholic's own contaminating history of lies, envy, or broken promises. In a group, individuals may come and go, but the meeting endures and is reliable.

Before one can begin to treat alcoholics in a group setting, one must have some answer for the question, "What is to be recovered in Recovery?" Patients and clinicians alike often assume that what is recovered is the practice of a clean and sober lifestyle. What is recovered, however, is not a chemical state, but rather the capacity for human intimacy. A career in addiction inevitably takes place against the backdrop of lost relationships, lies, and betrayals, all of which can be small or large. Over time chemicals consume more and more waking hours. Although a few medications (disulfiram, naltrexone, and acamprosate) may reduce the overall risks of relapse, state-of-the-art treatment today seeks to put people back into their regular lives. If the goal is to restore capacities for human interrelatedness in the context of sober living, many individuals become "dry" or "sober" without ever entering recovery proper. Recovery proper is best reserved for individuals who are able to respond to the illness of alcohol dependence by changing in very fundamental ways.

Group therapy works because it allows the creation of a transitional space between pathological self-sufficiency and true intimacy, in which progressively more intimate relationships develop for patients who have an impaired capacity for human relations. Therapy groups and self-help groups enhance support and individual defenses against the intolerable personal and interpersonal experiences that make the patient feel profoundly "out of control." Paradoxically, it is not simply the base emotions of rage, envy, or humiliation that make one feel "out of control," but also tender feelings of longing, compassion, and affection. In early recovery, group treatments provide the necessary safety in numbers against the vicissitudes of intense individual relationships and the feelings produced by them.

THE ROLE OF INSIGHT

Insight is not required to achieve initial abstinence. If the therapist has a full appreciation of largely nonverbal or preverbal developmental issues and is willing to establish a well-structured "holding environment" prior to engaging in dynamic exploration, an object-relations perspective can help the therapist to manage the patient in early abstinence. Groups form the basis of such "holding environments" in most clinical treatment programs.

Early treatment must emphasize a change in behavior over a change in thinking. Many alcoholics, particularly well-educated ones, are convinced that they drink for deeper underlying reasons and that exploratory psychotherapy is their best promise for a cure. The patient's wish to cure an underlying cause of his or her alcoholic drinking is well met by the psychodynamically oriented therapist's belief in the power of unconscious conflicts to produce a wide variety of behavioral symptoms; these conspire together to create a potential therapeutic misalliance in which both the patient and the therapist neglect changing behavior, friends, and habitual modes of spending time in favor of the verbal aspects of therapy.

The patient's fundamental desire is to achieve *control over alcohol* rather than to maintain a lifetime of abstinence, for a lifetime of abstinence represents a lifetime in a sick and devalued role. The patient hopes to drink in a normal manner, that is, to become a "controlled" or "social drinker." Premature psychotherapy will frequently lead to relapses if the patients have come to believe that their new insights have restored them to normality, if they cannot tolerate their emerging internal experiences (e.g., shame or guilt), or if the emergence of strong transferential feelings becomes far too anxiety-producing to endure without chemical assistance.

The crucial personal changes in early recovery are changes in behavior followed by painful shifts in identity, rather than learning psychologically convincing details (viz., "why" one drinks). In early treatment psychotherapy is best reserved for those patients who require additional support or additional working through of resistances to behavioral change and program participation. In more advanced recovery, psychotherapy can often be quite useful as patients struggle with their new identity and with their remorse.

Alcohol dependence treatment has a life and course of its own, which may be understood from a developmental perspective. Early treatment must look different from treatment in advanced sobriety. In this chapter, the language of a developmental perspective includes the metaphoric concept of interpersonal "closeness," the patient's fear of strong feelings, and the recovering patient's never ending struggle for a sense of personal control over fundamentally uncontrollable substances (alcohol), feelings (affects), and relationships (people), at times resembling obsessive-compulsive disorder. The tendency toward externalization and blame may make patients appear character-disordered or sociopathic. Depression and social isolation can produce schizoid clinical presentations. However, because these clinical presentations can improve dramatically over time, it is prudent to reserve making Axis II diagnoses until the patient is further into recovery. Alcohol dependence can produce profound regressions in ego function, and individuals with antecedent character pathology are well known to misuse alcohol and drugs.

A PHASE MODEL OF RECOVERY

Recovery from alcohol dependence may be theoretically conceptualized as a continuing process that recapitulates other, earlier tasks in human development. This chapter describes a psychodynamic phase model of recovery developed by the author. This model is comprised of the following four phases: *crisis, abstinence, sobriety,* and *recovery.*

For the patient, each phase of recovery calls for the solution of phase-specific tasks. In addition to behavioral maintenance of abstinence, recovery tasks inevitably include the need to repair and reconstruct damaged personal relationships. In long-standing alcohol dependence, the interpersonal damage has often been too great to repair and advanced therapeutic tasks center on the working through of loss, grief, guilt, and remorse.

For the individual and group therapist, each phase requires shifts in technique appropriate to the tasks of that phase. Phase progression depends on task completion, not on time in program. Early phases emphasize behavioral management and the completion of intensive program requirements. More advanced phases progressively introduce additional psychotherapeutic elements, although insight-oriented psychotherapy is always conceptualized as a risk factor for relapse.

Recurring technical problems in group therapy include a high dropout rate, "drunkalogues," a lack of spontaneous feeling, verbal intellectualization, "super-normal" behaviors, and poor cohesion. In addition, the group therapist must be prepared to handle inebriation and characterological acting-out in a consistent manner. Abstinence is frequently disillusioning because recovering patients find that character defects remain, as do depressive feelings and irreconcilable losses. Family and co-workers quickly lose interest in abstinence as a laudable achievement. Facing psychological conflicts and persistent difficulties at home and at work, most sober alcoholics will sooner or later ask, "Is this all there is?" Feelings of loss, remorse, depression, and guilt may be difficult for the patient to verbalize and to work through. Initially, using the psychodynamic phase model, a group is conceptualized as a transitional object, lying in an intermediate place between pathological self-reliance and true object relations. Group therapy is utilized, not as a venue for confrontation, but as a holding environment for the largely nonverbal processes of identification with other recovering individuals.

In the phase model, relapse is conceptualized as a failure of treatment structure rather than as a failure of the patient. It is axiomatic that with maximum structure (e.g., hospitalization) abstinence can be ensured. Relapse, therefore, can be seen as proof that an individual patient's level of structure is inadequate to the task. Relapse leads to an intensification of treatment through reassignment to an earlier, more highly structured, phase of treatment. This concept of phase progression and phase regression in groups solves one of the most difficult conundrums in alcohol dependence treatment—"what to do with the intoxicated or relapsing patient?" Patients are not kicked out of treatment; they are asked to return to early phase groups, which meet more often, have more behavioral requirements, and focus more on staying sober than on relationships.

Alcoholics Anonymous has always maintained that its program was a program for living and not merely a method for achieving abstinence. The program's twelve steps contain a latent developmental model of personal change. It is important to realize that, of the twelve steps, only the first mentions alcohol; the rest ask that AA members confront their excessive self-reliance and their wrongdoing and gradually turn selfishness into relations with others, and, eventually, into altruism. Movement through the twelve steps may be partially understood as a developmental progression from pathological self-sufficiency to full object-relatedness.

Until recently the most common professional model of alcoholic decline and recovery has been Jellinek's inverted horseshoe model of "hitting bottom" and a mirror image ascent into recovery (Jellinek 1952). However, recovery is never the simple opposite of drinking. The Jellinek model does not take into account phases of decline or phases of recovery. Moreover, the Jellinek model graphically supports the illusion that recovery can somehow undo the damage done during drinking. People may stop drinking but not necessarily do anything about changing their personality. Thus, certain things in life, once lost, can never be recovered.

Alcoholics often rely heavily on immature defenses. Many practitioners believe that these defenses (viz., denial) are obstructive to therapy. However, as John Wallace (1985) explains:

> In working with alcoholics, we must realize that the denial is there for a purpose. It is the glue that holds an already shattered self-esteem system together. And it is the tactic through which otherwise overwhelming anxiety can be contained. (p. 32)

When drinking, alcoholics manifest prominent narcissistic features. When newly sober, on the other hand, they manifest obsessive-compulsive defenses against their impulses. Common defenses in these patients are externalization, acting-out, and splitting, which are more primitive than such neurotic defenses as reaction formation, rationalization, and sublimation. Following Anna Freud, George Vaillant (1994) has proposed a hierarchy of defenses according to developmental maturity. Vaillant's long-term prospective studies on the natural history of alcohol dependence and adaptation to life have helped reverse the classic psychoanalytic belief that alcohol dependence is caused by character pathology. His studies strongly support the idea that alcohol dependence causes character disorder or, put another way, that chronic drinking will tend to push anyone into using less mature defenses.

A developmental model assumes that there are critical phases in recovery and that each phase requires a differentiated treatment approach. It is assumed that the core tasks for patients will change over time and that each patient moves at a different pace. The early phases of treatment rely on a high level of program structure as the central therapeutic element, whereas advanced phases more closely resemble traditional group psychotherapy.

Crisis, Abstinence, Sobriety, and Recovery

In this context, the term "recovery" implies a process of psychological change, whereas "abstinence" and "sobriety" refer to behaviors without change in psychological structure. Each phase of treatment adds a new clinical focus without, however, neglecting those of the preceding phases (see Table 4.1 for a description of the different

TABLE 4.1. Description of Treatment Phases

Phase	Treatment Program	Comments
1. Crisis		
Drinking	• Triage clinic	• Daily, walk-in program • Immediate, supportive response • Housing placement
Withdrawal	• Inpatient detoxification • Outpatient detoxification	• High medical risk patients • Day-by-day prescriptions for benzodiazepines, contingent on blood alcohol concentration (BAC) = 0%
Transition	• Day hospital • Inpatient hospital	• Daily group meetings • Ambulatory detoxification • Treatment placement • Stabilization • Differential diagnosis • Family intervention • Treatment placement
2. Abstinence	• Structured requirements • Required AA and education meetings • Routine use of Breathalyzer	• Three to five groups per week • Emphasis on behavior • Relapse prevention • Task completion criteria for advancement to next phase • Treatment of Axis I dual diagnosis
3. Sobriety	• Affective focus • Alexithymic features	• Emphasis on cognition • Relapse prevention • Treatment of depression, grief, remorse • Acceptance of losses
4. Recovery	• Interactional therapy	• Emphasis on relationships • Individual psychotherapy, if indicated • Psychotherapy may be contingent on twelve-step participation • Treatment of characterological problems

phases). The *crisis phase* is very much one of problem solving. The clinical focus is on the patient's behavior. The working assumption is that program structure combined with the patient's own ego will suffice to maintain abstinence. How much program is "enough" is determined empirically. The *abstinence phase* adds an additional focus on cognition. In this phase, relapse-prevention techniques are especially useful. The *sobriety phase* is an advanced phase for which most patients are not ready in the first year. The added focus here is on the danger of feelings, particularly those of depression, self-hatred, grief, and remorse. Finally, the *recovery phase* is defined as the first fully interactional and psychodynamically oriented phase of group treatment. It resembles interactional group psychotherapy in its emphasis on relationships and the "here and now" nature of in-group relationships.

Phase 1: Crisis

To stop drinking is not a matter of insight or willpower, but requires a change in behavior. It is not "talking the talk"; it is "walking the walk." Most alcoholics know what it takes to get sober for the short term. Permanently remaining sober proves difficult. "Hitting bottom" may not be necessary for all newly abstinent patients, but some kind of psychosocial crisis is usually required to motivate alcoholics for recovery-oriented treatment. This may be a lengthy blackout, an episode of gastrointestinal bleeding, court pressures following drunk driving arrests, or employer pressures. Spouses and families who have "had enough" and who are capable of firm confrontation are also responsible for sending many individuals to treatment.

In the *crisis phase* of treatment, it is important to *formulate* clearly the nature of the psychosocial crisis and to *assist* the patient with it as soon as possible. This is not necessarily the same as assisting with detoxification; the patient may require family, workplace, or legal assistance. Both individual therapy and group support are required. For example, employment may be salvaged if the therapist writes a letter to the employer about the initiation, nature, and duration of appropriate treatment. The extent of the problem must match the amount of treatment structure recommended. Some patients might require hospitalization, while others may require a course of benzodiazepines to reduce withdrawal symptoms. Group work in this phase is highly supportive and helpful. It is essential to have groups or individual modalities capable of tolerating and assisting patients who are still "wet."

The immediate postwithdrawal period constitutes an important transitional time. After leaving the "wet" phase, the patient enters into the succeeding "dry" phase of treatment. Relief and euphoria about achieving abstinence may combine to make the patient discount the need for continued treatment and participation in AA. For others, becoming sober without having the additional concomitants of change in one's lifestyle and without the support of treatment or twelve-step structures necessarily leads to the resumption of drinking. The essential intervention is to assist the patient in bonding to other recovering patients, preferably those with somewhat more advanced sobriety. Referrals alone do not seem to work very well. Introducing patients to staff, and, whenever possible, the establishment of personal bonds among patients are often effective.

In group therapy, one channels dynamic process into, rather than out of, the group, discouraging personal pairings in order not to skew the group process. In recovery groups, personal ties should be supported, but sexual intimacy should be discouraged.

Phase 2: Abstinence

The primary focus in this first "dry" phase of recovery treatment is on the patient's behavior. Although it sounds preposterous, most patients wish to be relieved of their alcohol dependence without changing how they live. Few noticeable behavioral changes indicate a poor prognosis. To remain abstinent, patients must eliminate something in their pattern of socializing (viz., with whom they spend time). In addition, they must initiate something new, such as attendance at AA. In this phase, brief relapses to drinking and many kinds of acting-out behaviors are common.

Clinicians must monitor behavior rather than motivation or commitment. Outcome in alcohol dependence treatment has long been known to be best predicted by the social class factors of the patient. Clinical assessments of motivation do not predict eventual outcome. What alcoholics do with their minds and attitudes is of little importance. Confession of alcohol dependence is *not* the task of this phase of treatment but, rather, "the task ... is to shift identity and change behavior" (Brown 1985, p. 116). While the former occurs via identification, the latter occurs via imitation. The clinician must routinely assess what the patients are actually *doing* with their time and with their bodies, whether that is to change their friends, their haunts, take disulfiram, attend ninety AA meetings in ninety days, or move to a halfway house. As long as the patients attend, it does not matter whether they define themselves as alcoholics or merely as problem drinkers. Compliance and imitation, at this stage, are more important than insight.

Relapse prevention. During the past twenty years, clinical researchers have developed numerous, largely group-oriented, relapse prevention techniques (see Chapter 9). These techniques are especially important to the *abstinence phase* of treatment. In their influential works on relapse prevention, Marlatt and colleagues (Marlatt and Tapert 1993) conceptualize addiction as a set of habits that have been reinforced by drugs and social factors. Relapse prevention techniques that they explore include drug education, high-risk states and warning signs of relapse, coping skills training, and homework assignments for new lifestyle behaviors. Their work on the abstinence violation effect has led to a distinction between "slips" and full-blown "relapses." In the phase model, brief drinking episodes constitute "slips" and are learning experiences to be reviewed in a group setting. Relapses are treated as extended episodes that require a return to an earlier, more highly structured phase of treatment.

Structure is itself an important treatment in the *abstinence phase*. How to keep a highly structured abstinence phase treatment program from devolving into ritualization and the treatment equivalent of lesson plans is the crucial design question. It makes little sense to discontinue treatment during drinking episodes. It is axiomatic that anyone who relapses does not have sufficient treatment structure to maintain abstinence. A phase model of treatment permits the clinican to return a patient to an earlier, more intensive and more highly structured phase of treatment in lieu of terminating the treatment.

Attendance in the program needs to be scrupulously monitored and clinic settings need routine procedures in order to produce prompt responses to patient absences, such as attending a minimum number of treatment groups, AA groups, and education sessions—no matter how long it takes. In the phase model, patients are required to attend meetings in the clinic three to five days per week. Patients may not graduate to the next phase until they complete a minimum of twenty-four group meetings, thirty-six AA (or other self-help) meetings, and six education sessions. Refractory patients, who have had drinking episodes in this phase, may be asked to take disulfiram or naltrexone in addition to the other requirements. Although medications may diminish an internal sense of efficacy, relapse prevention counseling will foster internal attribution and sustained maintenance of change.

Patients are ambivalent and obsessed with weighing the pros and cons of an alcoholic identity. If one confronts "denial," rather than allowing the expression of the desire to drink, the patient will be driven into silence and this treasured, but unusually persistent, wish will remain unsatiated. Accepting the sick role permits a useful dependence on treatment, but at the risk of increasing self-disgust over being an alcoholic. Rather, accepting self-definition as a "problem drinker" may prove less damaging until the patient can more fully come to terms with his or her illness. Patients invariably fall back to understanding their problem in terms of a moral model, which suggests that they are weak or defective.

Treatment centers often sponsor the idea that the primary defense of the alcoholic is denial, but alcoholics have many other available defenses. One patient who blames others and another patient who rationalizes are both poorly understood if they are reductionistically seen to demonstrate "denial." Both have unique defensive systems, organized according to their levels of ego development and level of ego regression. By far the most prevalent ego defense mechanism at this stage is externalization. A primitive patient may have frankly paranoid features. For a more maturely organized patient, externalization will tend to be more plausible, more intellectual, and more glib. Blaming others is, in part, the cause of apparent disordered or sociopathic character in so many patients during early recovery. Patients with addictive disorders cannot bear to prematurely internalize their misbehavior because this can lead to renewed cycles of self-loathing and self-destructive acting out.

At this stage, patients are likely to have impaired learning capacities, defects in memory, and persistent sleeping disorders. Education sessions may be moved to more advanced phases of recovery when cognitive capacities have improved.

Patients in the first few months of abstinence frequently present a sense of general defeat coupled with an unrealistic disavowal of craving or of an interest in resumed drinking. They can appear to be alexithymic ("without words for feelings"). Strong affects "in group" tend to be anxiety-provoking and tend to increase the occurrence of missed sessions. It is not merely the "base" emotions (e.g., resentment, rage, or envy) that are treated as if they are dangerous, but also "noble" emotions (e.g., tenderness, pity, and longing).

During active drinking, alcohol acts as the primary object of relationship at the cost of the family and other human relationships. It is an inanimate substance imbued with the personification of human traits. AA says alcohol is "cunning, dangerous, and powerful." Although alcohol remains largely predictable and reliable, human relationships in the alcoholic's life become increasingly unmanageable. Alcoholics simultaneously animate inanimate chemicals (alcohol) with human properties such as comfort, friendship, and reliability, as they de-animate and neglect personal relationships. In treatment, this apparent replacement becomes observable in the alcoholic's reluctance to trust a therapeutic relationship. Using the preferred defenses of externalization and projective identification, newly abstinent alcoholics will tend to see clinicians as contemptuous, disdainful, disappointed, superior, or angry. Conversely, however, they may see clinicians as all-knowing, parental, and charismatic.

Group sessions in early treatment often have an "as if" quality. The patients are clean and hopeful; their lives are improving dramatically. Very often, they cannot find any sense of craving or desire to drink. They present all of this material sometimes with perplexity, sometimes with triumph, but they are reluctant to ask for help in deeply meaningful ways. Having lived a life of humiliation, the recovering patient now wants support and admiration from his or her group. This tends to make the therapist appear incidental to the process. Group interaction at this stage is probably better understood as a form of phase-appropriate oversimplification of relationships in the service of safety and stability.

Group meetings must, above all, regularly and reliably convene. The diffusion of personal ties in groups makes group treatment settings safer than individual psychotherapy and more tolerable for people whose capacity for intimacy has been damaged by a career in drinking.

The single most dangerous therapeutic experience for a patient in the abstinence phase is to develop a powerful, emotionally strong transference reaction to an individual therapist. This kind of relationship is simply too close and therefore, uncomfortable, as it leaves little room for the preferred defense of externalization.

The patients continuously struggle to achieve a pathological degree of self-sufficiency as a kind of antidote to their previous dependence. They do not want to depend on people such as therapists, or on medications such as disulfiram or, indeed, on other drunks who know no more than they about how to live in balance. However, a kind of dependence must be fostered in abstinence; although this dependence, driven by other, more defensive etiological factors, is applied to somewhat depersonified and abstracted entities such as AA, the clinic, or the Wednesday evening group.

All patients resist treatment. They resist group work because they cannot fully believe they can learn from people who are as ill as they are. They resist AA because they tend to confuse it with religion, which may grandly be seen as yet another dependence. Over time, however, in later phases, comes a gradual shifting toward structures, which allow a more personal, more permanently satisfying, approach.

Phase 3: Sobriety

The *sobriety phase* of treatment may be considered a transitional phase between mere abstinence and stable recovery. It is ideally defined by a shift in preferred ego defenses following a prior shift in behavior. This phase requires a far deeper "coming to terms" with one's identity than do the large behavioral changes of the preceding phase. Alcoholics Anonymous (Emrick 1993; McCrady and Miller 1993), Brown (1985), and others argue that such a shift is the result of a spiritual conversion necessary to proceed to true recovery rather than "white knuckle sobriety." This experience is variously called surrender, working the first and second step, or changing one's worldview. A contrary view holds that it is the mere passage of abstinent time that allows the individual to return to previous, higher levels of functioning.

Once patients have achieved relatively stable abstinence, they face a difficult and prolonged transition to stable recovery. In fact, many patients experience depression and intense disappointment in themselves and in the "promise" of recovery. Some patients may benefit from antidepressant medication.

Patients feel deep despair about lost time and lost loves and an inability to find (or recover) the playful, imaginative aspects of experience. Issues in group treatment now turn tentatively to the examination of the quality of relationships. Prospects for repair or reconciliation are sought while anxieties about new relationships are eased. Group therapy initiates this kind of practice, for in a group, others are available to rehearse social relationships.

The *sobriety phase* is characterized by overreaching perfectionism. Patients engage in self-improvement projects such as smoking cessation, weight loss, and improved personal appearance. Unexpected absences from treatment are less frequent. At this phase, many patients study normality, yet feel that they are merely pretending to be like normal people. Often, the free flow of the group process is hampered by correct or idealized responses, by the lack of deep affect, and the smothering presence of "normality." In order to deny the previous chaos in their drinking behaviors, patients turn toward orderliness and ritual and exemplary behavior.

A gradual transition from a reliance on externalization to overuse of intellectualization and abstraction is seen. These patients are extremely interested in rooting out the "underlying causes" of their drinking. At this point, relapse prevention in treatment is particularly important because, for the first time, certain insights may be useful for relapse prevention. Specifically, analyzing factors associated with previous slips and relapses can be very helpful for learning about relapse triggers. The risk of all this intellectualization, however, is the possible emergence of a pseudologic of self-control. As Stephanie Brown says, "I am an alcoholic and didn't drink tonight. But because I was able to abstain, I must not be an alcoholic and therefore can have a drink" (Brown 1985, p. 140).

In group therapy, the influence of AA is paramount, and patients support the injunction against "crosstalk." Interpersonal confrontations often take the form of telling parables, as problems are described personally but made generic, using abstraction and intellectualization. Members show a tremendous interest in "solving" other's problems, relying on simple rules, advice, and dogma.

After the "pink cloud" of exhilaration often experienced in early abstinence, recovering patients often are increasingly depressed. Families can often be unforgiving, even after the alcoholic has achieved abstinence. Clinical effort at this point concentrates on distinguishing the psychological work of grief and personal reconciliation from that of medically treatable depression.

The patient eventually learns that "feelings make you drink." In fact, many patients will henceforth unconsciously elect to organize their affective life around sentiments (social platitudes) rather than be open to spontaneous emotions. Drinking dreams return and can be very alarming. Patients "in group" begin to identify alarming "dry drunk" experiences in which they have behaved alcoholically, without any drinking.

Patients who need psychotherapy during the sobriety phase often flee to AA, and patients who need AA often seek refuge in therapy. Patients unconsciously activate profound resistances to further change (and pain). There is an inability to locate anything wrong in one's emotional life. Experiencing unaccountably strong feelings, good or bad, about the therapist or another group member is disconcerting, yet patients in this phase cling stubbornly to excessively idealized and unrealistic views of the therapist (combined with a subtle devaluing of one another).

Drinking is not a failure of the patient but a failure of the holding environment. If a patient drinks, the relapse represents an inadequate degree of internal and external structure; therefore, he or she is sent back a phase. Thus relapses lead to phase regression, "flunking a grade," not to termination.

Phase 4: Recovery

In the *recovery phase* much of the psychotherapeutic work resembles ordinary psychotherapy, with the caveat that alcohol and obsession with self-control remain touchstone themes. Only a minority of patients in this phase actually require or need psychotherapy. Many patients aspire to engage in psychotherapy but do not have the ego structure capable of enduring the upsurge of emotion and transference that might ensue. Most patients will improve simply by undergoing the twelve-step program and by attending clinic-based group therapy.

CORE CONFLICTS

In considering the process of recovery, it is essential to be aware of the core conflicts commonly seen in alcoholics (and common in alcohol abusers as well). These core conflicts must be understood and addressed in the course of treatment for the process of recovery to have a successful outcome.

Poor Self-Esteem, Self-Hatred

Patients need to abandon their conception of being normal and adopt the discomforting realism of being "sick," that is, an alcoholic, with all of the negative, painful associations attached. Calling alcohol dependence an illness, like diabetes, helps only a little.

Affect Intolerance

According to Brown, "In transitional and early recovery phases, affect may be diffuse and overwhelming, absent, or contained" (Brown 1985, p. 57). Similarly, in the phase model, feelings are the spontaneous, largely unpredictable, and often overwhelming experiences generated in human relationships; sentiments are ritualized, somewhat trite, and mostly appropriate ideas that people exchange at powerful social moments.

The Struggle for Control

Alcoholics invest years in failed attempts to control three of the most uncontrollable aspects of human experience—drinking, feelings, and people. At first, the natural history of recovery includes years of strategies to cut down or to stop drinking. Patients also commonly experience spontaneous feelings as particularly disorganizing and dangerous. Last, the patients will have difficulties returning to a disappointed or angry family, and run into perplexing resistances against their best efforts to help and to rejoin active family life.

Active/Passive Traumatization

Alcoholics are not only the victims of trauma, they are also often victimizers of others. It is now well known that alcohol dependence is highly correlated with early sexual or violent traumatic victimization. Alcoholics are also frequently victimizers; they have shameful histories replete with lying, petty theft, domestic abuse, and irresponsible child care. Many, of course, are both victims and victimizers in a time-worn pattern of repeating early life experiences. Ideally, group therapy will facilitate an individual's ability to identify both with the victim and with the victimizer of past traumas. Inevitably, actual reparative actions are required. If amends cannot be made, then good works for others may be needed to restore some inner peace. This is far from the standard psychotherapy approach that emphasizes the internal world at the expense of the outer. Self-forgiveness is neither easy nor necessarily desirable. Accumulated remorse and grief inevitably must be endured by any advanced phase recovery group.

Grief, Loss, Bereavement

Experiencing grief is an essential part of the advanced phases of recovery. Too much guilt and rumination too early in treatment is a powerful stimulus for drinking. However, too little guilt and a refusal to accept responsibility for one's actions does not bode well for future progress. George Vaillant (1994) has observed that one of the natural, nontreatment factors in recovery is the establishment of new love relationships. New relationships cannot easily be made without a prior phase of grieving the loss of individuals (viz., divorced spouses and estranged children), job opportunities, and, above all, the loss of youth dedicated to drinking. The past must not be rewritten; it must be accepted exactly as it happened. Others cannot take the blame. For the alcoholic, the past continues to influence the sober future.

The Drinking Patient

Psychotherapy patients traditionally come to treatment to discuss their symptoms and the behavioral repetitions that create life problems. The alcoholic (and many alcohol counselors) turn this model onto its head. Alcoholics come for treatment when they are doing well and stay away when they are doing badly. The success of abstinence is, then, a public activity, while the failure, or drinking, is a private secret. The tendency to hide while drinking turns group therapy into a kind of historical exercise. In order to work with an actively relapsing patient without demoralizing the rest of the group, a special level of care, sometimes called a "wet phase," can be offered. Needless to say, intoxicated patients are especially difficult to work with. The focus of therapy should be simple so that it is comprehended. Interruptive, hostile, incoherent participation need not be tolerated. The patients need to cooperate to increase the overall structure of their abstinence plan.

The Role of Confrontation

Confrontation is a term that has widely divergent meanings in the addiction treatment community. Actively aggressive confrontational techniques in addiction treatment were developed in therapeutic communities such as Phoenix House, Daytop Lodge, and Synanon in the 1960s (Casriel 1963; Rosenthal and Biase 1969; Shelly and Bassin 1965; Yablonsky 1965). To some extent, aggressive aspects of the Synanon "game," "the haircut," or "attack therapy" have found their way into many other kinds of treatment settings.

Such active methods have a cathartic and expressive focus. Therapists encourage patients to get in touch with their feelings and to let their anger out. Although some evidence indicates that intensive confrontation methods may change behaviors in alcohol and drug addicts (MacDonough 1976), such techniques are best left for self-help settings where they are not confused with medical/psychiatric treatments. These methods have no place in psychiatric treatment, for they are punitive, manipulative, disrespectful, and they exaggerate charismatic characteristics of leaders. There is a place for straight talk in alcohol dependence treatment, in which confrontations are relatively neutral observations about how one behavior (i.e., drinking) appears to be linked to another (i.e., resentment).

Common Errors in Group Treatment

Greif (1996) has identified a number of errors in conceptualization and techniques frequently made in the course of the group treatment of alcoholics. These errors can interfere with the course of treatment and the achievement of recovery. These potential errors include inappropriate self-disclosure, failure to clarify group rules, and failure to make proper use of the group.

SUMMARY AND CONCLUSIONS

The use of a four-phase developmental model of group therapy, which has phase-specific tasks and allows for inconsistency in the patient's clinical course helps address many of the potentially complex issues in recovery.

REFERENCES

Brown S. *Treating the Alcoholic: A Developmental Model of Recovery*. New York: John Wiley & Sons, 1985.

Casriel D. *So Fair a House: The Story of Synanon.* Englewood Cliffs, NJ: Prentice-Hall, 1963.

Emrick CD, Tonigan JS, Montgomery H, Little L. Alcoholics Anonymous: What is currently known? In *Research on Alcoholics Anonymous: Opportunities and Alternatives,* edited by McCrady BS, Miller WR. New Brunswick, NJ: Rutgers Center of Alcohol Studies, 1993, pp. 41-76.

Greif GL. Ten common errors beginning substance abuse workers make in group treatment. *Journal of Psychoactive Drugs* 28(3):297-299, 1996.

Jellinek EM. Phases of alcohol addiction. *Quarterly Journal of Studies on Alcohol* 13:673-684, 1952.

MacDonough TS. Evaluation of the effectiveness of intensive confrontation in changing the behavior of alcohol and drug abusers. *Behavior Therapy* 7(3):408-409, 1976.

Marlatt GA, Tapert SF. Harm reduction: Reducing the risks of addictive behaviors. In *Addictive Behaviors Across the Life Span: Prevention, Treatment, and Policy Issues,* edited by Baer JS, Marlatt GA. Thousand Oaks, CA: Sage Publications, Inc., 1993, pp. 243-273.

McCrady BS, Miller WR (eds.). *Research on Alcoholics: Opportunities and Alternatives.* New Brunswick, NJ: Rutgers Center of Alcohol Studies, 1993.

Rosenthal MS, Biase DV. Phoenix House: Therapeutic communities for drug addicts. *Hospital and Community Psychiatry* 20:26-30, 1969.

Shelly JA, Bassin A. Daytop Lodge: A new treatment approach for drug addicts. *Corrective Psychiatry* 11:186-195, 1965.

Vaillant GE. Ego mechanisms of defense and personality psychopathology. *Journal of Abnormal Psychology* 103 (1):44-50, 1994.

Wallace J. Critical issues in alcoholism therapy. In *Practical Approaches to Alcoholism Psychotherapy,* Second Edition, edited by Zimberg S, Wallace J, Blume SB. New York: Plenum Press, 1985, pp. 23-36.

Yablonsky L. *Synanon: The Tunnel Back.* New York: Macmillan, 1965.

Chapter 5

Self-Medication Theory and Modified Dynamic Group Therapy

Mark J. Albanese
Edward J. Khantzian

INTRODUCTION

The self-medication hypothesis (SMH) of addictions explains substance abuse as a self-regulation disorder. Although affective dysregulation is at the core of addictive behavior, there are other areas of dyscontrol as well. This chapter will review the key components of the self-medication hypothesis, then go on to describe Modified Dynamic Group Therapy (MDGT), a therapeutic offspring of the SMH.

THE SELF-MEDICATION HYPOTHESIS: SUBSTANCE ABUSE AS A SELF-REGULATION DISORDER

The SMH starts with the notion that deficits in the character structure of substance abusers leave them with self-regulation impairments. Deficits in affect regulation are compounded by related impairments in self-care, self-esteem, and relationships.

Khantzian has written that substance-abusing patients experience their affects in the extreme, feeling too much or too little (Khantzian, Halliday, and McAuliffe 1990; Khantzian 1997; Khantzian, Golden, and McAuliffe 1995). That is, there can be defects in affect tolerance, distress, tension, rage, shame, and loneliness, and/or a readiness to respond with activity or passivity in relationship to the environment. In other cases, the vagueness and confusion around feelings are such that patients are either unable to give words to them (alexithymia) or hardly seem to have feelings at all (disaffected) and defensively fight rather than feel. Some of these people find that substances of abuse can relieve the painful affect states (Khantzian 1997). At the same time, these patients suffer from deficits in self-care; that is, in potentially dangerous situations, they think and feel differently from non-substance abusers. This view has been influenced by a developmental perspective in that Khantzian and co-workers have been able to ascertain and identify with patients how they have suffered with lifelong vulnerabilities around self-care. This has been evident in patient histories (predating and postdating their substance abuse) of accidents and preventable medical, dental, legal, and financial difficulties in which there has been a persistent inability to worry about, anticipate, or consider consequences of their action or inaction. This also occurs with regard to involvement with drug-related environments and ultimately the drug use itself. These relapses in self-care are the symptomatic reflection of deficits in psychological structures and functions that normally protect us from harm and danger. Whereas most people fear or avoid the many dangerous aspects of drug use, addicts fail to show such worry or caution. The combination of affect dysregulation and impaired self-care results in greater likelihood for harmful substance use and relapse.

In addition to affect and self-care difficulties, substance abusers exhibit self-esteem deficits. Specifically, they lack adequate self-comforting skills. As a result, individuals who already suffer from an impairment in affect regulation, when confronted with uncomfortable affect, do not have the internal mechanisms to comfort themselves. Substances of abuse represent an external means of providing such comfort. Finally, because of their difficulties with both affect regulation and maintenance of self-esteem, substance abusers experience trouble in relating to others. They switch between being selfless and being demanding. Early relationship experiences in childhood provide a sense that one can feel validated from within, or can reach out easily when necessary, for nurturance and validation. The deficits in these abilities that are so often present in substance abusers produce extreme and uneven patterns in satisfying needs around dependency, self-worth, and comfort. As a consequence, they alternate between seductive and manipulative attitudes to extract satisfaction from the environment, and disdainful, aloof postures of independence and self-sufficiency that dismiss the need for others.

Specific Drug Effects

Faced with uncomfortable affects and an inability to regulate them, patients make the discovery that alcohol and other drugs offer a solution to this self-regulation deficit. Moreover, the choice of drug is not random. Substance abusers match drug choice specifically to the affect experienced. Often, patients struggle especially with a particularly painful affect and have developed a "drug of choice" or "king drug" to deal with this predominant affect that is especially painful or unbearable.

Opiates

Opiate abusers frequently describe histories, predating their addiction, of a difficulty with rage and violent behavior. This is often in the context of brutal home settings. They discover that opiates can counter the internally fragmenting and disorganizing effects of rage and the externally threatening and disruptive aspects of such affects to interpersonal relations.

Cocaine and Other Stimulants

Patients who have histories of depression discover the activating and energizing properties of the psychostimulants. Likewise, people with hypomanic symptoms find that the stimulants act as augmenters to their expansive, overactive lifestyles. Finally, stimulants act paradoxically to calm the hyperactivity and counter the attention problems of those suffering with ADHD.

Alcohol and Other Central Nervous System Depressants

People with rigid defenses producing feelings of isolation and emptiness and related tense/anxious states and masking fears of closeness and dependency find that alcohol and other sedative-hypnotics, by softening rigid defenses, temporarily ameliorate states of isolation and emptiness.

Order and Disorder

As outlined previously, the SMH posits that substance use is a means of bringing order to an unregulated internal affective world and related chaotic external interpersonal world. Using cocaine as an example, we can now briefly look at how a drug can bring temporary relief to a disordered individual, but lead to subsequent exacerbation in dysregulation.

In cocaine abusers, depressive symptoms are frequently noted to be a source of distress, which is overcome by the stimulating action of cocaine. Cocaine abusers exhibit vulnerabilities and deficits in narcissism leading to a fragile sense of self-worth. Thus, they exhibit concerns about performance and achievement and exaggerated needs for acceptance and approval. Cocaine produces a sense of well-being and empowerment. In relating to others, cocaine abusers can be uneven and inconsistent, alternating between being charming and aloof. Cocaine makes relating to others exhilarating and exciting. Finally, deficits in self-care functions prevent cocaine abusers from adequately considering the potential dangers of cocaine use. Also, because of their self-esteem and relational deficits, cocaine abusers can develop compensatory postures such as counterdependence and counterfearfulness, which override concerns about self-care.

In summary, developmental deficits in cocaine abusers leave them with a diminished capacity to self-regulate feelings, self-esteem, relations, and self-care. They discover that cocaine can temporarily bring order to their disordered internal and external worlds. These deficits and this discovery, when tragically combined with a genetic predisposition to cocaine abuse, result in a vicious cycle. The end result is ultimate worsening in self-regulation, as already limited self-regulatory mechanisms atrophy because of prolonged use of cocaine as a regulatory crutch.

The Cause-Consequence Controversy

The SMH maintains that it is subtle, syndromal dysphoric affects that people self-medicate with substances. Clearly, this hypothesis does not argue against the well-demonstrated evidence that substances can cause dysregulation in anxiety, depression, and mania that might contribute to the subsequent development of a full-blown Axis I syndrome. Furthermore, the SMH has never been about self-medicating an Axis I disorder, but about a person's attempt to regulate painful affect states that are often as elusive as they are unmanageable. Recent studies have provided evidence that subjective distressful feelings can precede the onset of substance use (McKenna and Ross 1994; Milin et al. 1992).

Further evidence suggestive of the relationship between distressing affect and use of substances comes from recent literature that describes the emergence of depressive symptoms during alcohol recovery. Treatment of the depression alleviates this disorder and prevents reemergence of the substance use disorder.

Recent Applications

Since its inception, the SMH has been applied to many different clinical situations. Three areas of application, recently reviewed by Khantzian (1997), include the possibility that nicotine-dependent individuals started using nicotine to alleviate dysphoria, dysthymia, and depression (Breslau, Kilbey, and Andreski 1993; Glass 1990). Similarly, schizophrenic patients may use substances as a means of coping with the subjective distress associated with the negative symptoms (Albanese et al. 1994; Noordsy et al. 1991). Finally, patients suffering with post-traumatic stress disorder may use substances to alleviate the distress of both affective flooding and emotional numbing (Kosten and Krystal 1988).

MODIFIED DYNAMIC GROUP THERAPY (MDGT): GENERAL BACKGROUND

Group therapy has emerged as a preferred treatment modality for patients with psychoactive substance use disorders. Modified Dynamic Group Therapy (MDGT) has roots in contemporary psychoanalytic theory. It was developed as part of a National Institute on Drug Abuse (NIDA)-sponsored project comparing behavioral and psychodynamic models in group treatments of cocaine addicts. MDGT was manualized in the book *Addiction and the Vulnerable Self: Modified Dynamic Group Therapy for Substance Abusers* (Khantzian, Halliday, and McAuliffe 1990).

Development

Contemporary psychoanalytic theory stresses the centrality of affect, problems with self-other relations, safety, and the psychological functions that regulate them. Developmental vulnerabilities are seen as defects of self, both intrapsychic and characterological, that can lead to addiction in an attempt by the person to regulate and medicate the distress caused by the defect (Kohut 1977; Meissner 1986; Wurmser 1978). Khantzian has addressed the particular psychological and narcissistic vulnerabilities of the potential "addict."

Rather than encouraging the expression of painful affects and the exploration of unconscious material, as in traditional psychodynamic treatment, modified dynamic group therapy, under the leadership of an active and friendly therapist and with the help of a supportive group, encourages and facilitates patients to look at four areas of ego deficits noted earlier: affective regulation, self-care, self-esteem, and interpersonal relationships. These four structural deficits are examined as they play themselves out in the group and in the patients' lives. Through this experience, group members discover alternative ways of seeing, experiencing, and exonerating themselves, thus allowing for greater flexibility and awareness of choice in their lives (Khantzian et al. 1995).

Assumptions

Group Leader and Members

In MDGT, the group leader facilitates interactions that foster sharing and comparing of experiences, empathy, and expanding awareness. Group leaders are trained to actively provide structure, ensure safety and comfort, and specifically key on the patients' issues and reactions related to feelings, relationships, self-esteem, and self-care problems. Although clarification and interpretation are provided, equal emphasis is placed on empathy, involvement, and support.

A group creates a special interpersonal context of relationships and experiences among the members and leader that allows a forum for examining and modifying members' problems. In group therapy, therapists are not the only curative agent, and they constantly foster the realization that members, as well as therapists, are aware, insightful, supportive, understanding, and corrective. At the same time, group leaders must be aware of their special position in the group and know that they will be targeted repeatedly with needs that are central to the members' dysfunctions. Given substance abusers' special difficulties with self-regulation, they are more likely than members of other groups to turn to the leader for comfort, protection, clarification, admiration, and guidance. The leader's skillful management and response to these requirements will balance the legitimate need for assistance and support from the leader with the need for further exploration of these themes by the group members. This, in turn, will lead members to discover that they can also provide what is needed for themselves and one another. When a group temporarily becomes fragmented, overwhelmed, stuck, or inhibited, the leader may need to provide what the group and its members cannot provide for themselves.

The Interpersonal Context

While MDGT was designed specifically to examine, modify, and compensate for the self-regulatory ego deficits of addicts, it rests on interpersonal factors described in the contemporary literature (Brown 1985; Vannicelli 1992). MDGT builds on the interpersonal context to provide a more specific focus on self-regulation deficits and the associated characterological patterns.

Putting the "Modified" in MDGT

Unlike groups that focus on interpersonal factors, MDGT places a greater emphasis on the understanding of one's structural deficits as these emerge during the group (Khantzian, Halliday, and McAuliffe 1990).

In contrast to classic psychoanalytic theory, which emphasizes the person's uniqueness psychodynamically and developmentally, MDGT encourages identification of commonalities in the service of overcoming the feelings of isolation, aberration, and shame that addicts share. Also, because the symptom of substance abuse is life-threatening, group requirements for safety become paramount. Thus, the modification of fostering a shared goal of control or abstinence as a requirement for treatment imposes a greater degree of homogeneity than is usually encountered in psychoanalytic group psychotherapy. Finally, although MDGT aims to elucidate and modify individual psychodynamics, a generic concept of "dynamic" is employed. This concept assumes that in addition to individual psychodynamics, the structure, context, and aims of any group also generate their own dynamics that cannot be explained or understood by the summing of the individual psychodynamics alone.

MDGT: FOCUS AND TECHNICAL CONSIDERATIONS

An Overview

MDGT stresses a focus on certain key deficits to guide the therapist and patients in appreciating particular aspects of their lives and behaviors involved with their disabilities. MDGT provides a context to elaborate and identify the deficits and compensatory mechanisms that perpetuate maladaptive responses, including substance use. The leaders and members are encouraged repeatedly to observe and describe in one another how difficulties in recognizing and regulating feelings, self-esteem, relationship, and self-care problems have been and are intimately related to their susceptibility to drug use, relapse, and drug effects. Constant attention is directed to monitoring self and others about drug use, exposure, and related activities.

The nature of affect disturbances that cause substance abusers to seek substances as a remedy is complex, and group leaders and members need to appreciate these disturbances to avoid premature conclusions about or impatience with a patient's affect life and related reliance on substance effects. Stress is placed on the defects in peoples' apparatus that cause them to experience their emotions in the extreme, feeling too much or too little. Also, as articulated in an earlier section, these patients might match a specific drug to a given affect state (e.g., opiates and rage).

An appreciation of some of these complexities can help group members develop a repertoire of responses to their dysregulated affects after they experience and process their feelings with one another. Some meetings might emphasize empathy and staying with individual or group distress. A leader might use such an occasion to acknowledge how such states lead to avoidance or drug craving and use. At other times a group might have to help a person label and describe the feelings that a certain life event might evoke. At these times groups help individuals to see that they sometimes use even the distressing and confusing disruptive effects of drugs as a controllable substitute for their feelings, which they experience as uncontrollable and even more confusing. At other times it is useful to point out how a specific affect state evoked in group treatment leads to a craving for a specific effect provided by a particular drug.

Two other deficits described earlier that substance abusers exhibit are their inability to feel good about themselves and their relationships with others. In the group setting, these patients display their failure to adequately internalize the part of development that allows one to sustain the comforting, admiring, and being admired experiences of childhood. Many of the interpersonal aspects of groups provide some of the curative responses for the self-esteem and relationship problems in an ongoing way through the shared, universal aspects of group, the support, acceptance, and instillation of caring, respectful modes of listening and interacting. Beyond these general elements, the group leader can point out and foster responses that allow more precise examination of the self-esteem and relational issues that contribute to the patients' posturing in extreme and characteristic ways. Key areas to focus on include self-defeating behaviors, compensatory attitudes of self-sufficiency, disavowal of need, bravado, and counterdependency.

Finally, in terms of the self-care deficit, alliance building with our patients is more likely if we help them see that their use of substances is a developmental vulnerability, and not evidence of self-destruction, a commonly invoked explanation. Group leaders and members can get to this vulnerability by cultivating an empathic understanding of the patients' inability or periodic failure to exercise caution when they report the typical mishaps, slips, and disasters that occur as a result of this problem. Patients can be taught to observe the characterological symptoms—counterphobia, hyperactivity, aggressive posturing, denial of danger, bravado—associated with the self-care deficit. In sum, we place great emphasis on identifying the self-defeating and self-destructive consequences of patients' self-care deficits and how this has left them susceptible to addiction. We clarify to patients that they have not necessarily intended to be self-destructive, but rather that their self-care susceptibilities have caused them difficulties in reacting appropriately to potential harm or danger, especially involving drugs.

Orientation to Group

Pregroup Preparation

Pregroup preparation for new members is beneficial in that it reduces premature treatment dropouts and increases their motivation for psychotherapy. The MDGT method of orientation was initially dictated by research concerns about minimizing no-shows and early dropouts. As many of the potential group members were new to treatment, we sought to familiarize them with the workings of a psycho-therapy group especially adapted to address their specific psychological vulnerabilities and characterological stances. Before the MDGT group meets as a whole, the group leader meets with the new members in a group format in order to provide a brief explanation of the group process, to anticipate the misconceptions and resistance they may have, and to engage them actively in the treatment process as a collaborative experience. The therapist's task in the preparatory phase is to diminish fears, clarify misconceptions, provide support, and discuss the MDGT group process.

The basic tasks of the brief preparatory phase are to make the new members feel safe, welcome, and valued; to reduce fears and misconceptions about the group and psychotherapy; to outline the rules and expectations regarding participation; to set an optimistic, hopeful tone regarding the likely benefits to the member; to state what the focus of the group will be; and to encourage members to begin to reflect on some of their difficulties in living.

Orientation and Screening of Prospective Members

Prospective members participate in the first part of a regularly scheduled MDGT meeting. They have the opportunity to ask questions and voice concerns. Current group members have an opportunity to describe how they have had similar struggles, and how the group helps them.

The leader always seeks to head off the premature revelation of traumatic material in these orientation sessions. Also, no prospective or current member is permitted to monopolize the time. When prospective members seek to compare this group approach to others, the leader responds by indicating how this approach differs positively from the ones mentioned, and does not conflict fundamentally with other approaches.

Structure

Structure is provided in a number of ways. First, the group contract initially serves to organize the group. Also, shared norms, explicitly stated and reiterated, provide structure. Abstinence from the addictive behavior, a commitment to talking about feelings and problems rather than acting on them in the group, and agreement about the goals of the treatment are important (Golden, Khantzian, and McAuliffe 1994).

Safety

Safety considerations in the group include immediate physical safety during the group meetings, ensuring safety for therapeutic exploration and change by establishing the norm of abstinence, and promoting an atmosphere of enough interpersonal comfort and psychological security for the interactive work of the group to proceed. Physical safety is a consideration in selection of the meeting place, the group leadership, and the strongly upheld norm of putting thoughts into words instead of actions (Golden, Khantzian, and McAuliffe 1994).

One of the four foci of the MDGT group is safety. Within the group, safety is maintained by keeping alert for signs of psychological relapse, such as the company patients keep and potentially risky environments. At the same time, the group leaders act as interventionists, catalysts, and modulators to ensure optimal interaction and to discourage member overactivity or premature self-disclosure and/ or defensive posturing. In doing so, the group leader creates conditions for listening, empathy, participation, and patience for the invariable excesses and resistances that occur, as well as toleration for the anxiety and discomfort that group participation can evolve (Khantzian, Golden, and McAuliffe 1995).

Confrontation versus Support

Confrontation is often employed in substance abuse groups to force individuals to face their self-destructive behaviors. In our opinion, this may foster defensiveness or seeming compliance and might be counterproductive.

In contrast, MDGT encourages an understanding of addictive behavior as an attempt to deal with unmanageable feelings and experiences and as an adaptation that has outlived its usefulness. In their resistance to change, group members are guided to appreciate how their ways of coping and the crises they precipitate are linked to the past. They need to acknowledge their painful feelings from the past and in the present, and to support one another in finding alternative ways to cope with their painful feeling states and problems in living. In other words, the group members, although they are held responsible for their choices and actions and are asked to look squarely at themselves, are not blamed and judged (Khantzian, Golden, and McAuliffe 1995).

The Early Group

The Leader

In contrast to traditional psychoanalytic psychotherapy, MDGT leaders are more active, firm but caring, directive and focused in their roles, especially early in the group's history.

Since MDGT is designed to focus on vulnerabilities in regulating feelings, self-esteem, relationships, and self-care, the leader helps the group to focus on these themes by clarifying any one of them and appropriately labeling them when necessary. Beyond labeling, clarification sometimes provides "words-for-feelings" when members cannot do it for themselves; at other times clarification is provided through instruction and explanation. Over time, members begin to clarify and label important themes for one another. However, the group leader continues to play a role by providing and demonstrating support, clarification, and interpretation.

The group leader plays an important role in modeling and encouraging certain group norms and behaviors that foster group cohesiveness and treatment effectiveness. The leader also acts to inhibit and discourage other responses and behaviors that reduce the group's cohesiveness and effectiveness. The group leader serves as a model by trying out new behaviors with the members, by maintaining a non-judgmental, open, and honest attitude. The leader deals directly with disruptive and inhibitive factors such as absences, divisive pairings, and scapegoating. The leader heads off and redirects verbal abuse or attacks, while discouraging multiple conversations and premature or excessive psychological probing.

The group leader in MDGT must be flexible as the group unfolds. He or she helps to move the group and keep them on track. A leader can often be extremely helpful by encouraging an embarrassed, ashamed member to give voice to painful issues never before shared or acknowledged with others. This can be accomplished by tactfully disclosing and elucidating on a personal reaction of her or his own that touches on the patient's experience.

The Group Members

In order for members to support one another and understand the characteristic difficulties that precipitate and maintain substance abuse, they need to get to know one another. Self-revelation occurs in a context of comfort, familiarity, and acceptance. Members talk about their past and present experiences and their reactions to one another in the group. Eventually they reveal deficits, dysfunctions, and conflicts about feelings, self-esteem, relationships, and self-care. Such difficulties characteristically and characterologically play themselves out, inside and outside group, around themes involving work, family, and friendships that precipitate and perpetuate reliance on drugs.

As often as group members reveal the bases of their psychological vulnerabilities, they just as often, and for long periods of time, remain defensive about these vulnerabilities and resist any awareness of their problems. Dynamic groups serve as excellent contexts for individuals to identify with one another the character styles and traits that mask and yet are symptomatic of their vulnerabilities. For example, problems with recognizing and verbalizing feelings are often masked by excessive preoccupation with activity and the logistical details of what happened around emotionally evocative experiences; this has been referred to as alexithymia. Members with low self-esteem and conflicts over dependency often adopt attitudes of disavowal and counterdependency. Patients deny self-care problems through counterphobic attitudes and activities. Again, members are encouraged by leader modeling and support to respectfully explore with one another what heightens, aggravates, and evokes these qualities inside and outside the group. In so doing, they gradually identify and understand the vulnerabilities that govern their character traits and styles. In some instances the group leader takes the initiative in pointing out these traits and their origins.

Resistance is to be expected and not prematurely or excessively challenged, and members are allowed to set their own pace in joining the group. The character traits and defenses mentioned previously are usually heightened at the outset of the group and are one of the main ways members manifest their resistance. The task for the leader and the group members in the early phase is to support and/or accept these defenses without imposing restrictive goals or premature confrontation on these resistances. Despite resistance, the leader can adopt an active, directive, and even managerial style to demonstrate to the group members that they can relatively quickly form a cohesive group, become interactive and supportive with one another, foster a climate of mutuality, and begin an interactive phase of work that does not depend solely on the leader.

Group members should share with the leader responsibility for respecting members' defenses by not prematurely or on any one occasion excessively exposing a member's vulnerabilities and shortcomings. Although it soon becomes apparent that substances are used to mask and overcome painful feeling states and problems with self-esteem and dependency, these vulnerabilities need to be revealed gradually so that excessive defensiveness can be avoided, and members can develop an awareness of and a capacity to tolerate painful affects. While MDGT is supportive, it is designed to be expressive, and this is to be done in a manner and at a rate that preserves self-respect. The goal, then, is to maintain self-esteem and to try to focus gently and gradually on underlying painful affects and associated defenses rather than to insist that such defenses be surrendered.

MDGT: PHASES OF THE GROUP

MDGT was designed to be a time-limited group psychotherapeutic experience occurring twice per week for twenty-six weeks. Because new participants are joining as others are completing the therapy, there is some movement between phases. The general tone, however, is set by the intermediate and senior members. While MDGT can be a short-term group (e.g., twenty-six weeks), as was the case for the Harvard Cocaine Recovery Project, it can alternatively be employed as a long-term group therapeutic approach. As a consequence, timing of the "phases" we discuss can be interpreted flexibly.

Beginning Phase

The wish to be liked and accepted significantly influences the type and quality of responses in this phase of the group's interactions. The therapist carefully attempts to help members become aware of emotions, characteristic attitudes, and assumptions that operate automatically and, often as a consequence, deleteriously, in their lives. In some instances members resist acknowledging the real pain in their lives; in others they are not in touch with their feelings or have difficulty putting them into words. Members should not be left to flounder or withdraw; the group leader can be more active drawing out and labeling reactions. In addition, the group leader underscores the idea that people are not alone with their feelings of anxiety and embarrassment, and helps members understand that others share these concerns.

Even as members begin to acknowledge that problems are within themselves and not outside, the group leader often can become a target, for example, of anger. The leader acknowledges frustration, reality-tests extreme distortions, and facilitates interactions that help members to realize they can generate answers among themselves. The group leader also helps members appreciate that the frustration, fear, and other reactions that occur both inside and outside the group can become opportunities in group for understanding and modifying their life problems.

Middle Phase

As group members feel increasingly involved and connected to the group and begin to experience attachments to one another, they begin to evoke special and often troubling feelings and perceptions about self and others. Members assume a more active and reflective role, but the leader remains alert for lapses in sensitivity when members demean, derogate, or overlook troublesome verbal and nonverbal communications about self and others.

In this phase more habitual, characterological ways of interacting are evident, and members find their own ways of positioning themselves in the group. They progressively see themselves as more worthy of attention and more self-accepting as they internalize the accepting, supportive attitude of the leader and other members. Also during this phase the group leader encourages group members to elaborate on experiences both inside and outside the group that typify the feeling, self-esteem, relationship, self-care, and character problems that lead to drug dependency and other self-defeating solutions to problems in living.

Advanced/Termination Phase

Crises can occur at this phase. Skillful management of the crises by the leader will preserve the group's existence and further its progress. Often crises are precipitated by poor attendance, the threat of premature termination, use of drugs or alcohol, inability to regulate affect in the group, the scapegoating of a group member, inappropriate extra-group contact among members, narcissistic crises, and issues external to the group that place a member in personal crisis.

The group is always at risk of psychological relapse, which is more dangerous than symptomatic drug relapse. As treatment advances, members should gain a better knowledge of their character structure, a stronger sense of how they have managed in the past to deal with central self-regulation issues, and a greater flexibility in their responses. Group members slowly realize that the search for external and magical solutions to the problem of the self does not yield a long-lasting resolution. The MDGT group is the road back to oneself.

The group leader needs to be vigilant for manifestations of psychological extremism and intolerance of ambivalence. These two tendencies both give rise to crises and prevent their constructive resolution. It is easier to quit, storm out, get high, sulk, and act out than to understand what is going on. The middle ground is not familiar to group members. They glorify extreme positions, although this leads repeatedly to a sad and vicious adaptation to life.

Although self-defeating, this way of looking at situations is ego-syntonic, comfortable, and automatic. The leader focuses on the extremism, and surveys the middle ground in members' lives, contrasting the ordinary aspects and demands of life with the extraordinary experiences sought through substances. Frequently, the work of the group is to understand better how one can find genuine pleasure and satisfaction in ordinary life.

When one member places the group in crisis, the leader has an opportunity to help all members find common ground. In a typical crisis, the seemingly central issue of group attendance quickly becomes peripheral as the group explores various conflicts such as vulnerability, dysfunctional patterns of self-care, and core relationship themes. While the group initially forms around the common ground of substance dependence, the leader moves the group to other sources of commonality: the psychological and life experiences in the four dimensions MDGT emphasizes.

SUMMARY AND CONCLUSIONS

MDGT is rooted in a human psychological understanding of the suffering that is at the heart of addictive vulnerability. Patients with substance use disorders do not use or rely on drugs to seek pleasure or to destroy themselves. They take drugs because substances of abuse act specifically to relieve painful affects or to give release to feelings that are nameless, cut off, and confusing. Besides difficulties in regulating their emotions, they also suffer because of deficits in regulating their self-esteem, relationships, and self-care.

MDGT, in the context of a supportive and semistructured format, allows for a natural unfolding of the ways individuals suffer with their self-regulation vulnerabilities and the ways that such individuals adopt characterologic defenses and use drugs to counter their inability to deal with their suffering and take care of themselves. MDGT places a premium on control, contact, comfort, and safety. The leaders are empathic at the same time they are focused and directive. The leader may act as catalyst, analyst, activator, and modulator. The constant challenge for the leader and members is to identify the human basis of individuals' addictive vulnerabilities to help them understand the extremes they have adopted to deal with their distress, and to discover in the presence of a caring leader and group members more mature middle ground alternatives to express and satisfy their human needs for comfort and a better sense of well-being.

REFERENCES

Albanese MJ, Khantzian EJ, Murphy SL, Green AI. Decreased substance use in chronically psychotic patients treated with clozapine. *American Journal of Psychiatry* 151:780-781, 1994.

Breslau N, Kilbey MM, Andreski P. Vulnerability to psychopathology in nicotine-dependent smokers: An epidemiologic study of young adults. *American Journal of Psychiatry* 150:941-946, 1993.

Brown S. *Treating the Alcoholic: A Developmental Model of Recovery.* New York: John Wiley & Sons, 1985.

Glass R. Blue mood, blackened lungs: Depression and smoking. *JAMA* 264:1583-1584, 1990.

Golden SG, Khantzian EJ, McAuliffe WE. Group therapy. In *The American Psychiatric Press Textbook of Substance Abuse Treatment,* edited by Galanter M, Kleber HD. Washington, DC: American Psychiatric Press, 1994, pp. 303-314.

Kessler RC, Crum RM, Warner LA, Nelson CB, Schulenberg J, Anthony JC. Lifetime co-occurrence of DSM-III-R alcohol abuse and dependence with other psychiatric disorders in the national comorbidity survey. *Archives of General Psychiatry* 54:313-321, 1997.

Khantzian EJ. The self-medication hypothesis of substance use disorders: A reconsideration and recent applications. *Harvard Review of Psychiatry* 4:231-244, 1997.

Khantzian EJ, Golden SJ, McAuliffe, WE. Group therapy for psychoactive substance use disorders. In *Treatment of Psychiatric Disorders,* Volume 1, edited by Gabbard GO. Washington, DC: American Psychiatric Press, 1995, pp. 832-839.

Khantzian EJ, Halliday KS, McAuliffe WE. *Addiction and the Vulnerable Self: Modified Dynamic Group Therapy for Substance Abusers.* New York: The Guilford Press, 1990.

Kohut H. Preface. In *Psychodynamics of Drug Dependence,* edited by Blaine JD, Julius DA. (NIDA Research Monograph Number 12; Department of Health, Education, and Welfare Publication Number ADM 77-470). Washington, DC: United States Government Printing Office, 1977, pp. vii-ix.

Kosten TR, Krystal J. Biological mechanisms in post-traumatic stress disorder: Relevance for substance abuse. *Recent Developments in Alcoholism* 6:49-68, 1988.

McKenna C, Ross C. Diagnostic conundrums in substance abusers with psychiatric symptoms: Variables suggestive of dual diagnosis. *American Journal of Drug and Alcohol Abuse* 20:397-412, 1994.

Meissner WW. *Psychotherapy and the Paranoid Process.* New York: Jason Aronson, 1986.

Milin R, Loh EA, Wilson A. Drug preference, reported drug experience, and stimulus sensitivity. *American Journal on Addictions* 1:248-256, 1992.

Noordsy DL, Drake RE, Teague GB, Osher FC, Hurlbut SC, Beaudett MS, Paskus TS. Subjective experiences related to alcohol use among schizophrenics. *Journal of Nervous and Mental Disease* 179:410-414, 1991.

Vannicelli M. *Removing the Roadblocks: Group Psychotherapy with Substance Abusers and Family Members.* New York: Guilford Press, 1992.

Wurmser L. *The Hidden Dimension: Psychodynamics of Compulsive Drug Use.* New York: Jason Aronson, 1978.

SECTION II:
SPECIFIC TREATMENT SETTINGS
AND GOALS

Chapter 6

Outpatient Groups at Different Stages of Substance Abuse Treatment: Preparation, Initial Abstinence, and Relapse Prevention

Arnold M. Washton

INTRODUCTION

The types of therapeutic interventions that work best in the treatment of psychoactive substance use disorders often depend on the person's place in the process of change. Patients attempting to give up alcohol and other substances progress through a series of definable stages as they move from active use toward sustained abstinence and recovery. Accordingly, treatment programs are often divided into several sequential components or stages, each focusing on specific tasks and goals most relevant to that particular stage.

There are a number of benefits to dividing a treatment program into discrete, if arbitrary stages:

1. It focuses the therapeutic work within each stage.
2. It provides predefined progress markers that give patients a sense of personal accomplishment.
3. It makes it easier for individuals to identify and relate to the content material being addressed at a particular stage and to bond with others who are dealing with the same or similar issues.
4. It facilitates placement into a level of care best suited to meet the patient's individual needs at a given point in the recovery process.

5. It encourages specificity in treatment goals and therapeutic interventions to be utilized at each stage.

The first stage of treatment can be defined as a *preparatory* or
prerecovery stage in which the individuals are typically ambivalent,
unsure, and questioning whether their substance use is a problem and
whether treatment is really necessary. Treatment interventions at this
stage enhance the person's motivation and readiness for change. Crisis intervention and medical detoxification may also be required at
this stage. In the *initial abstinence* or *active quitting* stage the person
makes a deliberate attempt to stop using substances and change other
behaviors to support abstinence. Primary goals are to interrupt the cycle of compulsive alcohol/drug use, counteract impulses and cravings
to resume use, and enhance commitment to ongoing change. In the
relapse prevention stage the major goals are to secure and maintain
abstinence, and to develop a satisfying lifestyle free of alcohol and
other drugs. Critical tasks include learning how to recognize and
safely respond to early warning signs of potential relapse, how to reliably counteract desires to "self-medicate," and on acquiring coping
skills. For some individuals, this stage may also need to address psychological issues including problems with relationships and affect
management.

Stages of Change

In recent years, the notion that therapeutic interventions must be
matched to stages in the process of change or recovery has gained
widespread acceptance with proliferation of the *stages of change*
model described by Prochaska and DiClemente (1986). This model
defines certain stages of change that people move through as they attempt to modify (overcome) problem behaviors such as psychoactive
substance abuse. The model also describes the types of interventions
that are most likely to be effective within each stage and to promote
movement into the next stage. For example, in the *precontemplation*
stage, the person is generally unaware that the behavior in question is
a "problem." In the *contemplation* stage, the individual begins to experience ambivalence or conflict about the behavior that is now perceived by him or her as possibly a problem, but takes no action. In the
determination or *decision* stage, the balance tips in favor of change
and the person decides to take some type of action, but has not yet de-

cided what method to employ. The *initiation* or *action* stage begins when the person has chosen a change method and now actually does something to modify the problem behavior. In the *maintenance* stage, the primary goal is to maintain progress and prevent backsliding or relapse. *Relapse* in this model is defined as regression (i.e., movement backward) from any given stage of change to an earlier one.

Applying this model to the stages of treatment previously described suggests that preparatory or prerecovery interventions are best suited for individuals in the stages of precontemplation, contemplation, or decision; early abstinence techniques are most appropriate for individuals in the initiation (action) stage; and relapse prevention techniques are most appropriate for individuals in the maintenance stage. Interventions not properly matched to the process of change are likely to be ineffective or harmful.

Motivational versus Confrontational Approaches

In motivational approaches a deliberate effort is made to adapt treatment interventions to fit the needs of the patient, whereas in the traditional system the patient is required to fit into the needs or requirements of the program. A good deal of skillful and tolerant preparatory work may be needed to mobilize the individuals' motivation so that they see treatment as desirable and are ready to make a beginning level commitment to change. In the current treatment system the tendency is to blame the patient's lack of motivation for failure to engage in treatment, rather than acknowledge that perhaps clinical interventions are significantly mismatched to the patient's current needs (Martin et al. 1996).

Fortunately, there are now alternatives to all of this. The recent influx of mental health professionals into the field has brought an enhanced appreciation for the clinical value of psychotherapeutic approaches in the treatment of addiction, and has stimulated efforts to adapt psychotherapeutic techniques to improve treatment effectiveness (Bean and Zinberg 1981; Khantzian, Halliday, and McAuliffe 1990; Vannicelli 1995; Washton 1989, 1995; Zweben 1989). For example, an issue of central importance in psychotherapeutic approaches is formation of a strong therapeutic or working alliance between patient and therapist. This alliance is seen as an essential vehicle for promoting therapeutic change. Psychotherapeutic approaches emphasize flexibility, collaboration, and negotiation when dealing with patient resistance, especially in the early stages. Since early dropout is the norm rather than exception in addiction treatment, a crucial task is to retain patients long enough to form at least the beginnings of a working alliance and gain sufficient therapeutic leverage to coax them forward in the process of change. The goal is to work *with,* not against, the patient's resistance in order to bring about change. Understanding transference and countertransference dynamics can be very helpful in minimizing power struggles and avoiding other destructive interactions that may unwittingly drive patients out of treatment (Imhof 1995; Zweben 1989).

In recent years, a significant advance in adaptation of psychotherapeutic approaches to treating substance abuse has been the development of motivational interviewing techniques by Miller and associates (Miller and Rollnick 1991). Within the stages of change model previously described, these motivational techniques combine Rogerian principles of patient-centered therapy with a variety of cognitive-behavioral interventions to help patients free up their own motivations so they can move forward in the process of change.

How to incorporate such motivational strategies into group treatment approaches to increase a substance-dependent patient's motivation, readiness, and ability to sustain change is the primary focus of the present chapter. Although these strategies have been designed and utilized as pretreatment interventions, they are useful in all stages of treatment. A chemically dependent patient's ambivalence, reluctance, conflict, and vacillating commitment to change are recurrent issues and themes that surface throughout the course of treatment.

The present chapter describes stage-specific outpatient groups for each of the three treatment stages previously described: (1) preparatory or prerecovery stage; (2) initial abstinence stage; and (3) relapse prevention stage. Discussion of relapse prevention groups can also be found in Chapter 7, written by Rawson and Obert.

Group approaches to early stage patients are of interest because motivational interviewing techniques have been designed primarily, if not exclusively, for use in individual rather than group session formats. (A recent article by Martin et al. [1996] titled "Group Interventions with Prerecovery Patients" is the only exception the author could find in the current literature.)

GROUP TREATMENT FOR PRERECOVERY PATIENTS: SELF-EVALUATION GROUP (SEG)

The Self-Evaluation Group (SEG) is a motivational intervention designed for individuals who are in the precontemplation, contemplation, or decision stage. The purpose of the group is to facilitate an accurate self-evaluation of each person's involvement with psychoactive substances to enhance the person's motivation and readiness to change. Individuals enrolled in the SEG are deliberately referred to as "participants" or "group members" rather than "patients" in keeping with the fact that they have not yet decided whether they want or need treatment.

The primary goals for each group member are as follows:

1. To evaluate past and present *involvement* with psychoactive substances
2. To evaluate *consequences* or problems related to alcohol/drug use
3. To enhance motivation and readiness for change
4. To develop a specific plan that includes goals and methods for initiating change, including formal treatment where indicated

The approach utilized in the SEG is motivational, consistent with techniques previously described. In contrast to standard approaches for dealing with ambivalent, wavering patients, no attempt is made to convince participants that they must accept the identity of "addict/alcoholic" or their substance use as a "disease." For example, the group leader carefully refrains from using interventions that

1. selectively emphasize or catastrophize negative consequences associated with substance use;
2. seize upon information suggesting that a group member's substance use is more extensive and more problematic than he or she is willing to acknowledge;
3. label discrepancies between the group member's view of his or her substance use and that of other observers as evidence of his or her "resistance" or "denial"; and
4. suggest that anyone with an alcohol/drug problem who does not go into treatment is headed for disastrous consequences.

Rather, the SEG actively encourages elucidation of facts concerning an individual's substance use through a process of self-evaluation and by offering objective feedback. The group leader's role is to structure each session, focus and guide the discussion, offer feedback, and teach participants how to provide helpful feedback to one another.

The tone and atmosphere of the group is very critical to accomplishing the desired goals. The group leader is respectful, nonthreatening, noncoercive, and encourages self-revelation and open, honest reporting. Although aggressive confrontation is categorically avoided, therapeutic confrontation is most certainly used. This often takes the form of pointing out discrepancies between the individuals' perceptions of their behavior and perception of that behavior by other group members and/or the group leader, and between the individuals' behavior and their stated values/goals.

Group Structure and Format

An individual's participation in the SEG is scheduled to last four consecutive weeks. The group meets twice per week. Each participant attends seven consecutive ninety-minute group sessions plus one individual session at the end (i.e., after the seventh group session). Newcomers are admitted to the group at any point in the program. Group membership is usually held to a maximum of eight people at any given time in order to ensure that all members receive sufficient, personalized attention.

A urine sample for drug testing is taken at each visit. Group members are asked to abstain at least temporarily from using alcohol and all other psychoactive substances during their four-week tenure in the group even if abstinence is not their desired goal and they have no intention of maintaining abstinence after leaving the group. They are told that temporary abstinence provides the best opportunity to acquire an accurate assessment of the role of substance use in one's daily (weekly) life. No one is expelled from the group for a positive urine as long as they are not under the influence of psychoactive substances (and not hungover, "crashing," or in withdrawal) during any of the group sessions.

Each group session focuses on a specific topic, using a set of guidelines, including content material and a brief questionnaire. The guidelines are intended to provide the basic structure, focus, and tone for each session and to ensure that certain important issues are properly addressed.

Patient Selection Factors

The SEG is intended for individuals

1. who exhibit behavioral and/or physical signs (e.g., employer/ family complaints, positive urine test) of substance use but do not perceive their use as a "problem";
2. who are questioning whether they really have an alcohol/drug "problem";
3. with mild to moderate levels of use who show little or no evidence of psychosocial dysfunction;
4. who currently appear to meet criteria for substance *abuse* (not dependence) and are at risk of developing a more serious alcohol/drug problem; and
5. those who clearly meet criteria for substance *dependence* (including chronic relapsers).

The SEG can and has been effectively used with voluntary as well as mandated people (Berg and Miller 1992). It is a structured intervention that essentially "starts where the person is" instead of engaging in a no-win power struggle intent on pressuring people to accept the therapist's or program's view of their behavior.

Individuals least suited for this approach include those with serious psychiatric illness, significant cognitive impairment, and/or active risk factors (e.g., suicidality). Participation in the SEG requires the individual to be at least moderately functional and, perhaps more important, to show up reliably for the scheduled sessions. Essentially, the SEG is best suited for individuals in the stages of *precontemplation, contemplation,* or *decision,* to move the person forward, where appropriate, into the *action* stage. Upon completing the SEG, people exercise their choice either to enter or not enter formal treatment.

Specific topics covered in each of the seven SEG group sessions and a final individual (eighth) session are described below. More detailed protocols can be found elsewhere (Washton 1995). Each group session includes

1. presentation of introductory material by the group leader,
2. review of a written exercise or questionnaire,
3. focused discussion of the topic related directly to each participant's own personal situation.

These sessions are designed to engender lively discussion and to involve all participants in the process of giving and receiving helpful feedback. The following is a brief description of each session. For an extensive resource book and compendium of assessment instruments, see Allen and Columbus (1995), a publication of the National Institute on Alcohol Abuse and Alcoholism.

Session 1: Your Personal History of Substance Use

The goal of this unit is to help members provide a complete and accurate history of their involvement with psychoactive substances.

Session 2: Your Family History of Substance Use

The primary goal is to obtain a history of substance use in the person's family members and any significant others.

Session 3: Risks and Consequences of Use

Participants formulate a complete and accurate accounting of consequences associated with their substance use.

Session 4: Perceived Benefits of Use

Participants identify perceived benefits of their substance use and address concerns or conflicts about quitting (including anticipated problems associated with *not* using). The group leader points out at the beginning of this session that the positive mood-altering effects make alcohol/drugs attractive and desirable in the first place. It can also be very useful to define the connection between an individual's substance use and certain feelings or moods.

Session 5: Distinguishing Between Use, Abuse, and Dependency

This session addresses the different patterns of use and the behavioral indicators of abuse and dependency. Participants describe their substance use along several dimensions, including

1. frequency,
2. chronicity,
3. intensity/amount,
4. route of administration,
5. compulsivity/obsession,
6. impulsivity and impaired control,
7. "triggering" events or precipitants of use,
8. context of use,
9. developmental course including evidence of progression or intensification over time.

Session 6: The Pros and Cons of Quitting

This session explores the perceived costs and benefits of quitting. Concerns about quitting are often linked to fears about how one will fare in certain situations without benefit of the substance's mood-altering effects.

Session 7: What Type of Help Is Available?

This session explores the various forms of help that are available for those who want to stop their alcohol/drug use, such as professional treatment, self-help, and medication. Those attending their seventh and final group session are asked at this point to schedule an individual session with the group leader (see below).

Session 8: (Individual Session) Formulating a Plan

The purpose of this eighth and final session is (1) to review and summarize what the individual has learned from participating in the SEG, (2) to discuss whether the individual is ready to make a commitment to abstinence or wants additional help in making this decision, and (3) for those who come to a decision that they do want to stop their alcohol/drug use, to formulate a specific combination of treatment and self-help. Those who elect not to enter treatment or self-help are assured that the door remains open, and they are encouraged to come back for a follow-up or "check-in" visit within the next ninety days.

Limitations, Pitfalls, and Required Skills for the SEG

The SEG is not intended as a launching pad into recovery and/ or treatment for every participant. For some individuals heightened awareness of their substance use and its related problems may be enough to convince them of the need to reduce or completely stop using. Many individuals with abuse or dependence have successfully achieved and maintained abstinence on their own with professional treatment or attendance at self-help meetings. The clinician's level of experience is probably less important than his or her compassion, flexibility, and skills of self-examination. At every step of the process one questions whose agenda is being serviced by a given statement or intervention, especially when it elicits and exacerbates defensiveness or simply does not produce the desired outcome. Good clinical supervision can also help a great deal to act as a sounding board in order to maintain the therapeutic posture and perspective required to appropriately lead the SEG.

THE INITIAL ABSTINENCE GROUP (IAG)

The Initial Abstinence Group or IAG is for individuals who are in the initiation or action stage and ready to make behavioral changes necessary to stop using all psychoactive substances—at least temporarily. Among patients seen as appropriate for the IAG are those who meet DSM-IV criteria for substance dependence and agree to at least a "trial period" of total abstinence. Individuals at this stage usually see no reason to give up using substances other than their drug of choice, especially if these substances have caused them no obvious problems. The clinician should accept rather than attack the patient's ambivalence about this matter, and form a therapeutic alliance around conducting an "experiment" with total abstinence. Learning the value of maintaining total abstinence is seen as a goal and not as a prerequisite to entering the IAG.

Simply stated, the primary goal of the IAG is to move patients through the initiation stage until they arrive at the maintenance stage, where the focus shifts from stopping alcohol/drug use to staying stopped. The IAG helps patients initiate and stabilize their abstinence. In Relapse Prevention Group (RPG), the next stage of treatment, the primary task is to help patients to maintain abstinence and counteract forces that may lead toward relapse.

Group Structure and Format

The IAG meets four times per week for ninety minutes each. One session per week is devoted to psychoeducation, as described below. The other three sessions are regular recovery groups that do not necessarily focus on a predetermined topic, but always deal with the "here and now" of establishing and securing abstinence. Newcomers are required to attend six consecutive weekly education sessions. Thereafter they attend only the recovery group sessions, which are held three times per week.

There is no predetermined length of stay in the IAG that works best for all patients. Completion or "graduation" from the group is based on completing a number of specific tasks and goals, defined as follows:

1. A period of at least six to eight weeks of uninterrupted abstinence (as verified by frequent urine and Breathalyzer tests), stable psychosocial functioning, and no intense cravings or urges
2. A reasonably accurate, realistic view of his or her psychoactive substance use and its resulting consequences
3. Openness and responsiveness to assistance offered by others
4. Significant progress in working through ambivalence and resentment about giving up alcohol/drugs
5. Progress in acquiring some of the most essential coping skills needed to support and protect abstinence; e.g., avoiding "high risk" situations, responding effectively to cravings and urges, and reaching out for help when needed
6. Reliable participation in group with honest self-disclosure
7. Attendance in at least several self-help (AA, CA, NA) meetings which are shared with the group

Most group members spend somewhere between eight and twelve weeks in the IAG. All of the above goals are not likely to be attained by the time of graduation from the IAG, but it is expected that significant progress will be clearly evident in most areas. Sometimes a patient's stay in the IAG is restricted by outside factors such as managed care. In some cases, a patient spends only several weeks rather than the more usual two to three months in a three to four times per week IAG before transitioning into a once per week Relapse Prevention Group. Clinical observation indicates that some patients do quite well with less-than-usual lengths of stay in the IAG while others do not. It appears that patients who leave the IAG prior to attaining the most basic goals (e.g., stable abstinence and reasonably normalized psychosocial functioning) are the ones most likely to relapse shortly after leaving the group.

Throughout the IAG, every group member's progress is reviewed weekly in the group, including self-assessment and feedback from other group members and the group leader. The review helps to identify the specific changes needed in order to successfully transition to the next stage of treatment.

Group Rules

The group leader discusses the group rules (see below) with each newcomer before the first session. Every patient must read, sign, and agree to these rules as a prerequisite to entering the group (Washton 1989):

1. Come to group sessions completely "straight," not intoxicated, "crashing," hungover, or under the influence of alcohol or any other mood-altering substances.
2. Abstain from the use of alcohol and all other mood-altering chemicals during your participation in the group. In the event of any alcohol/drug use, you must bring up this issue for discussion at the *beginning* of the next group session. "Slips" will be viewed as potential learning experiences, but you will not be able to continue in the group if you slip repeatedly, since this is destructive for you and for your fellow group members. If you are removed from the group due to slips, you

will be given the option, where appropriate, of individual therapy to help you reestablish at least two consecutive weeks of uninterrupted abstinence (verified by clean urines) as a prerequisite to coming back into the group.
3. Attend all scheduled sessions and arrive on time without fail. This may require you to rearrange other obligations and perhaps even postpone vacations while participating in the group.
4. Preserve the anonymity and confidentiality of all group members.
5. Remain in the group until you have completed the program. If you have an impulse or desire to leave the group prematurely, you will raise this issue for discussion in the group before deciding to leave.
6. Refrain from becoming involved romantically, sexually, or financially with any other group member during your participation in the program.
7. Acknowledge that you will be immediately terminated from the program if you offer alcohol/drugs to any member of the group or use together with another group member.
8. Have your telephone number(s) added to the contact list distributed to all group members.
9. Give a supervised urine sample at least twice a week and whenever the group leader may request it.
10. Discuss in the group any issue that threatens your own or another member's recovery. You will not keep secrets regarding another member's alcohol/drug use or other destructive behavior.

Urine Testing

Frequent urine testing is an important component of outpatient group treatment not only in the IAG, but in all subsequent phases. Urine testing creates a "safety net" by establishing behavioral accountability for any alcohol/drug use that may occur. This can be a strong deterrent to acting on an impulse to use and a desire to conceal from others any instance of use. Urine testing provides an objective indicator of alcohol/drug use or the absence of use (i.e., verification of abstinence), and also provides an objective, concrete marker of an individual's progress in treatment. The motivational value of urine test results can be significant. Patients often point to a continuous period of "clean urines" as concrete evidence of their motivation and ability to sustain abstinence, as do concerned others.

Implementing a urine testing procedure of clinical value requires adherence to several important guidelines. These include the following:

1. All samples should be "supervised" (witnessed) in order to prevent falsification.
2. Urine samples should be taken routinely at least every three to four days so as not to exceed the sensitivity limits of standard laboratory testing methods.
3. Samples should be tested by enzymeimmunoassay (EIA) or radioimmunoassay (RIA) methods to ensure accuracy, and all positive results should be confirmed by a second test using a different method than the first test.
4. Samples should be tested routinely for all of the most commonly used psychoactive substances.
5. Patients should be tested throughout the entire treatment program and not be taken off urine testing until solidly in recovery. Even then, sporadic testing is useful.

Achieving Initial Abstinence

The first and foremost goal of the IAG is immediate cessation of all psychoactive substance use and rapid integration of the newcomer into the group. To break the addictive cycle, the patient's habitual alcohol/drug use must be replaced with habitual attendance at the group. Attending group sessions three to four times per week can provide at least some of the much-needed structure and behavioral accountability in the early stages. The group provides a ready-made support network that, for some patients, is the only opportunity they have to interact with peers who are not actively using or intoxicated. Individual sessions, when indicated, are also helpful, especially for those who are apprehensive or anxious about entering a group. Faithful attendance at group sessions is an essential part of recovery. When patients miss a session, it is critical that group members and the group leader call to express concern and communicate that the person's absence did not go unnoticed, to help prevent dropouts.

The group provides a forum for social support, positive role-modeling, peer identification, mutual sharing of experiences, and for acquiring crucial information about the importance of mastering the basics such as avoiding triggers and other high-risk situations.

Education Sessions

Education and skill development are important components of group treatment, especially in the early phase when dropout rates tend to be highest. Teaching specific coping and problem-solving skills can enhance the person's effectiveness in dealing with a wide variety of situations that could easily lead back to alcohol/drug use. Abstinence is very tenuous and fragile at this stage and is repeatedly tested by impulses, cravings, social pressures, and easy access to a wide variety of substances. Education sessions help to ensure that a certain core of essential information including basic "survival skills" is transmitted to all group members.

Each education session follows a set of general guidelines. After giving a brief introductory lecture, the group leader facilitates a discussion in which all members are asked to discuss the relevance of the topic directly to their personal experience. Among the topics covered in these sessions are

1. finding your motivation to stop using;
2. identifying, avoiding, and coping with your high-risk situations;
3. dealing with cravings and urges;
4. reasons for total abstinence;
5. early warning signs of relapse;
6. tips for handling slips;
7. how to have fun without using alcohol/drugs;
8. managing anger and frustration;
9. how your family and friends can help; and
10. the combined roles of treatment and self-help, and how to get the most out of each (see Washton and Stone-Washton 1990; Washton 1995).

Support and advice from established group members who have dealt successfully with these issues can help the newcomer resist habitual impulses to "self-medicate" in the face of seemingly unresolvable problems that have taken them by surprise.

Self-Help Involvement

The twelve-step programs of AA, CA, and NA have facilitated the recovery of countless thousands of individuals throughout the world and it is generally a good idea to encourage all patients to attend at least several meetings as a way to get started.

Managing Ambivalence and Resistance to Change

An issue that typically consumes a great deal of the group's attention is the ambivalence and reluctance of certain members to make the most essential changes needed to support abstinence, accepting that returning to controlled use is not a viable option. It can also be difficult to accept that personal determination and willpower alone are not sufficient to successfully stop alcohol/drug use. Resistance is to be expected, especially in the early stages of quitting. Prematurely or excessively confronting an ambivalent newcomer may do more harm than good by raising rather than lowering the person's defenses and driving him or her out of treatment. It is essential that every group meeting devote meaningful attention to as many members as possible, although it is unlikely that within any one session the needs of all in attendance will be completely met.

Responding to "Slips"

It is preferable to deal with a group member's "slip," should it occur, as a mistake and motivational crisis rather than tragic failure or willful noncompliance. When group members report that they have slipped since the previous session and/or a positive urine test indicates that this is so, the group must give immediate priority to a detailed therapeutic group discussion of the slip (Washton and Stone-Washton 1990). When a member repeatedly slips and fails to make use of the group's prior recommendations, the group may become intolerant. The group leader must guard against the group's tendency to scapegoat or alienate a member who has experienced multiple slips.

Protecting the group's integrity against the destructive influences of a repeatedly slipping member should be given priority over the individual's stated desire to stay in the group. It is important for the group to appropriately share concerns and offer recommendations to the person whose group membership is in jeopardy. It can be counter-productive to short-circuit this process by adopting an inflexible rule such as "three slips and you're out of the group." If the final decision is to at least temporarily suspend the individual from participating in the group, this can be done with the stipulation that he or she can gain reentry after attaining at least two weeks of total abstinence as veri-fied by urine tests.

Group Composition

Much is to be said in favor of treating those suffering with different primary addictions within the same group as long as the program spe-cifically addresses those issues that are clearly substance-specific and essential to recovery. This can help patients realize that different substances usually lead to the same destructive behaviors and that the process of recovery is nearly identical for each.

Closed versus Open Membership

Without open membership it may be impossible to maintain ade-quate group size because some members inevitably drop out of the group before completing the program. Optimal group size is usually eight to twelve members. New members are added as others complete treatment or drop out. There are both benefits and drawbacks to open membership (Spitz 1987). From the standpoint of a newcomer to the group, having immediate access to a ready-made support network of recovering peers who are eager to share knowledge and lend emo-tional support is seen as one of the major advantages of group treat-ment.

THE RELAPSE PREVENTION GROUP (RPG)

It is often said that stopping an addictive behavior is not nearly as difficult as staying abstinent over the long term. Relapse is a well-known and frequent occurrence in the treatment of alcohol/drug de-pendence. Relapse during and after treatment may be the norm rather than exception. Approximately two-thirds of relapses occur in the initial three months of abstinence (Daley and Lis 1995). Relapse prevention (RP) strategies, as formulated by Marlatt and Gordon (1985), include a wide range of cognitive-behavioral interventions that incorporate skills training, cognitive reframing, and lifestyle interventions, including psychoeducation, identification of high-risk situations, developing coping and stress management skills, and enhancing self-efficacy. RP strategies have been adapted and expanded to accommodate a variety of patient populations and treatment settings including inpatient treatment of alcoholism and outpatient treatment of heroin addiction (Zackon, McAuliffe, and Chien 1993) and cocaine dependence (Carroll, Rounsaville, and Keller 1991; Rawson et al. 1990; Washton 1989; Washton and Stone-Washton 1990).

Group Structure, Content, and Goals

The RPG is for graduates of the IAG and others who have achieved at least two to three months of stable abstinence. There is the option of a once or twice weekly RPG group, depending on stability and longevity of the patient's abstinence. Patients who may be better off with the twice weekly RPG include those who are still experiencing frequent and/or intense cravings, those with inadequate support systems, those who have previously relapsed, and those who are still struggling with strong conflicts and ambivalence about maintaining abstinence.

The intended length of participation in the RPG for most patients is approximately twelve weeks, although some require longer stays to achieve their desired treatment goals. Attainment of the most essential goals of the RPG are evidenced by the following patient behaviors:

1. Reliably identifies and responds appropriately to relapse warning signs
2. Reliably anticipates and avoids high-risk situations
3. Remains open, receptive, and nondefensive in response to advice and suggestions
4. Is regularly and meaningfully involved in self-help and/or other support systems
5. Has made significant progress in developing a reasonably balanced lifestyle that includes healthy leisure activities
6. Has strengthened his or her personal resolve and commitment to maintaining abstinence

There is also an extended RPG for patients who want and need recovery-oriented group psychotherapy over a longer period of time.

Similar to the IAG, RPG group sessions consist of a mixture of education, peer support, and recovery-oriented therapy. Most sessions address issues raised by group members such as coping with stressors, counteracting desires to self-medicate, anticipating and avoiding high-risk situations, and learning more effective and adaptive ways to deal with negative emotions, moods, and interpersonal problems, which are interwoven with the ongoing work of the group (Washton 1989; Washton and Stone-Washton 1990).

Relapses that occur after several weeks or months of stable abstinence are often caused not so much by environmental triggers (which is more typical during early abstinence) as by failure of the patient to cope adequately with problems of daily living or unexpected stressors that generate negative emotions. Research on the relapse process (Marlatt and Gordon 1985) indicates that the major precipitants of relapse are negative mood states, interpersonal conflict, and social pressures to use drugs. Identifying the specific areas of vulnerability in each patient allows the group leader to prioritize which issues warrant current attention in the group.

Explaining the relapse dynamic (Washton 1989) as a progressive process that is set in motion long before the person returns to alcohol/drug use empowers group members to formulate plans to interrupt the process and prevent relapse from occurring, even many months after stopping alcohol and drug use.

In the extended RPG, group sessions address psychodynamic issues that go beyond the basic cognitive and behavioral factors that may contribute to relapse (Murphy and Khantzian 1995). The ultimate goal of the extended RPG is not merely acquisition of self-knowledge and insight, but fundamental change in the individual's characteristically maladaptive patterns of thinking, feeling, behaving, and interacting.

Coordination between individual and group therapy is especially vital here. Moreover, whenever such sensitive, highly charged issues are being discussed the group leader must be especially mindful of the possibility that group members may be at increased risk of relapse. The group leader must make a special effort to end each session with some closure and on a reasonably positive, optimistic note.

FINAL COMMENT

This chapter has described outpatient groups designed to address specific issues, tasks, and goals that define each stage of treatment and recovery. Groups are cost-effective and clinically effective interventions that continue to be the preferred modality of addiction treatment by patients, clinicians, and third party payers alike. The aggressive push toward cost containment has made outpatient treatment the modality of first choice for treating addiction and this has, in turn, created increased demand for improved treatment specificity and patient-treatment matching. The adaptation and expansion of motivational techniques for use in group settings, as described in this chapter, may facilitate more widespread acceptance and application of these techniques, especially in structured outpatient programs. This could help fill what is now a sizeable gap in the current system for substance abuse treatment. Structured, stage-specific group approaches for the initial abstinence and relapse prevention phases of treatment, such as those described here and in the chapter by Rawson and Obert (Chapter 7) may also help to enhance treatment specificity and patient-treatment matching.

REFERENCES

Allen JP, Columbus M (eds.). *Assessing Alcohol Problems: A Guide for Clinicians and Researchers.* Treatment Handbook Series 4 (NIH Publ No 95-3745). Bethesda, MD: National Institute on Alcohol Abuse and Alcoholism, 1995.

Bean MH, Zinberg N (eds.). *Dynamic Approaches to the Understanding and Treatment of Alcoholism.* New York: The Free Press, 1981.

Berg IK, Miller SD. *Working with the Problem Drinker: A Solution-Focused Approach.* New York: Norton, 1992.

Carroll KM, Rounsaville BJ, Keller DS. Relapse prevention strategies for the treatment of cocaine abusers. *American Journal of Drug and Alcohol Abuse* 17(3):19-26, 1991.

Daley DC, Lis JA. Relapse prevention: Intervention strategies for mental health clients with comorbid addictive disorders. In *Psychotherapy in Substance Abuse: A Practitioner's Handbook,* edited by Washton AM. New York: Guilford, 1995, pp. 243-263.

Imhof J. Overcoming countertransference and other attitudinal barriers in the treatment of substance abuse. In *Psychotherapy and Substance Abuse: A Practitioner's Handbook,* edited by Washton AM. New York: Guilford, 1995, pp. 3-22.

Khantzian EJ, Halliday KS, McAuliffe WE. *Addiction and the Valuable Self: Modified Group Therapy for Substance Abusers.* New York: Guilford, 1990.

Marlatt GA, Gordon J. *Relapse Prevention.* New York: Guilford, 1985.

Martin K, Giannandrea P, Rogers B, Johnson J. Group intervention with prerecovery patients. *Journal of Substance Abuse Treatment* 13(1):31-41, 1996.

Miller WR, Rollnick S (eds.). *Motivational Interviewing: Preparing People to Change Addictive Behaviors.* New York: Guilford, 1991.

Murphy SL, Khantzian EJ. Addiction as a "self-medication" disorder: Application of ego psychology to the treatment of substance abuse. In *Psychotherapy and Substance Abuse: A Practitioner's Handbook,* edited by Washton AM. New York: Guilford, 1995, pp. 161-175.

Prochaska JO, DiClemente CC. Toward a comprehensive model of change. In *Treating Addictive Behaviors: Processes of Change,* edited by Miller WR, Heather N. New York: Plenum, 1986, pp. 3-27.

Rawson RA, Obert JL, McCann MJ, Smith D, Scheffey EH. Neurobehavioral treatment of cocaine dependency. *Journal of Psychoactive Drugs* 22:283-297, 1990.

Spitz HI. Cocaine abuse: Therapeutic group approaches. In *Cocaine Abuse: New Directions in Treatment and Research,* edited by Spitz HI, Rosecan JS. New York: Bruner/Mazel, 1987, pp. 156-201.

Vannicelli M. Group psychotherapy with substance abusers and family members. In *Psychotherapy and Substance Abuse: A Practitioner's Handbook,* edited by Washton AM. New York: Guilford, 1995, pp. 337-356.

Washton AM. *Cocaine Addiction: Treatment, Recovery, and Relapse Prevention.* New York: WW Norton, 1989.

Washton AM (ed.). *Psychotherapy and Substance Abuse: A Practitioner's Handbook.* New York: Guilford, 1995.

Washton AM, Stone-Washton N. Abstinence and relapse in outpatient cocaine addicts. *Journal of Psychoactive Drugs* 22:135-148, 1990.

Zackon F, McAuliffe WE, Chien JM. *Recovery Training and Self-help: Relapse Prevention and Aftercare for Drug Addicts.* U.S. Department of Health and Human Services (NIH Publ No 93-3521). Rockville, MD: National Institute on Drug Abuse, 1993.

Zweben J. Recovery-oriented psychotherapy. *Journal of Substance Abuse Treatment* 3:255-262, 1989.

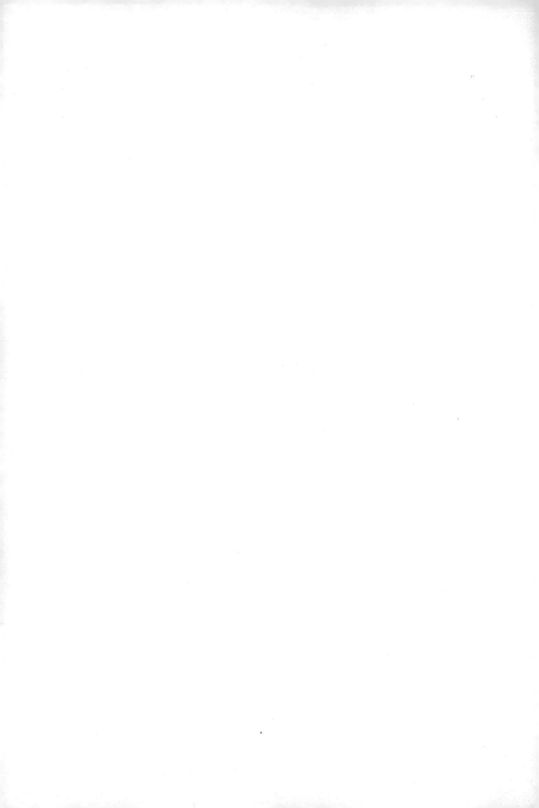

Chapter 7

Relapse Prevention Groups in Outpatient Substance Abuse Treatment

Richard A. Rawson
Jeanne L. Obert

During the 1950s and 1960s when therapeutic communities (TC) were the most widely recognized form of drug abuse treatment, the aggressive, boot camp-like techniques associated with Synanon were a commonly employed group method for treating drug abusers. During the 1970s and 1980s when the twenty-eight-day "Minnesota Model" became the de facto standard for alcohol dependence care, the emotion-eliciting, spiritually oriented twelve-step-based group approach was widely used. These two types of groups continue today to be depicted in the media as standard methods of group therapy for substance abuse treatment.

During the 1990s, outpatient approaches became widely employed as the first treatment of choice for substance abuse patients. In outpatient settings, emotionally based insight-oriented therapy techniques do not address patients' specific needs and may even be counterproductive in early recovery. Instead, techniques to address the needs of newly recovering people who are living/working in their substance-using environments have emerged. Within the last decade, the collection of techniques categorized as relapse prevention (RP) strategies have provided an organizing principle around which many outpatient treatment programs have been designed (Rawson et al. 1993). The use of groups has been the primary paradigm used for applying RP techniques.

This work is supported in part by Grants: (DA06185) and (DA09419) from NIDA to Matrix Center and Friends Research Institute.

THEORETICAL BACKGROUND OF RELAPSE PREVENTION APPROACHES

Common elements to the RP strategies are a cognitive behavioral framework and a theoretical basis in social learning theory (Bandura 1982). RP techniques are appealing to clinical researchers in the field of substance abuse treatment because they have a solid conceptual foundation and can be empirically evaluated. Use of these techniques in outpatient drug-free treatment allows for the systematic development of protocols that can be replicated. The term relapse prevention is defined by Marlatt and Gordon (1985) as a variety of strategies to prevent relapse to addictive behavior.

The purpose of this chapter is to review the use of RP groups in the treatment of substance abuse disorders.

THE FOUNDATION OF RELAPSE PREVENTION MODELS: MARLATT AND GORDON (1985)

The most conceptually well-constructed model of RP is the model described in detail by Marlatt and Gordon (1985). Although a synopsis of Marlatt's model is beyond the scope of this chapter, a number of noteworthy key points have given direction and impetus to the development of RP methods.

Marlatt provides a compelling conceptualization of addiction as a set of habit patterns that have been reinforced by pharmacological and social reinforcement contingencies. Consequently, addiction treatment is a process of habit change. The techniques that have been developed to facilitate this process have their roots in social learning principles. This view of addiction and addiction treatment is contrasted with the view of addiction as a disease. A second important issue discussed by Marlatt is the nature of relapse. He differentiates a "lapse," the initial episode of alcohol or other drug use following a period of recovery, from a "relapse," the failure to maintain behavior change over time (Annis and Davis 1989). His position that relapse is the result of a predictable series of cognitive and behavioral events that lead to a return to drug or alcohol use has been tremendously valuable in demystifying relapse. The observation that relapse has clear antecedents and warning signs has provided a perspective that allows the relapse process to be dissected and systematically studied.

Marlatt's work has provided a framework within which the situations and circumstances that put addicts and alcoholics at high risk for relapse can be studied. By describing a range of coping responses to these high-risk situations, he has given clinicians a broad range of behavioral strategies for addressing patient needs. His application of self-efficacy principles from the work of Bandura (1982) has given addiction researchers an approach for addressing the cognitive aspects of addiction. A related concept described by Marlatt is the abstinence violation effect. This phenomenon, explained in terms of attribution theory, presents a rationale for explaining why addicts and alcoholics often respond to a single lapse by returning to a full-blown readdiction episode. Marlatt has also emphasized the value of using education and information in the treatment process, and he suggests using metaphors for explaining addiction and recovery-related concepts. Finally, recovery from addiction is conceptualized as a type of lifestyle modification in which achieving balance and developing alternative behaviors are key ingredients. Marlatt's work has provided a foundation for much of the theoretical and empirical writings on RP. Most of the models described in this chapter have borrowed extensively from his writing. His contribution to the field is unmatched.

RELAPSE PREVENTION CONTENT AREAS

The techniques that have been used within the designation of the RP category include the following groups of strategies.

Psychoeducation

An important ingredient in most of the RP models is the use of information and education about a variety of addiction-related topics. Central among the issues taught to substance abusers during the course of treatment are the following topic areas: brain chemistry and addiction, conditioned cues and craving, drug and alcohol effects, addiction as a biological disorder, drug use and AIDS, addiction and the family, need for lifestyle change, and relationships between substance abuse and other compulsive disorders. The psychoeducational material is often presented in classroom format or group discussion and is integrated into individual therapy sessions. Many of the models use videotape and slide presentations and written materials to facilitate acquisition of educational concepts.

Identification of High-Risk Situations for Relapse and Warning Signs for Relapse

Patients are taught that there are behaviors and environments as well as cognitive and affective states that are associated with drug/alcohol use. Through individual and group discussion, as well as in homework assignments, they learn the specific set of conditions that have the greatest association with drug/alcohol use. Some examples of these conditions are:

- High-risk states—certain times of day, being around drug-using friends, bars, the presence of money, idle time, interpersonal conflicts
- Behavioral warning signs—"addict" behavior, compulsive and impulsive behavior, time with drug users, stopping recovery activities, returning to secondary drug use
- Cognitive warning signs—euphoric recall, relapse justification, drug dreams, rationalizations to justify discontinuing new recovery behaviors
- Affective warning signs—periods of emotionality previously associated with drug use, including positive affective states (e.g., excitement, arousal, celebration), and negative affective states (e.g., depression, loneliness, anger, boredom)

Development of Coping Skills

It is hypothesized in these models that substance abusers have maladaptive coping skills when placed in high-risk situations. Much RP group "therapy" is focused on teaching and reinforcing alternative responses that will not lead to drug/alcohol use. These new coping skills are discussed in group sessions. Options are explored and, in some cases, new skills are role-played and/or homework assignments are given to practice the new coping response. Examples of these coping skills include: saying "no" to an offer of drug/alcohol use, engaging in alternative behaviors during high-risk periods (e.g., exercising rather than going to "happy hour"), expressing affective states rather than using drugs or alcohol, and using new cognitive strategies, such as thought stopping, to avoid drug thoughts and craving.

Development of New Lifestyle Behaviors

Once drug/alcohol use has been reduced, it is considered useful to reinforce the development of alternative activities to serve as intrinsic reinforcers of abstinence. Group discussions and homework assignments are used to assist drug/alcohol users in acquiring and maintaining new leisure, recreational, and employment activities that will support a non–drug-using lifestyle. Exercise, hobbies, family activities, community activities, and self-help involvement are the types of activities that are reinforced by program staff and group peers.

Increased Self-Efficacy

Bandura's self-efficacy theory (1982) proposes that when people enter high risk situations for drug or alcohol use, they choose each response based upon their appraisal of their ability to cope with the situation. If they view themselves as competent they will abstain from using drugs or alcohol. If not competent, they are at increased risk to use. In order to facilitate the development of the self-perception of competence, patients are given homework assignments that involve entering high-risk situations and employing new responses. It is hypothesized that repeated success in coping with these situations in new, non-drug/alcohol using ways will increase the self-perception of competence and self-efficacy. The development of self-efficacy is viewed as critical to long-term abstinence. This method is typically employed in group settings, sometimes employing role-play and rehearsal, with homework assignments of gradually increasing difficulty as the essential treatment exercise.

Dealing with Relapse—Avoiding the Abstinence Violation Effect

Within these models, the reality of relapse is addressed. Patients are taught to view return to drug/alcohol use as "slips" or "lapses" that need not lead back to full blown relapse and readdiction. This cognitive reframing of a lapse from a catastrophe into a learning opportunity reduces the shame and failure often experienced in the event of a slip or lapse and can interrupt the return to an extended relapse episode.

Drug/Alcohol Monitoring

Although not specifically a RP technique, these models all make use of urine and breath testing to monitor drug and alcohol use. These procedures are viewed as critical for promoting accountability, and they serve as dependent measures of program effectiveness.

THE APPLICATION OF RELAPSE PREVENTION METHODS IN GROUP SETTINGS

There are a number of advantages in delivering RP materials in group settings. Studies show that the estimated recovery rate for chemically dependent patients treated in group settings is two to three times higher than for those who only receive individual psychotherapy (Kanas 1982; Yalom et al. 1978). Group settings allow patients to

1. interrupt the isolation that often develops along with a dependence on alcohol and other drugs;
2. interact with other people who are going through the same process;
3. experience a sense of acceptance and encouragement that may be lacking outside the group setting; and
4. learn (or relearn) how to communicate with others effectively.

The goals of the outpatient RP group are different from the goals of many group therapies used to treat chemical dependence in inpatient settings. Specific RP group goals are

1. to allow members to interact with other people in recovery;
2. to provide a forum for the presentation of specific relapse prevention materials;
3. to allow group members to learn from the experience of a co-leader;
4. to produce some group cohesion among members;

5. to allow the group leader to witness group members interacting interpersonally with other group members; and
6. to allow group members to benefit from participating in a long-term group experience.

RP groups resemble the interpersonal learning and change groups that encompass Yalom's psychotherapy groups and some forms of sensitivity training groups (Flores 1997). The nonjudgmental leader who serves as a directive guide to the group process is taken from this tradition. However, the focus of the RP prevention group is the dissemination and utilization of RP information by group members, in contrast to focusing on the feelings and emotional expressions of the group members as is characteristic in traditional substance abuse groups. The purpose of the RP group is to provide a forum in which people in substance abuse treatment can receive assistance with the issue of relapse. This is accomplished through the use of didactic materials and by exploring group members' immediate problems in achieving and sustaining abstinence. Patients who have come from treatment settings where they have experienced predominately emotionally oriented group experiences need an explanation of the rationale and goals of the RP group. Without this explanation, many confuse the reduced emotional tone of the group with a lack of group effectiveness.

THE RELAPSE PREVENTION GROUP

It is often useful to have patients enter the RP groups after they have achieved several weeks of abstinence. The skills and guidance needed to stop alcohol and drug use require a different focus than those needed to prevent relapse. The chapter in this book by Washton describes techniques that are complimentary to the RP groups and are often appropriate as abstinence initiation groups (see Chapter 6). If it is necessary to immediately induct patients into RP groups for practical reasons, they should spend the first several groups primarily listening to more senior members. As they establish some time being abstinent, they can begin to become more participatory group members. The RP group is most often an open group where information about relapse and relapse prevention can be shared. Impending relapses can be identified and interventions can be designed and encouraged. As in many other group therapies, the RP group is only as safe as the interactions between the group leader and the group members. Grotjohn (1983) described six essential qualities of a credible and effective group leader: reliability, spontaneity and responsiveness, trustworthiness, firm identity, humor, and fallibility. In addition to the leader, each RP group should ideally have a coleader who can serve as a role model for other group members and who has, ideally, six months more sobriety than the most senior group member. The coleader is preferably someone who has successfully integrated twelve-step participation with the more cognitive-behaviorally oriented RP principles. As a successful recovering person, he or she is in a position to address controversial, difficult issues from the perspective of "senior peer" and can share experiences in a manner that is less threatening and will create less defensiveness than a direct, confrontational assault or advice from the group leader.

The group coleader can be enlisted to provide positive role modeling and to reinforce suggestions and advice on the basis of personal experience. The following is an example of an interaction during a group session involving the use of the coleader, Paul:

LEADER: While we're talking about relapse, let me ask, did anyone have any problems over the weekend that involved, or might have involved, a slip or a relapse?

GROUP MEMBER: Well, I didn't relapse but I sure had a good time!

LEADER: What do you mean by that?

GROUP MEMBER: Well, my brother was in town. It was great to see him. I haven't seen him since I've been in this program and we used to hang out together all the time before he moved. He wanted to see some of our old friends, so we did.

LEADER: Then you and your brother went out together to see these friends?

GROUP MEMBER: Yeah. We went to the club where we used to go all the time. Most of the people he wanted to see hang out there on weekends. They were all there. It was great! I didn't realize how much I've missed those guys. I was avoiding going there because that's where I used to get high all the time but it was great. I was able to dance and have a great time without drinking or using. I didn't even have a craving. I think I may be able to hang out with those guys sometimes as long as I don't drink or use.

LEADER: Paul, I think I remember you having a similar experience when you first entered treatment. Do you remember that?

PAUL: Yeah, I remember that. My experience was different so, hopefully, the outcome will be different too. I really learned the hard way. I had a reunion about six weeks after I started treatment. I debated going but decided I wouldn't get another chance to attend the reunion, so I went. It was the first time I had been in a party-type situation since I stopped drinking. I was able to get through the night without drinking but I noticed that I felt different the next day about my recovery. I felt deprived and I thought more about alcohol than I had before. I wasn't as excited about the days I had sober. My head started telling me I might be able to be "normal" and do all the things I used to do—except, of course, I wouldn't drink. It was the beginning of the end for me. But this is just me. I went to a friend's house (a friend I had been avoiding before) and there were other people there. They were all drinking and I just decided to have one drink, no more. Somehow that one drink became two. Then I stopped. But the next day I was in the liquor store and I decided to buy a bottle. I really relapsed! I don't remember all of that night but I know it was hard to get myself back in here. I know, for me that is, I can't start down that slippery path. I don't have another relapse in me. I have to avoid those kinds of places altogether.

Each group is organized around a topic or topics. In some settings the topics are presented on worksheets and one participant may be asked to read the worksheet aloud and address questions posed by the worksheet. The topics are designed to communicate important information about addiction and recovery concepts and promote changes in behavior. In advance of the group, all materials (e.g., workbooks, handouts) should be prepared for all participants. Groups should start promptly on time. Details of this type are important in imparting the critically important message that the group leader is prepared and in control of the group situation.

Prior to beginning group each patient should have one individual introductory session with the therapist. This session establishes the interpersonal relationship necessary for the patient and the therapist to interact in the group setting successfully. In addition, patients need to be aware of the group rules prior to entering the group situation. A sample of the group rules employed at Matrix Center is included in Box 7.1.

Each group meeting begins with an introduction of all group members whenever there are new people joining the group for the first time. Participants are asked to identify their primary drug problems, the length of time they have been in treatment, and to share some brief personal information (e.g., reason for entering treatment, occupation, living situation, past treatment experiences, etc.). This brief

---

Box 7.1. Matrix Center Group Rules

Treatment participation requires some basic "ground rules." These conditions are essential for a successful treatment experience. Violations of these rules can result in treatment termination. Group members agree in writing to:

1. Arrive on time for appointments, and in each visit be prepared to give a urine sample.
2. *Abstain from all drug and alcohol use for the entire treatment program.* If unable to make this commitment, discuss other treatment options with the program staff.
3. Discuss any drug or alcohol use with the staff and group while in treatment.
4. Attend both individual and group sessions. Twenty-four hours will be given to reschedule individual appointments if necessary. *Group appointments cannot be rescheduled and attendance is extremely important.* Tell the therapist in advance if one needs to miss group, and telephone the therapist with "last-minute" absences or lateness.
5. Selling drugs or encouraging drug use by other group members will lead to termination of treatment.
6. Graphic stories of drug or alcohol use will not be allowed.
7. Agree not to become involved romantically or sexually with other group members.
8. Do not become involved in any business transactions with other group members.
9. Understand that all matters discussed in group sessions and the identity of all group members are absolutely confidential and will not be shared with nonmembers.
10. All treatment is voluntary. Discuss the decision to stop treatment with the staff.

introductory exercise encourages openness in sharing personal information in the group.

During the first fifteen minutes of the group, the leader presents a specific topic in a casual, didactic manner. If handouts or other written materials are used, one of the group members can be called upon to read through the material. A list of topics used in the Matrix Center RP materials are listed in Box 7.2.

The specific topic is discussed with the group for approximately thirty to forty-five minutes. The leader should ensure that the important matters relative to the specific topic are covered and that premature digressions from the main topic issues are avoided. Care should be taken to avoid directing any necessary negative feedback toward any person, but rather toward the addiction-based aspects of a group member's behavior or thinking. Group members with an "agenda" unrelated to the topic can be assured that they will have a chance to discuss their issues following the discussion of the weekly

---

BOX 7.2. Matrix Center Relapse Prevention Topics

Alcohol—The Legal Drug	*Relapse Justification I*
Boredom	Taking Care of Yourself
Avoiding Relapse Drift	Dangerous Emotions
Mooring Lines	Illness
Work and Recovery	Recognizing Stress
Guilt and Shame	*Relapse Justification II*
Staying Busy	Reducing Stress
Motivation for Recovery	Managing Anger
Truthfulness	Managing Money
Total Abstinence	Acceptance
Sex and Recovery	Making New Friends
Relapse Prevention	Repairing Relationships
Trust	Serenity Prayer
Be Smart; Not Strong	Compulsive Behaviors
Defining Spirituality	Dealing with Feelings
Taking Care of Business	Dealing with Depression
Recreational Activities	Patient Status Review
Looking Forward	Holidays and Recovery
Twelve-Step Programs	

topic. The leader wraps up the discussion period with a reiteration of the session topic and the important issues relative to it.

During the last thirty to forty-five minutes of each group session, group members are asked if they have any recent problems, or any matters they wish to bring up. Frequently, those who are quiet and noncommunicative may need to be coaxed to discuss concealed issues that should be elicited and dealt with.

Some groups will be very closely connected and integrated, while others will be less cohesive. The leader needs to maintain a focus and direction and be ready to assert control of discussions moving into redundancy, irrelevance, inappropriateness, or volatility. Fluctuations in group tone are normal, particularly with open groups, and occur cyclically regardless of the therapist's efforts. Either extreme can be problematic. A tightly connected group runs the risk of one member's relapse becoming "contagious" and causing a domino effect where many group members subsequently relapse. To avoid such an occurrence, group members should be encouraged to establish additional support systems outside the RP group (e.g., twelve-step meetings, church, etc.). These outside support systems will be helpful in preventing group members from feeling that their recovery is totally interdependent upon the recovery of other group members. The opposite problem occurs when group members feel that there is no one they can relate to in the group or that no one cares. In these circumstances the therapist's and coleader's attention to group members must be clearly expressed to ensure the continued participation of members in the group. Typically this situation will be short-lived as the commonality of the recovery process issues will typically promote a bond between group members.

Special Situations

At times the group leader may need to intervene aggressively in response to specific types of behavior in the group. This intervention may consist of quieting a member, limiting the member's involvement in the group, or removing the member from the group.

>*Behavior:* Perseverating on an issue.
>*Intervention:* Politely acknowledge the need to continue discussion and move on.

Behavior: Arguing a case for behavior that is counter to recovery (e.g., social drinking, dropping out of group, using "self-control" versus avoiding cocaine triggers, etc.) after receiving repeated feedback.

Intervention: Point out the futility of these sorts of approaches in light of the realities of addiction and the experience of others. If group members continue along the same lines, ask them to listen for the remainder of the group since the issues being presented should be discussed individually with a therapist.

Behavior: Making threatening, insulting, or personally directed remarks; behaving in a manner obviously indicative of intoxication.

Intervention: Ask the person to sit quietly through the rest of the group. If that is unsuccessful, leave the group with the group member, letting the coleader take over. Have a brief individual session, or have another therapist intervene. If necessary, see that safe transportation home is arranged.

Behavior: General lack of commitment to treatment as evidenced by poor attendance, resistance to treatment intervention, disruptive behavior.

Intervention: The group leader should consider removing the member from group sessions until behavior and/or attitude improvement suggests otherwise. It may be appropriate to see the person on an individual basis, if possible, or to have them participate in a motivational group as described in the Washton chapter.

End of Session

The leader summarizes the discussion and reviews the key points covered in the session. Unresolved issues may be acknowledged and discussion carried over to the next meeting. Individuals who brought up important issues relative to their recovery can be directed to discuss the issues in self-help meetings and with sponsors or therapists. The session should finish on time and, if possible, on a positive note. Group members who appear troubled, angry, depressed, or those who mentioned cravings during the session should be asked to stay afterward for a debriefing. Direct these people to speak with a therapist or sponsor or to attend a self-help meeting as soon as possible. It is also useful to conduct a brief (five-minute) debriefing session with the coleader to ensure his or her stability and to provide positive reinforcement for his or her participation.

EVALUATION OF RELAPSE PREVENTION METHODS

Researchers at Yale have created a protocol to evaluate the value of RP techniques for the treatment of cocaine abusers (Carroll, Rounsaville, and Keller 1991) and have conducted several well-controlled evaluations of RP protocols for the treatment of cocaine abuse. While these studies have been conducted in individual sessions, they do provide some of the best data on RP effectiveness.

In a later study comparing RP to a case management approach, the during-treatment data did not demonstrate an overall difference between RP and case management; however, the authors reported evidence that the more severe cocaine abusers and the more depressed subjects showed a superior response to the RP condition (Carroll, Rounsaville, and Gordon 1994). In addition, in a later report, at follow-up, the cocaine abstinence rate of RP group subjects was significantly higher than for the case management group subjects; the authors suggested that the RP procedures produced a delayed treatment effect (Carroll, Rounsaville, and Gordon 1994).

In another study, Wells and associates (1994) found few meaningful differences in cocaine treatment outcome between an outpatient RP protocol and a twelve-step–based protocol delivered in a group setting. Subjects in both groups reported a significant decrease in cocaine and other drug/alcohol use from pretreatment to posttreatment and follow-up. Although evidence showed that those subjects in the twelve-step group returned to alcohol use to a greater degree than did the subjects in the RP condition, no differences were found between the two groups on measures of cocaine use.

Integrated Outpatient Models

McAuliffe and Associates—Recovery Training and Self-Help Model

McAuliffe and associates have constructed an intensive outpatient treatment model combining RP strategies with self-help concepts, the Recovery Training and Self-Help Model (RTSH) (McAuliffe

1990; Zackon, McAuliffe, and Chien 1993). The RTSH model has been evaluated in a large, controlled trial with random assignment (McAuliffe 1990). In this study 168 detoxified opioid addicts were randomly assigned to either the RTSH program or a control condition that consisted of referral to another community-based aftercare program. This study, therefore, evaluated the RTSH model as an outpatient aftercare strategy and not as a stand-alone outpatient treatment approach. The RTSH program showed superior levels of opioid abstinence at six- and twelve-month follow-up points, and significantly more employment activity and less criminal activity during the twelve-month follow-up point. The RTSH group members found their treatment experiences more helpful than the control subjects found theirs, and the mean retention rate of four months by RTSH subjects suggests that the program was able to sustain the treatment involvement of this group.

It should be noted that although the RTSH approach demonstrated significantly better outcome on important clinical measures, the abstinence rate at twelve months was only 30 percent. This finding underscores the difficulty of treating opioid users with nonpharmacologic and non-residential treatment approaches. It is possible that the outcome with this model could be improved by combining the approach with a pharmacologic treatment such as naltrexone. Similarly, it is possible that the use of this model with other categories of drug users such as cocaine abusers or alcoholics might show higher rates of follow-up abstinence.

Roffman and Associates—Relapse Prevention Treatment for Marijuana Dependence

Roffman and colleagues constructed an RP approach that adapted material from Marlatt and Gordon (1985) for the specific needs of marijuana users. The treatment model was delivered in a group format consisting of ten sessions, which were scheduled over a twelve-week period. This treatment model has been evaluated in a controlled study comparing subjects receiving the RP model with a group receiving a social support procedure (Roffman et al. 1990). The results of the study suggested that the RP procedure produced a greater reduction of marijuana use than did the social support procedure. Subject reports from both treatment conditions indicated that the cessation of marijuana had very significant beneficial effects on their functioning.

Rawson and Associates—The Matrix Model

In 1983 the Matrix Center was established in Southern California to provide cocaine users with a structured outpatient treatment experience. The program was designed around cognitive behavioral principles using many of the RP techniques previously described. The treatment model referred to as the Matrix Model provides intensive treatment contact over the initial six months. Along with the RP group techniques, there is a significant amount of patient and family participation in psychoeducational sessions and individual therapy sessions. Urine testing is an integral part of the program and involvement in twelve-step programs is encouraged. The Matrix treatment model has been formalized into treatment manuals for the abuse treatment of stimulants (Rawson et al. 1989), alcohol (Rawson et al. 1991), and opiates. This standardization of the model has allowed for replication and evaluation.

Research evidence on the usefulness of the Matrix approach has been published in a number of articles. These include articles on the value of the approach for cocaine abuse treatment (Rawson et al. 1995; Shoptaw et al. 1994), methamphetamine abuse (Huber et al. 1997), and opiate dependence (Rawson et al. 2001). In all of these reports, treatments with these Matrix manualized protocols were associated with very significant reductions in drug and alcohol use and other associated improvements in functioning.

Much of the content of this chapter is based upon the materials and approach used at Matrix. The clear content, direct application, practicality, and effectiveness of the approach have promoted its adoption, and it has gained broad acceptance in the VA system, the Indian Health Service, county and state treatment interventions, and many local southern California treatment efforts.

SUMMARY

Clearly, the development and refinement of the RP approach was the major nonpharmacologic substance abuse treatment advancement of the 1980s. Since the techniques are clearly definable and replicable, systematic evaluation is feasible. Use of treatment manuals, which standardize protocols for replication and evaluation, has improved research methodology. The RP movement has provided a cognitive-behavioral foundation upon which drug-free outpatient substance abuse treatment systems can be built. Continued empirical testing of these techniques and models is essential to the development of this approach.

The RP techniques have been created to directly address substance abuse behaviors and the conditions leading to those behaviors. They provide tangible, understandable, directive, nonjudgmental tools for therapists to use with substance-abusing patients. The approach has provided the outpatient substance abuse treatment field with some clear guidelines and protocols, and in constructing controlled evaluations of treatment models for differing clinical populations. Outcome data are very preliminary, but the overwhelming attitude of clinicians and researchers is that this methodology of RP has given focus and standardization to a previously disorganized set of outpatient treatment techniques. Long-term follow-up data on the extended impact of these strategies will be necessary to assess their value to the field of substance abuse treatment.

REFERENCES

Annis HM, Davis CS. Relapse prevention. In *Handbook of Alcoholism Treatment Approaches,* edited by Hester RK, Miller WR. New York: Pergamon Press, 1989.

Bandura A. Self-efficacy mechanism in human agency. *American Psychologist* 37:122-147, 1982.

Carroll KM, Rounsaville BJ, Gordon LT, Nich C, Jatlow P, Bisighini RM, Gawin FH. Psychotherapy and pharmacotherapy for ambulatory cocaine abusers. *Archives of General Psychiatry* 51:171-181, 1994.

Carroll KM, Rounsaville BJ, Keller DS. Relapse prevention strategies for the treatment of cocaine abuse. *American Journal of Drug and Alcohol Abuse* 17(3):19-26, 1991.

Flores PJ. *Group Psychotherapy With Addicted Populations.* Binghamton, NY: The Haworth Press, 1997.

Grotjohn M. The qualities of the group psychotherapist. In *Comprehensive Group Psychotherapy,* edited by Kaplan HI, Sadock BJ. Baltimore, MD: Williams & Wilkins, 1983, pp. 294-301.

Huber A, Ling W, Shoptaw S, Gulati V, Brethen P, Rawson R. Integrating treatments for methamphetamine abuse: A psychosocial perspective. *Addictive Diseases* 16:41-50, 1997.

Kanas N. Alcoholism and group psychotherapy. In *Encyclopedic Handbook of Alcoholism,* edited by Pattison EM, Kaufman E. New York: Gardner Press, 1982, pp. 1011-1021.

Marlatt GA, Gordon JR (eds.). *Relapse Prevention: Maintenance Strategies in the Treatment of Addictive Behaviors.* New York: Guilford Press, 1985.

McAuliffe WE. A randomized controlled trial of recovery training and self-help for opioid addicts in New England and Hong Kong. *Journal of Psychoactive Drugs* 22:197-210, 1990.

Rawson RA, McCann MJ, Shoptaw S, Miotto K, Frosch DL, Obert JL, Ling W. Naltrexone for opiate addiction: The evaluation of a manualized psychosocial protocol to enhance treatment response. *Drug and Alcohol Review* 20: 69-80, 2001.

Rawson RA, Obert JL, McCann MJ, Ling W. Psychological approaches for the treatment of cocaine dependence: A neurobehavioral approach. *Journal of Addictive Diseases* 11:97-119, 1991.

Rawson RA, Obert JL, McCann MJ, Marinelli-Casey PJ. Use of relapse prevention strategies in the treatment of substance abuse disorders. *Psychotherapy* 30(2): 284-298, 1993.

Rawson RA, Obert JL, McCann MJ, Smith D, Scheffey EH. *The Neurobehavioral Treatment Manual: A Therapist Manual for Outpatient Cocaine Addiction Treatment.* Beverly Hills, CA: The Matrix Center, Inc., 1989.

Rawson, RA, Shoptaw SJ, Obert JL, McCann MJ, Hasson AL, Marinelli-Casey PJ, Brethen PR, Ling W. An intensive outpatient approach for cocaine abuse treatment: The Matrix Model. *Journal of Substance Abuse Treatment* 12(2):117-127, 1995.

Roffman RA, Stephens RS, Simpson EE, Whitaker DL. Treatment of marijuana dependencies: Preliminary results. *Journal of Psychoactive Drugs* 22:129-137, 1990.

Shoptaw S, Rawson RA, McCann MJ, Obert JL. The Matrix Model of outpatient stimulant abuse treatment: Evidence of efficacy. *Journal of Addictive Diseases* 13(4):129-141, 1994.

Wells EA, Peterson PL, Gainey RR, Hawkins JD, Catalano RF. Outpatient treatment for cocaine abuse: A controlled comparison of relapse prevention and twelve-step approaches. *American Journal of Drug and Alcohol Abuse* 20:1-17, 1994.

Yalom ID, Block S, Bond G, Zimmerman E, Qualls B. Alcoholics in interactional group therapy: An outcome study. *Archives of General Psychiatry* 35:419-425, 1978.

Zackon F, McAuliffe WE, Chien JM. *Addict Aftercare: A Manual of Training and Self-Help.* Rockville, MD: NIDA, 1993.

Chapter 8

Inpatient Groups and Partial Hospitalization

Andrew Edmund Slaby

INTRODUCTION: ASSESSMENT AND DIAGNOSIS

Screening

Substance abuse disorders are chronic illnesses with psychosocial, genetic, and environmental forces impacting their development, manifestation, and treatment. They are often progressive and sometimes fatal. Signs and symptoms may be periodic or continuous and include distortions in thinking and behavior (e.g., denial, impaired control over drinking, alcohol use in spite of adverse consequences, and preoccupation with alcohol). Those who are dependent show a typical pattern of heavy use in their twenties, followed by interference in multiple life areas in their thirties, and in their mid or late thirties evidence of bodily deterioration appears (Schuckit et al. 1993). Comparable data exists on the abuse of stimulants, opiates, hallucinogens, and sedative-hypnotics, indicating the need for early identification and aggressive treatment to prevent dire psychological, social, and medical consequences.

Medical History

A careful history should be taken of each patient prior to entry into a program. Attention should be directed not only to the severity and presence of one or more substance abuse disorders, but also to the presence of concurrent physical or mental disorders that might impact prognosis. In addition, assessments of factors such as work history, social supports, and expected compliance impacting treatment choice and outcome should be conducted.

Physical Examination

A physical exam should be performed on all patients preferably by a physician familiar with the consequences of substance abuse disorders.

Urine and serum drug screens serve to document the presence, as well as the extent, of substance abuse. Screens are routinely performed at the beginning of treatment and periodically thereafter, particularly if it is mandatory for the patient to comply with abstinence in order to maintain employment, professional licensure, or enrollment in school.

Differential Diagnosis and Diagnostic Criteria

Although alcohol dependence itself may be a neuropsychiatric disorder, which someday may be treated with a pharmacologically specific intervention, the effective treatment plan involves traditional group therapy and twelve-step interventions coupled with general or specific pharmacological interventions as directed by diagnosis and as indicated by complementary psychotherapeutic and sociotherapeutic management strategies. Polysubstance abuse entails a multimodality approach, while alcohol dependence alone, unattended by any other substance abuse, medical, or psychiatric disorder, may be managed by the Twelve-Step Program of Alcoholics Anonymous using a sponsor and an initial "ninety in ninety" program (viz., a patient attends ninety AA meetings in the initial ninety days of recovery).

In order to participate actively in the twelve-step program and its attendant group structure as an inpatient, as a day patient, or as an outpatient, one's medical status and specific psychiatric requirements need to be addressed. Substance abuse treatment does not cure the illness, but rather catalyzes a number of interventions that maintain remission. Substance-abusing patients must be initially evaluated and treated for any specific medical problems; nearly all can exacerbate anxiety and other psychiatric symptoms can threaten sobriety.

Comorbid psychiatric disorders are very common and can appear to be a manifestation of substance abuse as well as an ongoing impetus to relapse via self-medication. These factors can impede participation in outpatient recovery programs. Depression is particularly prevalent among alcohol-abusing populations. Alcohol can cause depression, and both alcohol and stimulants can be used to self-medicate depression.

Evaluation and Management of Suicide/Homicide Potential

Substance abuse reduces judgment and increases impulsivity, enhancing the risk of suicide. The initial evaluation of a patient who has a history of substance abuse should always include an assessment of the risk of self- and other-directed violence. In addition, continued vigilance for signs of increased homicide and suicide risk is necessary throughout the course of partial hospitalization and subsequent outpatient group psychotherapy.

DEVELOPMENT OF A TREATMENT PLAN

Contemporary substance abuse treatment entails a sophisticated understanding of the essential role of group psychotherapy in maintaining abstinence, the pragmatic use of other therapies including inpatient and partial hospitalization, the enhancement of social supports, and the reevaluation of suicide and homicide potential. One clinician should be responsible for coordinating all aspects of treatment and ensuring continued compliance.

Patients who comply with treatment have lower medical service use rates, fewer legal complications, and enhanced worksite performance. The treatment plan is patient specific depending on patterns of drug use, concurrent medical and psychiatric illness, and social support availability. Working with a patient's family, spouse, children, lover, friends, clergy, and/or employers increases the likelihood of adherence to a treatment program and attendance at partial hospitalization and outpatient group activities (Galanter 1997).

Including members of the patient's social support network in the treatment plan provides an excellent opportunity to learn about the process of addiction and the relative efficacy of interventions. Substance abuse disorders are family illnesses; recognizing the role of each individual involved in the healing process increases motivation for treatment. The identified patient and his or her family, broadly defined, must admit that there is a problem, understand the role of denial in the maintenance of the illness, and encourage compliance with group and other therapies.

Inpatient Treatment

Until recently, inpatient treatment was seen as the fundamental step in a program of continuing recovery. The once-popular Minnesota Model (so called because of the twenty-eight-day programs associated with treatment facilities in the Minneapolis-St. Paul area) is no longer accepted in the current medical-economic climate; moreover, its methods have become outdated. The critical components of such programs (Collins 1997) consisted of twenty-four-hour supervision, group and individual peer pressure, and education in a secure environment monitored by individuals who were, themselves, frequently in recovery and therefore sensitive to pitfalls such as recurrent denial. Self-help meetings coupled with urine and serum tests, for evidence of relapse, were given in most of these programs.

The group process plays a pivotal role in the maintenance of abstinence. Often this position develops during the inpatient phase for those who are hospitalized; however, it is not necessary to hospitalize all substance abusers in order to initiate them into the group process. Only the most recalcitrant of patients, having failed as outpatients, are hospitalized. Inpatient treatment, offered as the first step or simply as an element in the continuing outpatient group treatment, is usually designed to protect a suicidal/homicidal patient, minimize adverse events during detoxification, facilitate compliance with group treatment in the absence of adequate social supports, and treat a patient with serious, concurrent medical and psychiatric illness.

Some patients relapse several times before they become aware of the need for daily involvement in group treatment and for total abstinence. It is best to immediately involve patients in groups with which they plan to continue engagement following discharge. Most hospitals serve as sites for AA groups; however, on days when they themselves do not have a twelve-step meeting, patients are sent to attend groups outside the hospital accompanied by hospital staff. Only in cases when a patient's medical condition precludes attendance at an outpatient group (e.g., active psychosis, difficult withdrawal, suicide or homicidal risk, fear of elopement) does a patient abstain. In addition to AA, NA, and CA groups, family groups, sexual addiction groups, dual diagnosis groups, gay groups, men's groups, women's groups, psychoeducation groups, and sexual abuse groups are all part of inpatient programs. Individual therapy is also generally provided to further evaluate the psychiatric needs of the patient and to thwart denial. Psychopharmacotherapy is initiated to treat concurrent psychiatric disorders, to facilitate withdrawal, or to maintain abstinence. Patients at high risk for suicide or homicide require constant observation on a one-on-one basis if the threat is imminent.

Day Hospital Treatment

The goals of a partial or day hospital program are sustained abstinence and compliance with treatment. Participation in group therapy is essential to the success of such a program. Groups are open to entry at any time after admission. Ideally, they are open to all those in need and not restricted to those who require partial hospitalization. They should be flexible, allowing inpatients who are partially hospitalized, relapsed, and new outpatients to participate in order to facilitate continuity of care regardless of the required intensity of treatment. Topics discussed within the groups vary; however, they usually involve problems managing stress and anger, loss, and abandonment.

Although the groups used in day or partial hospital programs are the same as those used for inpatient treatment, inpatient groups tend to focus more on dual diagnosis issues. Ideally, if a patient proceeds from an inpatient setting to partial hospitalization, the difference in approach should simply be a change in lodging. The patient should continue participation in the same group program as was attended as an inpatient. The degree of participation should be lessened only if the patient's condition warrants, resources dictate, or the return to school or work requires. The greater the intensity of group involvement, the greater the likelihood of continued compliance with the treatment plan and sustained abstinence. The coping mechanisms that patients learn in a twelve-step program are basically cognitive therapy mechanisms for managing stresses.

The most conservative approach is consistently the most rewarding. A patient should strive to attend ninety meetings in ninety days, but should feel comfortable to attend more meetings if stresses and cravings dictate. There should be a concerted effort during both inpatient and partial hospital phases to provide a diversity of group activities. Step meetings should be supplemented regularly with speaker meetings, Big Book meetings, men/women groups, and shared autobiography meetings. During the partial hospital phase, an interim sponsor or continuing sponsor should be identified and used, and the recognition and acceptance of powerlessness over alcohol and mood-altering drugs should be affirmed (Step One). Movies, lecture sessions, and sharing sessions should also supplement group activities in both phases.

On leaving a structured inpatient or partial hospitalization program, the individual should be ready to accept outside help and to take a moral inventory. Patients are encouraged at all times to supplement inpatient and partial hospital groups with social support groups in the community, such as single parent groups, men's/women's groups, gay groups, AIDS support groups, and prayer groups.

Residential Treatment

A residential treatment program, to some degree, is a variant of partial hospitalization. Such programs may be so restrictive that until residents reach an advanced stage of recovery, they cannot leave the setting without supervision. In other instances, these programs serve as halfway or quarterway houses and so require residents to live in supervised settings, participate in daily in-house groups, take medication as prescribed, and submit willingly to drug screening to ensure compliance. When residents are permitted to work or go to school, they are expected to return to their program to participate in group meals, community meetings, group therapy meetings, and twelve-step group programs. These settings provide an obvious check on impulsive drug use and a support structure. Residential treatment can be particularly helpful for adolescents whose social milieu is beset by peer pressure to use recreational drugs and to neglect school or work.

Residential treatment is required only when a person comes from an environment that actively prevents recovery because of continued exposure to drugs and alcohol, pressures to use, or external stresses that considerably impede compliance with treatment. When residential treatment is necessary, ideally, the patients are allowed to contrive their involvement within a group program. Moreover, the location of treatment should be close to a patient's social support network, including his or her sponsor, to allow continued attendance at work or school.

Detoxification

A drug-free state is essential to achieve recovery from substance abuse. Therefore, detoxification is the first step, with recurrent episodes of detoxification if a relapse occurs and results in readdiction. Patients who are intoxicated at a time of a group activity, even if not readdicted, are usually asked to leave group. In such instances, a patient may require individual intervention to reinvolve them in the group process and obtain detoxification if needed. Concomitant involvement in groups during withdrawal and use of clinicians who are themselves recovering helps to minimize delays in achievement of sobriety (Slaby 1997).

Psychopharmacotherapy

In addition to specific psychopharmacologic intervention for dually diagnosed patients, a number of pharmacological interventions can facilitate group participation by serving as deterrents to impulsive drug use. Perhaps the best known of these deterrents is disulfiram, which inhibits aldehyde dehydrogenase, and rapidly causes an uncomfortable reaction in the patient when alcohol is ingested. Disulfiram therefore acts as a good deterrent for impulsive drinking, yet use of the drug requires a clear understanding by the patient of the risks involved in drinking while on disulfiram. Unfortunately, disulfiram use has not been found to impact the long-term prognosis of alcohol dependence (Wright and Moore 1990). Other drugs for treatment of dependence coming into more widespread use include naltrexone and buprenorphine.

Treatment of Concurrent Medical Disorders

Substance-abusing patients, as a group, tend to neglect medical problems. Such neglect can cause problems because illness complicates group treatment; the stress of the illness or attendant pain, either real or perceived, may cause absenteeism or relapse. A physical illness, no matter how relatively insignificant, may create a convenient excuse to miss a group meeting or to use an addicting substance to reduce pain.

GROUP PSYCHOTHERAPY

The basis of inpatient substance abuse treatment is undoubtedly the twelve-step self-help group. However, other forms of group therapy, to be discussed in subsequent sections, reinforce the themes of AA, NA, and CA by providing specific strategies for the specific problems associated with being an adolescent, woman, man, sexually abused person, gay, etc. Group therapies act as support systems. They instill hope for members to see how others have progressed despite earlier doubts and current stresses. Members do not feel isolated, as they find out how others have lied, stolen, and prostituted themselves to obtain drugs and maintain a habit. Coping strategies are shared and individuals help themselves by helping others (the Twelve Steps). Group members learn to be therapeutic for one another and to educate others about denial and the risks of substance abuse and benefits of sustained abstinence. Finally, groups facilitate interpersonal learning.

Alcoholics Anonymous (AA)

Involvement in Alcoholics Anonymous, or the correlates Cocaine Anonymous (CA) or Narcotics Anonymous (NA), is essential to any substance abuse recovery. The principles of these twelve-step programs are essentially a grassroots application in cognitive therapy. Alcoholics Anonymous is based on peer support and spiritual growth. Alcohol dependence is accepted as a medical illness and recovery is predicated on a process of growth associated with an increased ability to make healthy choices (Minkoff 1997). Rates for continuous abstinence as great as 80 percent are achieved by a year of continuous treatment, attendance at Alcoholics Anonymous meetings (Harrison, Hoffman and Streed 1991), use of a sponsor, leadership at meetings, and working on the twelve steps (Emrick et al. 1993). Continued involvement in AA is critical to one's success.

Cocaine Anonymous (CA), Narcotics Anonymous (NA), and Pills Anonymous (PA)

The basic assumption underlying the group process of Alcoholics Anonymous applies also for Cocaine Anonymous (CA), Narcotics Anonymous (NA), and Pills Anonymous (PA). Peer support is provided for those willing to profess helplessness in managing their addictions as they progress from a state of denial to a state of spiritual growth. When an addiction-specific meeting is not available, individuals can attend any of the other meetings and receive support for their recovery and desire to maintain abstinence. There are obviously different symptoms with different drug use, but the principles and dynamics of the self-help groups are the same. Sadly, some groups will attempt to persuade those who are in need of prescribed psychotropic drugs to remain totally drug free. Physicians prescribing medication for these patients should make them aware that some extremists may attempt to have them discontinue these medications that allow them to participate in the group and to comply with their specific treatment plan.

Family Therapy and Multifamily Groups

All illnesses are family illnesses. When a person hurts, pain is felt by all who are emotionally tied to that person. Security of the family unit is disrupted by addiction. Thus individual family therapy and multifamily groups help those individuals in a recovering person's supportive network to recognize in themselves, and in other family members, denial, codependence, enabling, and other similar addictions.

While individual family sessions are important for intensive family-specific work, the general themes of denial, coping with a family member's substance-abusing behavior, codependency, enabling, financial strain, and physical and sexual abuse are issues that multifamily groups are better equipped to resolve (Nageotte and Amato 1997). Members of different families can help educate one another about the treatment process and direct one another to community resources such as Alateen, Al-Anon and Adult Children of Alcoholics (ACOA) groups. These groups supplement inpatient and partial hospital work during the period of relative confinement and, subsequently, upon discharge.

Adolescent Groups

Treatment of substance-abusing adolescents is a particularly difficult task. Attempts to self-medicate psychiatric symptoms involving issues of emerging sexual identity, anxieties over separation from parents, and stresses attendant with the development of intimate relationships with another person may give rise to substance abuse. Peer pressure (Patton 1995) to experiment with drugs and alcohol is rampant. Sadly, normal adolescent development can be retarded, or even arrested, during periods of drug use. An adolescent who uses marijuana daily will not be cognitively or emotionally available, and so will be unable to explore emerging sexuality and the drive for intimacy. In addition, heavy use of drugs, such as marijuana, often leads to an amotivational syndrome that retards academic and career achievement, leads to low self-esteem, and creates a sense of helplessness. Because adolescents are so sensitive to peer pressure, a positive peer group can model healthy stress reduction strategies to counteract pressure to self-destruct.

Couples Therapy

No matter how loving, a life partner may unwittingly be co-dependent or enabling. Couples groups allow those who are more adept at identifying such traits in themselves and others to serve as catalysts for concurrent, individualized couples therapy. Some couples, like individuals, are better able to discuss their own struggles in private, individual settings.

Al-Anon and Alateen Meetings

Al-Anon and Alateen self-help meetings provide support to the family members of alchoholics/substance abusers who are confused and pained as they attempt to cope with a loved one's suffering. Adults and teenagers learn about the illness of alcohol dependence (or comparable substance abuse disorders), their own limited ability to ensure a family member's compliance with treatment, and the means to cope with the illness in a supportive group structure. Those who are genetically related to alcoholics learn how to identify and manage their own drive to abuse substances during times of stress.

Physical/Sexual Abuse Groups

Substance abusers as a group are more likely to abuse others physically and sexually when under the influence. Often they, themselves, have been physically abused by substance-abusing family members such as grandparents, parents, aunts, and uncles. Groups for victims of abuse help survivors effectively manage symptoms of early abuse. In fact, group psychotherapy is well recognized as essential in the treatment of those suffering post-traumatic stress disorder. Members learn new ways to manage violent impulses and to avoid those items that contribute to the risk of abuse (viz., substance use).

Sexoholics Anonymous

Use of alcohol and, especially, cocaine impacts sexual drive and behavior. Both sex and cocaine are powerful reinforcers of human behavior and can lead to cross addiction and the need for management of sexual addiction to prevent relapse of cocaine addiction. The twelve-step group approach serves to guide the sex addict from a stage of denial to spiritual growth, with the help of a sponsor and other group members. Sexual abstinence ideally spans a year (unless a person is in an enduring committed relationship) to minimize relapse.

HIV Groups

Support groups for HIV-positive patients are common to both inpatient and partial hospital substance abuse programs. Issues discussed in HIV groups often overlap with those discussed in gay and lesbian groups; however, the primary focus of HIV-positive groups should be to define constructive ways of coping with AIDS and the fear of developing a disabling illness.

Lesbian/Gay/Bisexual Groups

Both men and women who identify themselves as gay stand as great a risk of developing a substance abuse problem as they do of becoming suicidal. HIV groups and men's or women's groups may be attended concurrently. Lesbian/gay/bisexual groups provide an understanding of the development of substance abuse in the context of an ambivalent sexual identity.

Men's Groups and Women's Groups

Some examples of specific problems related to the use of alcohol are sexual promiscuity among women and sexual impotency among men. However, there are a number of issues, in addition to sexuality, that gender-specific substance abuse treatment groups address.

Guilt is a predominant issue of discussion among women whose use of alcohol or cocaine during pregnancy caused neuropsychological retardation in their infant (Raskin 1997). Women may also discuss feelings of guilt associated with physically abusing a child or spouse while intoxicated, or by their inconstant ability to mother due to their substance use. Men, on the other hand, more frequently discuss the shame and guilt associated with sexual abuse. Ironically, although many men and women discuss the guilt and shame they feel about their behavior toward their children, they also tend to express depression and rage about the abuse they experienced as children of alcoholics.

Men and women alike discuss issues such as the lack of security in their sense of gender, fears of intimacy, and the inability to develop a bonded emotional relationship. During periods of abuse, development is often arrested resulting in patterns of behavior that are age-inappropriate. Since the use of recreational drugs impairs normal psychosocial development, men and women in their late twenties and even forties who have abused alcohol and drugs since childhood tend to discuss the same issues as would normal adolescents.

Stress Reduction Groups

Stress reduction groups are part of any inpatient or partial hospitalization group therapy program. Patients learn how to minimize resentment and anger by changing their expectations and accepting more freely those things they cannot, never will, and never have been able to control. Stress reduction is part of the twelve-step program. Techniques for coping with adverse life events, cognitive therapy, and learning social skills should be the basis for these groups.

Relapse Prevention Groups

Genetically determined, biological vulnerability to addiction will remain constant, making the goal of treatment prevention of relapse. Total cure is not realistic. Relapse prevention group participation commences within the inpatient and partial hospital phases and continues throughout recovery with more activity when drive, stress, or behavior dictates. Individuals learn, from more experienced group members, the skill to anticipate urges to use and to avoid settings of temptation (e.g., bars, sex with prostitutes, pornography). (See Chapter 9.)

The use of naltrexone and disulfiram, more frequent attendance (even three or four times a day) at AA, NA, or CA meetings, and more frequent contact with one's sponsor are sometimes required. The pragmatic use of other treatments may also be needed. After six months of treatment, most outpatient group work focuses on relapse prevention involving education in social skills to minimize anger and to promote the development of more effective communication.

There are two specific areas of relapse prevention in which peer groups are especially helpful. The first is in the identification of the signs of potential relapse; individuals who have a history of relapse tend to recognize indicators of denial better than clinicians, and can facilitate strategies to counter such tendencies. The second area is in the recognition of high-risk situations and of subsequent behavior development that often leads to anger and relapse (Nageotte and Amato 1997). Specific strategies to handle such situations include lifestyle changes, cognitive and behavioral interventions, and training in assertiveness (e.g., how to say no to an offer of drugs or alcohol) (Westermeyer and Isenhart 1997). Couples therapy is very helpful in counteracting relapse.

OTHER TREATMENT STRATEGIES AND TREATMENT-RELATED ISSUES

Community Meetings

Community meetings to discuss inpatient and partial hospital services are somewhat analogous to business meetings. More appropriate methods of intervention are addressed. Discussions focus on denial, how to identify an interim sponsor, and problems due to relapse.

Psychoeducation

Psychoeducation is part of all inpatient, partial hospital, and outpatient group programs. Movies, lectures, and autobiography sessions help those in the initial phase of recovery to learn about the effects of untreated and treated substance abuse.

Individual Therapy

Individual psychotherapy is an important adjunctive therapy to be used with group psychotherapy in selected patients. Cognitive therapy management of drug use, both within group and individual contexts, is predicated on the assumption that emotional distress that leads to drug use is due to an exaggerated, irrational, or distorted perception about circumstances and events (Westermeyer and Isenhart 1997). These irrational beliefs apply to the ideas individuals have about themselves, their self-worth, their capacity to deal with stress, and their use of drugs and alcohol. Drug and alcohol addiction recovery is seen as a lifelong process that requires a more rational management of the thoughts, behaviors, and events that trigger use. Individual therapy, therefore, fits into this scheme by educationally and pragmatically meeting an individual's specific needs and circumstances (DuPont 1997). (See Chapter 3.)

Creative Therapies

Creative therapies such as art, psychodrama, writing, and music therapy are directed specifically at using a creative process, in an adaptive way, to mollify the drive to use drugs.

Vocational and Educational Rehabilitation

Substance abuse frequently results in academic or career difficulties. Students may need to return to school or take their GEDs, and professionals may need to seek relicensure or even retraining. Group work should focus on helping a person move back into school and/or work.

Liaison with Employee Assistance Personnel and School Counselors

When possible, recovery should be facilitated by hospital-based clinicians in cooperation with school counselors and employee assistance personnel in order to facilitate the return of an employee or student to work or school respectively. Requirements, such as involvement in a viable group therapy outpatient program, periodic testing, and continued communication with a school counselor or employee assistance program (EAP), can ensure compliance and provide support during recovery.

Case Management

In an ideal situation, a case manager is employed to coordinate the movement of a recovering individual through inpatient, partial hospital, and outpatient treatment and daily attendance in AA and group therapy (ideally, ninety meetings in ninety days). A therapist skilled in substance abuse, group therapy, the twelve-step process, and spiritual issues can serve as a case manager as well.

CONCLUSION

Recovery from substance abuse is a lifelong process focusing on prevention of relapse through group support. Spiritual growth through the twelve-step process and effective management of concurrent physical and psychiatric disorders are the keys to success. Brief inpatient stays with a strong group component to the treatment plan are often essential to the attainment of stabilization of the addicted patient.

REFERENCES

Collins GB. Inpatient and outpatient treatment of alcoholism—essential features. In *The Principles and Practice of Addictions in Psychiatry,* edited by Miller NS. Philadelphia: WB Saunders, 1997, pp. 319-330.

DuPont RL. Psychotherapy in addictive disorders. In *The Principles and Practice of Addiction in Psychiatry,* edited by Miller NS. Philadelphia: WB Saunders, 1997, pp. 370-377.

Emrick CD, Tonigan JS, Montgomery H, Little L. Alcoholics Anonymous: What is currently known. In *Research on Alcoholics Anonymous: Opportunities and Alternatives,* edited by McCrady BS, Miller WR. Piscataway, NJ: Rutgers Center of Alcohol Studies, 1993, pp. 41-76.

Galanter M. Network Therapy: A practical approach to the office treatment of addiction. In *The Principles and Practice of Addiction in Psychiatry,* edited by Miller NS. Philadelphia: WB Saunders, 1997, pp. 378-383.

Harrison PA, Hoffman NG, Streed SG. Drug and alcohol addiction treatment outcome. In *Comprehensive Handbook of Drug and Alcohol Addiction,* edited by Miller NS. New York: Marcel Dekker, 1991.

Miller NS, Klamen DL, Hoffman NG. Abstinence-based treatment and depression. In *The Principles and Practice of Addiction in Psychiatry,* edited by Miller NS. Philadelphia: WB Saunders, 1997, pp. 351-358.

Minkoff K. Integration of addiction and psychiatric treatment. In *The Principles and Practice of Addiction in Psychiatry,* edited by Miller NS. Philadelphia: WB Saunders, 1997, pp. 191-199.

Nageotte CA, Amato JM. Treatment of addiction in adolescent populations. In *The Principles and Practice of Addiction in Psychiatry,* edited by Miller NS. Philadelphia: WB Saunders, 1997, pp. 268-278.

Patton LH. Adolescent substance abuse: Risk factors and protective factors. *Pediatr Clin North Am* 42: 283-293, 1995.

Raskin VD. Treatment of addictions in childbearing populations. In *The Principles and Practice of Addiction in Psychiatry,* edited by Miller NS. Philadelphia: WB Saunders, 1997, pp. 297-303.

Schuckit MA, Smith TL, Anthenelli R, Irwin M. Clinical course of alcoholism in 636 male inpatients. *American Journal of Psychiatry* 150: 786-792, 1993.

Slaby AE. Treatment of addictive disorders in emergency populations. In *The Principles and Practice of Addiction in Psychiatry,* edited by Miller NS. Philadelphia: WB Saunders, 1997, pp. 241-248.

Westermeyer J, Isenhart C. New and experimental psychosocial therapies in alcoholism and addiction. In *The Principles and Practice of Addiction in Psychiatry,* edited by Miller NS. Philadelphia: WB Saunders, 1997, pp. 359-369.

Wright C, Moore RD. Disulfiram treatment of alcoholism. *American Journal of Psychiatry* 88: 647-655, 1990.

Chapter 9

Groups in Therapeutic Communities

George De Leon

The group process is an important element of treatment found throughout the therapeutic community (TC) approach. Such a process unfolds formally in scheduled community-wide meetings, therapeutic groups, and educational groups, as well as informally in ad hoc collectives of residents who are engaged in conversation and rap sessions. Other smaller community groups address therapeutic and educational matters relevant to the individual members. In all of these formats and settings, the process for change is mediated directly and indirectly through interaction with other members of the community.

This chapter presents an overview of community groups in therapeutic communities. These groups are components of the general TC approach for the treatment of substance abuse.

THE THERAPEUTIC COMMUNITY APPROACH

The therapeutic community is a *drug-free modality* that utilizes a *psychosocial approach* in the treatment of drug abuse. The characteristic *setting* of a therapeutic community is a community-based residence, but TC programs have been implemented in a variety of other settings, residential and nonresidential (e.g., hospitals, jails, schools, halfway houses, day treatment clinics, ambulatory clinics). TCs offer a wide variety of *services* including social, psychological, educational, medical, legal, and social/advocacy services. However, these services are coordinated in accordance with the TC's basic self-help model. The distinctions between residential treatment and residential therapeutic communities, as well as the diversity of programs, characterize a *generic* therapeutic community approach. For this purpose, informal and formal accounts of TC theory and method can be found in much of the literature (e.g., De Leon 1995; Frankel 1989; Sugarman 1986; Kooyman 1993; Yablonsky 1989).

TCs are guided by a particular perspective on the person, substance disorders, recovery, and healthy living. Full accounts of this perspective are provided in many texts (e.g., De Leon 1994; De Leon and Rosenthal 1989); its main points are that substance abuse is a disorder of the whole person (see Box 9.1), and recovery is a self-help process of incremental learning toward a stable change in behavior, attitudes, and values of healthy living.

The quintessential element of the TC approach may be termed "community as method" (De Leon 1995). What distinguishes the TC

Box 9.1. The Therapeutic Community Perspective: Four Interrelated Views

1. *View of disorder:* Drug abuse is a disorder of the whole person. It may involve cognitive, behavioral, emotional, medical, social, and spiritual dimensions of a person's life. Physical dependency must be seen in the context of the individual's psychological status and lifestyle: "Problem is the Person," not the drug.

2. *View of the person:* Individuals are distinguished along the dimensions of psychological dysfunction and social deficits, rather than by drug use patterns. Some shared characteristics include poor tolerance for frustration/discomfort/delay of gratification, low self-esteem, problems with authority, problems with responsibility, poor impulse control, unrealistic expectations, coping with feelings, dishonesty/manipulation/self-deception, guilt (self, others, community), and deficits (reading, writing, attention, communication).

3. *View of recovery:* The goals of treatment are global changes in lifestyle and identity. Recovery is viewed as developmental learning, involving self-help and mutual self-help, and addresses motivation and social learning. Treatment is an episode in the recovery process.

4. *View of right living:* Certain beliefs are essential to recovery and healthy living. Examples include honesty, "here and now" focus, personal responsibility for one's destiny, social responsibility ("Brother's/Sister's Keeper"), and a moral code concerning right and wrong behavior. Work ethic is essential, and one must learn to develop economic self-reliance through community involvement, and to be a good citizen.

Source: De Leon 1995.

from other treatment approaches (and other communities) is its *purposive use of the peer community to facilitate social and psychological change in individuals.* In a therapeutic community, all activities are designed to produce therapeutic and educational change in its individual participants, and all participants are mediators of these therapeutic and educational changes.

The TC perspective and approach provide a conceptual basis for defining the *generic* TC program model in terms of its basic components. Boxes 9.2 and 9.3 abstract recent writings on theory and method (De Leon 1995). They list some essential concepts of "community as method," and basic program components of a generic TC model, which can be adapted in different ways and in various settings *(both residential and nonresidential).*

TC Groups and the TC Perspective

Conventional group psychotherapy may not be appropriate for the serious substance abuser. Fortunately, in a variety of ways, the TC perspective and approach reflects the particular needs of such substance abusers. Substance abusers in TCs cannot listen to or "behave for" others—not for parents, teachers, or mental health professionals. With the assistance of TCs, a unique and important element of mutual self-help in addiction recovery has been developed.

The psychosocial distance between the traditional mental health therapist and the substance abuser (and sometimes his or her social status) is often too great for an effective therapeutic alliance. An individual's acceptance of therapeutic authority and of the peer group, however, is grounded in the credibility of the membership, consisting of recovered staff and recovering peers. Based on common characteristics and experiences, residents "know one another" in ways the conventional "expert" therapist cannot. And once residents are committed to personal and social change, they act as most credible and effective people for fostering changes in one another.

Other critical elements inherent to TC peer groups strengthen the therapeutic alliance between the individual and the group. These elements of safety, continuity, and the history of the peer group also maintain the theme of trust and credibility, within the commonalities of behavior and experiences shared among residents.

Box 9.2. Community As Method: Nine Essential Concepts

Use of participant roles: Individuals contribute directly to all activities of daily life in the TC. This contribution provides learning opportunities by engaging the individual in a variety of social roles (e.g., peer, friend, coordinator, tutor).

Use of membership feedback: The primary source of instruction and support for individual change is peer membership and the shared responsibility of all participants.

Use of membership as role models: Each participant strives to be a role model of the change process. Members must also provide examples of how others can change.

Use of collective formats for guiding individual change: The individual engages in the process of change and recovery primarily with peers in a social context. Education, training, and therapeutic activities occur in groups, meetings, seminars, job functions, and recreation.

Use of shared norms and values: Rules, regulations, and social norms protect the physical and psychological safety of the community. However, there are beliefs and values that serve as explicit guidelines for self-help recovery and healthy living.

Use of structure and systems: The organization of work (e.g., the varied job functions, chores, and management roles), which is needed to maintain the daily operations of the facility, is a main vehicle for teaching self-development and responsible behavior.

Use of open communication: The public nature of shared experiences is used for therapeutic purposes. The private inner life experiences of the individual, feelings, and thoughts are matters of importance to the recovery and change process for both the individual and other members. Thus, all personal disclosure is eventually shared publicly.

Use of relationships: Friendships with particular individuals, peers, and staff are essential for encouraging the individual to engage and remain in the change process, and sustain recovery beyond treatment.

Use of language: The argot, or special vocabulary, used by residents reflects elements of the group's subculture, particularly its recovery and healthy living teachings. As with any special language, TC argot represents individual integration into the peer community. It also mirrors the individual's clinical progress. Thus, the residents' use of argot is an explicit measure of their affiliation and socialization in the TC community.

Source: De Leon 1995.

Box 9.3. Components of a Generic TC Program Model

Community separateness: TC-oriented programs have their own names, often given by their residents, and are housed in a space or locale separate from other agency or institutional programs. In such settings, residents remain free from outside influences twenty-four hours a day for several months before earning short-term day-out privileges. In the nonresidential "day treatment" settings, the individuals are in the TC environment for four to eight hours, and then they are monitored by peers and family. Even in the least restrictive outpatient settings, TC-oriented programs and components are firmly set, allowing members to gradually detach from old networks and relate with drug-free peers in the program.

Community activities: To be effectively utilized, treatment or educational services must be provided within a context of the environment of the peer community. Thus, with the exception of individual therapy, all activities are programmed within collective formats: at least one daily meal prepared, served, and shared by all members; a daily schedule of groups, meetings, and seminars; team job functions; organized recreational/leisure time; and ceremonies and rituals (e.g., birthdays, phase/progress graduations).

Staff roles and functions: The staff are a mix of self-help professionals and other traditional professionals (e.g., medical, legal, mental health, and educational professionals) who must be integrated through cross-training grounded in the basic concepts of the TC perspective and the community approach. Professional skills define staff function. However, regardless of professional discipline or function, the generic *role* of all staff is community member.

Peers as role models: Members who demonstrate expected behaviors and reflect the values and teachings of the community are viewed as role models. All members of the community are expected to be role models—roommates, older and younger residents, and junior, senior, and directorial staff.

A structured day: The structure of the program relates to the TC perspective, particularly the view of the person and recovery. Ordered, routine activities counter characteristically disordered lives and distract from negative thinking and boredom, which predispose to drug use. In general, structured activities of the community facilitate learning self-structure for the individual, in time management, planning, setting and meeting goals, and accountability.

Work as therapy and education: Consistent with the TC's self-help approach, all residents are responsible for the daily management of the facility (e.g., cleaning, activities, meal preparation and service,

(continued)

(continued)

maintenance, purchasing, security, coordinating schedules, preparatory chores for groups, meetings, seminars, etc.). In the TC, various work roles mediate essential educational and therapeutic effects. Job functions strengthen affiliation in the program through participation and skills development, and foster self-examination and personal growth through performance challenge and program responsibility.

Phase format: The treatment protocol is organized into phases, which reflect a developmental view of the change process. Emphasis is given to incremental learning at each phase, allowing the individual to move on to the next stage of recovery.

TC concepts: TC curriculum is formalized, but is also informal. It focuses on teaching the TC perspective, particularly its self-help recovery concepts and view of healthy living.

Peer encounter groups: The main community or therapeutic group is the encounter, although other forms of therapeutic, educational, and support groups are utilized as needed. The objective of the peer encounter is similar to that of TC-oriented programs—to heighten individual awareness of specific attitudes or behavioral patterns that should be modified.

Awareness training: All therapeutic and educational interventions involve raising individuals' awareness of the impact of their conduct/attitudes on themselves and the social environment, and, conversely, the impact of the behaviors and attitudes of others on themselves and the social environment.

Emotional growth training: Achieving the goals of personal growth and socialization involves teaching individuals how to identify and express feelings appropriately, and manage feelings constructively throughout the interpersonal and social demands of communal life.

Planned duration of treatment: The optimal length of time for full program involvement must be consistent with the TC goals of recovery and its developmental view of the change process. The duration of participation depends on the individual's phase of recovery; however, a period of intensive involvement is required to ensure internalization of the TC teachings.

Continuity of care: The completion of primary treatment is just a stage in the recovery process. Aftercare services are also essential in the TC model. Any aftercare program must be *continuous* with that of the primary treatment of the TC. Thus, the instruction of healthy living and self-help recovery and the use of a peer network are essential for enhancing the appropriate use of vocational, educational, mental health, social, and other typical aftercare or reentry services.

Source: De Leon 1995.

Groups and Community As Method

The community groups are critical, but not exclusive, components of the TC program. The groups are smaller units of the larger peer community. Thus, the therapeutic/educational effects of the group are enhanced by the myriad of community activities.

Residents living and working twenty-four hours a day in TCs engage in a variety of social roles through changing job functions and community status in their roles as mentors, tutors, students, and friends. The behaviors, attitudes, and emotions in these roles provide the data or subject matter that residents address in group. This learned behavior meets the objective and method of the TC approach, to use the peer community, its context, and expectations to change individuals.

GENERAL ELEMENTS OF GROUPS

There are three main community groups in the TC that have a clinical focus: encounters, probes, and marathons. There are also three main forms of educational groups: seminars, tutorials, and workshops. Workshops are special tutorials that involve selected residents, special themes or lessons, and special individual assignments. Seminars are also prominent assemblies in the TC, which often have both clinical and educational foci, yet their topics can also be discussed in facility-wide, regularly scheduled community enhancement meetings.

Any group can act as a setting for an individual to display intense emotions, gain insights, vicariously learn from others, and experience social relatedness and healing effects. All groups aim to increase self-awareness and self-understanding and foster healing experiences. The clinical groups stress the awareness of feelings and the development of new insight and coping behaviors. All educational groups stress input, understanding, information, and skills. In general, the standard components of TC are present in each kind of group: sharing, support, and the use of peers in learning skills.

Rationale for Different Groups

Although their common goal is to facilitate positive psychological change in an individual, groups differ in rationale, specific goals, and specific approach. These differences are instrumental in advancing the overall therapeutic and educational aims of the specific treatment. Clinical groups address different dimensions of the individual's problems and growth. Probes focus on personal feelings, personal exploration, biographical material, and past history. Marathons attempt to induce profound therapeutic experiences in a context that uses both people and the environment. Encounters focus on modifying behaviors and attitudes. Despite their different approaches, all groups share the common goal of promoting self-understanding and change.

Thus, the distinctive formats of the different groups ensure residents that there is an appropriate time and forum for dealing with practical, personal, and community business respectfully, effectively, and in a psychologically safe environment. This distinction provides staff with greater clarity for following the course of each individual's therapeutic progress.

The Rules of Group Process

General rules apply across all groups in the TC, as do guidelines for particular groups, which do not vary. These rules are presented in written material, in orientation sessions, and by peers, and they are usually announced before each group. These rules and guidelines are fundamental for the success of using community as a method to facilitate individual change. Psychological and physical safety plus strict confidentiality are cornerstones of the group process.

THE TOOLS OF CLINICAL GROUP PROCESS

Certain strategies and techniques of verbal interchange are used by all group participants to facilitate individual change. These tools are designed to penetrate denial, raise awareness, stimulate reactions (particularly expressions of feelings), to facilitate self-disclosure, and promote members' involvement in the group process.

There are two main classes of group process strategies: provocative and evocative. Provocative tools *challenge* an individual member to react or respond; they are generally less supportive and more confrontational. Evocative tools *encourage* the individual member to react or respond; they are more supportive and facilitative. Regardless of the type, however, residents learn that the use of any tool must be accompanied by *responsible concern* if it is to be effective.

Provocative Tools

These tools—hostility, anger, engrossment, ridicule, and humor—are most pointedly used to penetrate denial and destroy deviant coping strategies, such as lying. They must focus on specific behaviors and attitudes, and they are not to be used to address what cannot be changed nor to attack the "inner person." Because of their limitations, these tools are most often used in encounter groups.

Evocative Tools

These tools—compassion, identification, empathy, and affirmation—use various forms of emotional expression primarily to facilitate self-disclosure and participation. All groups use evocative tools, both formally and informally, to balance the use of provocative tools. If they are properly used, evocative tools can allow healing experiences for individual members.

Using Tools

Some tools, such as projection, "caroms," "lugs," and gossip, function to both provoke and evoke. They involve using various forms of indirect communication both to challenge and assist the individuals to break through their resistance to direct communication.

The use of tools—particularly the provocative ones, such as hostility, anger, or humor—must always reflect the element of concern for the individuals toward whom their use is directed.

THE MAIN CLINICAL GROUPS

This section provides a snapshot of each of the main clinical groups, including their main features, differences, and similarities. Specific details of implementation and processes can be found in other writings (e.g., De Leon 1994; Denson-Gerber 1973; Kooyman

1993). However, brief clinical examples illustrate the various formats or tools of the group process.

Encounter Groups

A variety of "encounter groups" emerged outside of addiction treatment in the human potential movement (see, for example, Lieberman, Yalom, and Miles 1973). However, as it is practiced in the TC, the encounter or confrontation group was developed by people in recovery from chemical dependency quite independently of the human potential movement, traditional counseling, or therapy groups utilized in the mental health field. Alcoholics and drug addicts in TCs spontaneously evolved a purely self-help group process to address their disorders, their personalities, their interpersonal conflicts, and their recovery.

Encounters serve as the foundation of the group process in the TC. The label "encounter" describes all forms of interpersonal exchange based on the direct reactions, both positive and negative, of the participants to one another's behaviors and attitudes. In the TC, encounter groups emphasize *confrontational* (primarily negative feelings) procedures in their approach. *Sharing* (primarily positive feelings) and compassionate conversation, responsible concern, and affirmatory interactions are equally essential to its efficacy.

Various forms of the encounter group utilize common procedures. The basic encounter is a peer-led group composed of twelve to twenty residents; it meets at least three times weekly, usually for two hours in the evening, and is followed by an additional thirty minutes for snacks and socializing. Although often intense and profoundly therapeutic, the basic encounter is modest and limited; it heightens individual awareness of specific attitudes or behavioral patterns that should be modified.

Typically there are three continuous phases of the encounter: *confrontation, conversation, closure*. These phases guide the encountered member to acknowledge the behaviors/attitudes to be changed, to recognize the impact of these behaviors/attitudes on the self and others, to hear practical suggestions for change, and to receive group support and affirmation for engaging in the process of change. Various group tools may be utilized to facilitate the objective of each phase of the encounter. For example, in Phase 1, confrontation, the group may use provocative tools such as engrossment or humor to penetrate the individual's denial of problem behavior or to weaken resistance to change.

Probes

Probes are six- to twenty-four-hour group sessions, conducted on an as-needed basis, whose purpose is to obtain in-depth clinical information concerning every resident in treatment. Probes are often employed with newer residents (two to six months in residence) to help surface personal aspects of the individual's life. Thus, the goals of the probe are to increase the openness and trust of new individuals and their identification with others, as well as to increase the staff's understanding.

The general approach of the probe is to explore at least one important life experience. Although the probe does not inhibit intense emotional expression, it is considered successful if the new member is able to acknowledge the importance of a particular experience—even without catharsis or emotional processing ("working through").

Probes can be viewed as extended encounters or mini-marathons. The probe differs from the encounter in its use of support, empathy, comfort, and identification of other group members with the individual's experience. A probe may begin with a staff person questioning a resident about general or specific themes. The aim of the initial stage is to reduce resistance through group questioning, using light challenges until relevant material surfaces. Staff and the group provide supportive pressure (e.g., encouragement, prodding) for the unrestrained expression of appropriate emotions. At this point, group support is freely provided in the form of physical comfort, expressions of identification, or empathic statements, all of which may lead to resolution (full release of emotion, new conceptualization or perspective on the theme) and be accompanied by calmness and a sense of peace.

Marathons and Retreats

Marathons are extended group sessions that initiate and facilitate the resolution of major life experiences and conflicts that have impeded an individual's growth or development. The marathon does not aim to cure long-standing emotional problems.

Generally residents in long-term TCs will participate in at least three marathons during their residential tenure. These marathons may be scheduled in accordance with program phase movement or may be ad hoc, implemented when clinically indicated. The duration of each marathon is rather long, ranging from eight to twenty-four hours and sometimes even longer in retreat versions.

The ambitious psychological goals and complex approach of marathons requires extensive preparation to be conducted by several experienced clinical staff members and senior residents. The general approach of the marathon is to dissipate defense and resistance by means of a variety of techniques—physical, psychological, and social. Participants may be deprived of the ability to smoke or to move around. Special environmental stimulation (music, lights) may be employed. The marathon is often set up as a theater, consisting of many scenes that replay the significant life events of membership. Thus, the marathon incorporates elements of psychodrama, primal therapy, and pure theater to produce its significant impact.

Retreats

Retreats are special variants of marathons; they are extended group sessions that utilize elements and methods from encounters, probes, and tutorials, integrated in specially programmed ways. However, a retreat differs from a marathon in several ways:

1. A retreat is usually convened away from the main residential facility.
2. It is organized around a particular theme, such as child abuse or gender issues, which dictates the composition of participants.
3. It incorporates techniques and strategies from varied sources, including physical exercises and spiritual readings.
4. Rather than utilizing continuous participation to induce a dissipation of defenses, the schedule is balanced with work, recreation, and sleep.
5. Although its explicit goal is similar to that of the marathon (to foster significant psychological experiences), its implicit goal is a social one—to strengthen affiliation and bonding, and renew commitment to the community.

SEMINARS, TUTORIALS, AND WORKSHOPS
FOR SKILL DEVELOPMENT

In accordance with the TC view of the whole person, educational and training groups focus upon cognitive and behavioral skills building. The groups unfold into three main formats: seminars, tutorials, and workshops.

Seminars

The seminar is both a community meeting and a form of group process in TCs. Seminars convene every afternoon assembling on the premises all residents of the facility and selected staff. The community goal of the seminar is to enhance affiliation and program management, and staff observation of the entire facility is regularized. The seminar meeting in the afternoon complements the daily morning meeting and the house meeting in the evening.

The primary *clinical goal* of the seminar is to strengthen the individual's cognitive and communication skills. Thus, among the various meetings and group processes in the TC, the seminar is unique in its emphases on altering thought by means of an educational information-sharing approach.

Tutorials

Tutorial groups meet on an ad hoc basis and generally involve selected residents. They can address any theme, but the three main types include tutorials that teach: (1) personal growth concepts (e.g., self-reliance, independence, relationships), (2) job skill training (e.g., managing the reception desk), and (3) clinical skill training (e.g., the use of encounter tools). Each form of tutorial group has a somewhat different format specific to its own objective.

Personal Growth Tutorials

In contrast to a formal classroom or seminar, the personal growth tutorial is completely informal. It requires a comfortable, supportive learning setting in which confrontation is absent. Participants may ask any question, particularly of the staff leader. The focus is on self-reliance and goal setting. The themes selected explicitly contain a relevant teaching value, attitude, and perspective. The implicit goal of a personal growth tutorial is to teach residents *how* to explore a question rather than choosing just to listen to a specific conclusion or position. Follow-up is a critical stage of the tutorial.

Job Skills Tutorials

These tutorials focus specifically on training residents in facility job skills. All residents of the house are involved, since everyone, at one time or another, will engage in every job function in the facility. Usually job skills tutorials involve role-playing in the real setting of the job. Senior residents, as well as clinical and facility support staff, are often the trainers and teachers of job skills tutorials involving TC work roles. These tutorials prepare the resident for on-the-job field training and build a certain quality control for facility operations.

The Clinical Skills Tutorial (Mock Encounter)

These tutorials are designed to teach specific clinical skills, the most common of which are those of the encounter. The objective of the encounter tutorial is to teach the specific tools used in that group by means of the "mock" or simulated encounter.

A critical difference between the mock encounter and the encounter proper is that the mock encounter does not proceed to the closure/resolution stage. Its goal is to train residents (and staff) in the encounter process.

Workshops

Workshops differ from tutorials for they involve selected residents, special themes or lessons, and special individual assignments. Workshops are generally more intensive than tutorials; they are often ongoing (over several weeks or months) and are led by an expert who is frequently not from the TC. They offer life skills in preparation for transition into the greater community. Other workshops, such as those that deal with the reduction of health risks and the dangers of alcohol, are more problem-oriented. Didactic and experiential formats, reading materials, videos, and other educational aids are included in presentations. Curricula reflect the life experiences, problems, issues, and perspectives of the residents.

Seminars differ from workshops because they meet on a regular schedule, include all the residents of the facility, are usually run by residents, and focus on topics relevant to the whole community. Workshops meet less frequently, involve smaller numbers, focus upon special themes, require active participation from all members (work), and are generally led by staff. Tutorial groups are primarily directed toward training specific skills or teaching verbal and nonverbal skills; they foster self-examination and understanding through ideas, contemplation, and conversation.

The intellectual and training objectives of educational groups contrast with the objectives of the clinical groups (to facilitate emotional change and psychological insight). Nevertheless, educational groups pursue clinical goals indirectly by emphasizing the cognitive and conceptual domains of the individual. The messages of self-awareness, self-examination, personal growth, recovery, and healthy living are implicit in all groups, regardless of their formats.

In summary, regardless of their specific differences, the main therapeutic and educational groups are viewed as *interrelated,* sharing the common goal of advancing an individual's recovery and healthy living. Each group focuses on a dimension of the individual—intellectual, emotional, behavioral, and even spiritual.

OTHER TC AND NON–TC-ORIENTED GROUPS

In addition to the main groups, a variety of other groups are offered in TC programs.

Special Theme Groups

Theme groups utilize the elements of the main groups. Their formats and clinical tools focus on specific issues of gender, race, age, sexual abuse, cultural relevance, alcoholic parents, etc. Other thematic groups may be geared to program stages.

Special groups are generally conducted by primary and clinical support staff, taking into account clinical criteria and program management objectives, i.e., to enhance retention in treatment.

There are a variety of family-oriented groups offered by TCs. These groups attempt to develop an alliance with the TC program, support significant others, educate using the TC perspective and method, and form a social network among different families.

Non–TC-Oriented Groups

TCs integrate various conventional group forms, which are ancillary to the main TC groups, into the treatment regimen. These integrated groups are generally conducted by clinical support staff or, on occasion, by invited experts from outside the agency. The most common examples of conventional formats used are psychodrama, Gestalt therapy, primal therapy, reality therapy, family therapy, and, more recently, relapse prevention and cognitive-behavioral groups.

The goals, formats, and materials of these groups are not unique to TCs and are utilized in TCs to enhance, or advance, the change process.

Most non–TC-oriented groups should not be introduced at early stages of the program when residents are working on affiliation with the community and commitment to the recovery process, as they can undermine the affiliation process. Moreover, at the reentry stage, in order to appropriately utilize conventional groups, residents must be sufficiently stable with their socialization changes.

The group leaders, or therapists, of these non-TC groups must have a thorough understanding of the TC approach. Specifically, they need to recognize and appreciate the specific purpose of their group, the nature of their group members, and the relevance and timing of the special group to the TC recovery process.

GROUPS IN MODIFIED TC PROGRAMS

This discussion of groups is drawn from the experiences of long-term residential programs, which adhere to the traditional TC approach. However, the TC is continually evolving in response to changes in population, research findings, funding, and health care policy. Understandably, such changes have impacted groups in TC-oriented programs in various ways.

This last section briefly summarizes some key adaptations of groups that serve special populations and special settings in modified

TC programs. Such groups support mentally ill chemical abusers, substance-abusing inmates in prisons, women and children, homeless substance abusers in shelters, and adolescents. One of the significant adaptations has been the inclusion of special theme groups, such as the "double trouble" (mental illness and substance abuse problem groups), the "triple trouble" (mental illness, substance abuse, and homelessness groups), HIV/AIDS groups, child abuse groups, and rape and violence groups.

Current evidence demonstrates the general effectiveness of modified TC programs for different populations and settings (e.g., De Leon 1997; Knight and Simpson 1997; Jainchill 1994; Graham and Wexler 1997).

CONCLUSION

Notwithstanding any modification, group process in the TC model must be viewed as an active treatment ingredient. The use of community as method to change individuals must be embedded in the TC approach. Despite the uniqueness and difficulties of this method, TCs must strive to maintain the method as they continue to move into mainstream human services.

REFERENCES

De Leon G. Therapeutic communities. In *The American Psychiatric Press Textbook of Substance Abuse,* edited by Galanter M, Kleber HD. Chicago: American Psychiatric Press, 1994, pp. 391-414.

De Leon G. Therapeutic communities for addictions: A theoretical framework. *International Journal of the Addictions* 30(12):1603-1645, 1995.

De Leon G (Ed.). *Community As Method: Therapeutic Communities for Special Populations in Special Settings.* Westport, CT: Greenwood Publishing Group, Inc., 1997.

De Leon G, Rosenthal MS. Treatment in residential therapeutic communities. In *Treatments of Psychiatric Disorders,* Volume 2, edited by Karasu TB. Washington, DC: American Psychiatric Press, 1989, pp. 1379-1396.

Denson-Gerber J. *We Mainline Dreams: The Story of Odyssey House.* Garden City, NY: Doubleday Press, 1973.

Frankel B. *Transforming Identities, Context, Power, and Ideology in a Therapeutic Community.* New York, NY: Doubleday Press, 1989.

Graham WF, Wexler HK. The Amity Therapeutic Community Program at Donovan Prison: Program description and approach. In *Community As Method: Therapeutic Communities for Special Populations in Special Settings,* edited by De Leon G. Westport, CT: Praeger, 1997, pp. 69-86.

Jainchill N. Co-morbidity and therapeutic community treatment. In *Therapeutic Community: Advances in Research and Application* (NIDA Research Monographs No 144, NIH Publ No 94-3633), edited by Tims FM, De Leon G, Jainchill N. Rockville, MD: National Institute on Drug Abuse, 1994, pp. 209-231.

Knight K, Simpson DD, Chatham LR, Camacho LM. An assessment of prison-based drug treatment: Texas' in-prison therapeutic community program. *Journal of Offender Rehabilitation* 24:75-100, 1997.

Kooyman M. *The Therapeutic Community for Addicts: Intimacy, Parent Involvement, and Treatment Success.* Rotterdam, the Netherlands: Erasmus University, 1993.

Lieberman MA, Yalom ID, Miles MB. *Encounter Groups: First Facts.* New York: Basic Books, Inc., 1973.

Sugarman B. Structure, variations, and context: A sociological view of the therapeutic community. In *Therapeutic Communities for Addictions: Readings in Theory, Research and Practice,* edited by De Leon G, Ziegenfuss JT. Springfield, IL: Charles C Thomas, 1986, pp. 65-82.

Yablonsky L. *The Therapeutic Community.* New York: Gardner Press, 1989.

Chapter 10

Time-Limited Groups

William E. Piper
Anthony S. Joyce

INTRODUCTION

This chapter focuses on some recent developments in time-limited group interventions (TLGI) for persons experiencing problems associated with substance abuse. There are a number of reasons to consider TLGI as a promising approach for people with substance abuse problems. Some issues concern economics, efficiency, and effectiveness. In an era characterized by rapidly rising health care costs, treatment for substance abuse has been a major contributor (Welch 1992). Although the interventionist policies of managed care have created considerable resentment among health care providers, there has been general recognition that changes are needed and that people should not be overtreated. TLGI are among the most efficient approaches because they involve the simultaneous treatment of entire groups of patients.

Reviews of research literature have documented the efficacy of TLGI for patients with substance abuse (Fuhriman and Burlingame 1994; Piper and Joyce 1996). Reviews have also revealed comparable outcomes for group and individual time-limited treatment approaches.

Objectives of TLGI include both modification of substance abuse behaviors and improvement in problem areas, e.g., coping skills, social skills, problem-solving skills, maladaptive interpersonal patterns, and reduction of depression and anxiety. However, there are limitations associated with what can be accomplished. TLGI may represent one of a combination of treatment approaches that are part of an integrated program.

Time-limited means that both the patient and the therapist know that the total amount of time and number of sessions will be limited. TLGI and short-term treatments are not synonymous. Short-term treatments usually involve twenty or fewer sessions. For serious substance abuse problems, the number of sessions may be extended to 100 sessions or more. A series of time-limited treatments may occur over the course of the patient's life span. As Budman and colleagues (1996) have emphasized, long-term time-limited treatment is time-efficient if it is provided in group form and it prevents more costly alternatives such as repeated emergency room visits, hospitalizations, and individual treatment.

In the present chapter, due to space limitations, we assume a selective approach to covering types of abused substances and types of TLGI. For alcohol, opioids, and cocaine, major areas of treatment are covered. Given that abusers often use multiple substances, our chapter sections refer to the predominant substance. TLGI are often embedded in multimodal treatment programs. This limitation, in combination with the lack of large-scale clinical trials that compare the efficacy of different TLGI, compelled us to include approaches that appear to be promising rather than only those that are well-differentiated and validated.

ALCOHOL ABUSE

Cognitive-Behavioral Orientation

A variety of TLGI originating from a base of social learning theory (Bandura 1997a; 1997b), have emerged, often with a cognitive-behavioral orientation to teach the patient new cognitive skills that in turn will effect changes in affective experience and drinking behavior.

Cognitive-behavioral approaches frequently align themselves with the stage model of recovery developed by Prochaska and DiClemente (1986). Assertion or social skills training (SST) approaches are commonly oriented to treatment during the action stage, i.e., when the patients are seeking to free themselves from the addiction. Relapse prevention (RP) approaches are commonly associated with the maintenance stage, i.e., when the patient seeks to prevent a return to addictive behavior.

Social learning theory provides a framework for specifying treatment goals and validating treatment components (Mackay, Donovan, and Marlatt 1991). The perspective regards addictions as acquired behaviors with multiple biopsychosocial determinants. During the active stage of recovery, the development of social skills and coping behaviors are the aims of therapy. In terms of maintenance of abstinence or controlled drinking, relapse prevention strategies are the focus of intervention.

Social Skills Training (SST) Approaches

Time-limited, group-oriented skills training approaches have been employed in inpatient programs as a focus of aftercare following inpatient treatment (Kadden et al. 1989), and as a freestanding outpatient approach (Monti et al. 1989). Skills training approaches, in particular modeling, rehearsal, and feedback, have more power in a group setting. "Rehearsal with and feedback from peers are likely to be more realistic than in individual treatment" (Mackay, Donovan, and Marlatt 1991, p. 474) and generalize more readily to the patient's social environment. The group environment also provides a source of social support.

Representative Approaches and Empirical Research

There have been a number of investigations of the SST approach using groups. For example, Sandahl and Rönnberg (1990) reported differential effectiveness for an SST approach as a function of the alcoholic patient's level of functioning. A hybrid social skills training and discussion group plus "regular medically oriented support" (Sandahl and Rönnberg 1990, p. 459) was compared to the regular support treatment. Patients formulated treatment goals of controlled drinking or total abstinence. The group treatment involved eight structured ninety-minute sessions; the focus was the development of the patients' feeling of self-efficacy in high-risk drinking situations. Cognitive-behavioral techniques and discussion of problematic feelings were featured. At one-year follow-up, treated patients showed better control over drinking behavior than prior to treatment and relative to the comparison sample. Evidence showed that the skills-discussion group was more effective for patients who had a shorter career as alcohol abusers, a later onset of uncontrolled drinking, and better social and personal stability.

Eriksen, Björnstad, and Götestam (1986) replicated earlier work and reported similar findings: patients in the SST condition drank less, had double the number of days of sobriety and employment, and were abstinent longer than controls in the year after inpatient treatment. However, when SST patients did drink they consumed twice as much alcohol as controls. This finding suggested that the SST approach helped to postpone but not prevent a return to addictive behavior.

Jackson and Oei evaluated time-limited SST approaches for alcoholic patients in a series of studies (Oei and Jackson 1980; Oei and Jackson 1984). Comparing the effects of different kinds of group interventions, they found that modifications of the patients' maladaptive cognitions had greater long-term efficacy than the direct modification of overt behavior. They concluded that the group environment could produce rapid change through the utilization of a cognitive approach, and that manipulation of cognitive factors was important in the maintenance of behavioral gains (see also Rugel 1991).

The Relapse Prevention (RP) Approach

A number of different clinical approaches have been developed to maintain changes and minimize relapse (Rawson et al. 1993). Most of these approaches adhere to the model developed by Marlatt and Gordon (1985). However, outcome research has not kept pace with the activity devoted to the development of clinical programs.

Relapse prevention approaches are characterized by a combination of psychoeducation, behavioral coping skills and self-control training, cognitive intervention techniques, and, in group-oriented programs, the provision of peer support. The goals of RP are to increase the patient's adaptive coping and problem-solving skills, enhance the patient's sense of self-efficacy, and assist the patient to deal effectively with urges to drink. In the early phases, the abstinent alcoholic is helped to become aware of intrapersonal, interpersonal, and situational factors that increase the risk of relapse. Cognitive and behavioral coping skills training is provided to assist the patient in dealing with these risks more effectively. Later, the focus shifts toward developing more general stress management skills and achieving a more balanced lifestyle. Finally, patients are taught about predictable after-effects of a drinking lapse and methods to cope.

Representative Approaches and Empirical Research

A representative group-oriented RP treatment approach for alcohol abuse disorders has been described by Annis and colleagues (Annis and Davis 1989). The treatment is provided during a twelve-week period. Assessment identifies categories of high-risk situations for each patient. The Inventory of Drinking Situations and the Situational Confidence Questionnaire assess risk and perceived ability to cope with alcohol-related situations, respectively. The rationale for the Annis RP approach is that once high-risk situations for drinking are identified, it is possible to teach alcoholics to resist the temptation. The treatment consists of eight ninety-minute outpatient sessions, each session involving one hour of group and thirty minutes of individual counseling. The group sessions are used to discuss problem drinking situations, construct homework assignments, and review progress. Homework is the central technique and assignments are individualized and made progressively more difficult. Assignments include planning and implementing alternative coping responses in high-risk situations, increasing alternative activities to drinking, improving interpersonal competency, increasing social interactions, testing personal control, and attempting to resolve interpersonal problems. The model holds that repeated exposure to high-risk settings without the use of alcohol increases feelings of competence and self-efficacy.

In a comparative trial of the Annis RP approach, eighty-three employed alcoholic patients who had completed a three-week inpatient program were randomly assigned to receive relapse prevention training or outpatient counseling. Patients with differentiated profiles showed less alcohol consumption after six months of RP treatment than after traditional counseling. The patient-treatment matching effect accounted for over 30 percent of the variance of alcohol consumption (Annis 1990).

Summary Comment

Social skills training and relapse prevention are allied with the cognitive-behavioral orientation. In addition to the teaching of more adaptive social skills, both emphasize modifying the patient's cognitive appraisal of situations. In the case of SST, "cognitive restructuring" came to be seen as a necessary component for maximizing long-term benefits. In the case of the relapse prevention, addressing the patient's cognitive evaluation of drinking risks formed the basis of the model. Both approaches have relied on a group format as a source of social support.

The research that has been conducted on SST and RP has identified certain patient characteristics that interact with the treatment approach. At the action stage of recovery, SST appears particularly useful for the more chronic and impaired alcoholic patient. Higher functioning alcoholics show equivalent benefit from SST or supportive (discussion) group treatments. RP treatments appear to be particularly effective with alcoholics who face a risk of returning to drinking in specific situations.

Psychodynamic Orientation

Historically, there have been few examples of dynamically oriented TLGI for substance abuse. Most psychodynamic group approaches have been time-unlimited and long-term. Character pathology related to long-term conflicts is viewed as the underlying problem, and substance abuse is regarded as the symptom.

In a recent review of group therapy for alcoholics, Flores (1993) identified a major change in thinking regarding the necessity of abstinence prior to participation in dynamically oriented group psychotherapy. According to this view, addiction is the primary condition. It requires initial modification, followed by character pathology and symptomatology. Once the substance abuse is under control, the group therapist can focus on uncovering chronic conflicts that are associated with character pathology, maladaptive interpersonal behavior, and symptomatology. A number of experienced group therapists have advocated this sequence (Khantzian, Halliday, and McAuliffe 1990; Matano and Yalom 1991; McAuliffe and Albert 1992). However, most of these authors have maintained an open-ended, long-term format. An exception is advocated by Khantzian (see Chapter 5).

Khantzian's approach, which is called modified dynamic group therapy (MDGT), is a six-month, time-limited treatment with rotating membership. Emphasis is given to the substance abuser's developmental deficits and vulnerabilities in four areas: affects, relationships, self-care, and self-esteem. Pathological character, maladaptive interpersonal patterns, and substance abuse itself are viewed as attempts to compensate for these vulnerabilities. Accordingly, MDGT attempts to modify the vulnerabilities (Halliday 1993).

Other Approaches

Certain applications of TLGI to alcohol abuse treatment are not clearly cognitive-behavioral or psychodynamic. Some are strictly behavioral. Gamble, Elder, and Lashley (1989) indicate that group behavior therapy is promising. Foy, Nunn, and Rychtarik (1984) compared a four-week broad spectrum behavioral treatment program with and without a controlled drinking skills component. Other applications have incorporated TLGI with individual therapy or attempted innovations with the group modality. Duckert, Amundsen, and Johnson (1992) utilized social learning theory; Matulis (1985) describes a treatment format in a short-term inpatient unit, utilizing a "family relations group" operating without the patient to establish a revised perception of the alcoholic's social network. Also "multiple family groups" include the patient and operate "to stimulate better mutual understanding in order to insure the patient's continued well-being after discharge" (Matulis 1985, p. 138). Finally, Martin and Privette (1989) describe a brief, combined process- and skills-oriented group addressing issues of loss in an intensive one-month alcohol rehabilitation program. The alcohol problem is assumed to represent a pathological bereavement reaction.

Partial Hospital Approaches

Partial hospital (PH) approaches to the treatment of alcohol abuse require that the patient commute for treatment daily. In many instances, the PH program is identical to the treatment provided to inpatients. The advantage of the PH is reduced restrictiveness: patients are allowed to work while in recovery treatment.

A typical time-limited PH treatment approach relies on cognitive-behavioral group techniques, and addresses several areas of patient functioning: drinking behavior with abstinence as the goal; concurrent psychopathology; coping abilities and adaptive cognitive problem-solving skills; and environmental alteration to develop social support for maintenance.

Research on PH treatments has commonly addressed questions of efficacy and cost-effectiveness relative to inpatient treatments. The findings of this research are consistent: PH treatments are equivalent to inpatient care in terms of effectiveness, and costs per patient are commonly one-third to one-half the expenditure for inpatient admissions. McKay, Alterman, McLellan et al. (1995) reported no outcome differences after comparing twenty-eight-day PH and inpatient treatments, but PH patients were more likely to enter aftercare programs.

COCAINE ABUSE

Psychodynamic Orientation

As indicated, one of the few explicitly formulated TLGI for cocaine abuse from the psychodynamic orientation is Khantzian's modified dynamic group therapy (MDGT) (Khantzian, Halliday, and McAuliffe 1990). (See Chapter 5 of this text for further details on the MDGT format.) (See also Campbell and Brasher 1994.)

In a chapter on group treatment and research directions for cocaine abuse, Spitz (1987) outlines a series of patient objectives in group therapy. These include: detoxification, achievement of emotional equilibrium, addressing life issues, self-monitoring, and development of problem-solving skills. Each can be viewed as representing a stage of treatment. Progression through the stages requires time. It is conceivable that a longer term, time-limited group program would allow the progression to be completed. Treatment can be presented as a series of time-limited segments that requires periodic recontracting.

Partial Hospital Approaches

Intensive day hospital treatment for cocaine abusers is a common multimodal approach. Alterman et al. (1994) conducted a randomized trial comparing one-month day hospital treatment and one-month inpatient treatment for inner city African-American male veterans. The day hospital program consisted of twenty-seven hours of primarily group treatment per week (Monday-Friday). A combination of medical, educational, psychotherapeutic, and self-help interventions were included. Significant improvements in substance abuse, psychosocial functioning, and health status were found at seven months postadmission. Although there were minimal differences in improvement between the day hospital and inpatient participants, the cost of inpatient treatment was 1.5 to 3.0 times greater.

OPIOID ABUSE

Perhaps more than other substance abuse disorders, heroin addiction is regarded as a chronically relapsing disease (Alterman, O'Brien, and McLellan 1991). The distinction between rehabilitation and aftercare is consequently not as clear. Treatment has usually been methadone maintenance or antagonist drug treatment. Alternative treatments, such as residential therapeutic communities or outpatient drug-free programs, usually require initial detoxification. Alternative treatments commonly record attrition rates of 40 to 50 percent during the first three months, in contrast to 14 percent for well-run methadone maintenance programs (Alterman, O'Brien, and McLellan 1991).

Outpatient programs and therapeutic community programs utilizing TLGI will be briefly reviewed. The cognitive behavioral orientation predominates in outpatient treatments, all of which place emphasis on skills training and/or relapse prevention techniques. Outpatient treatment approaches borrow from the therapeutic community tradition and place a premium on peer support and encouragement.

Cognitive-Behavioral Orientation

Skills Training Approaches

The TIPS (Training in Interpersonal Problem Solving) program is a group cognitive-behavioral approach to problem-solving skills training (Platt, Husband, and Taube 1991) used for the aftercare maintenance of detoxified heroin addicts. The group treatment has a psychoeducational focus.

Relapse Prevention Approaches

McAuliffe (1990) discussed the Recovery Training and Self-Help (RTSH) program as a multicomponent aftercare treatment for detoxified addicts that adheres to the relapse prevention model (Marlatt and Gordon 1985). The six-month program stresses skills training to systematically address predictable causes of relapse, and the development of group factors to provide motivation and support for continued abstinence and social reintegration.

Psychodynamic Orientation

Dore (1994) advocates a short-term, time-limited group therapy model of aftercare for male addicts in recovery. Men's issues, e.g., masculine identity, "fatherlessness," and gender role strain, are the foci of the group. The assumption is that drug addiction develops as an attempt to cope with the conflicts associated with these issues.

Groups consist of eight men meeting weekly for two hours, with intensive weekend retreats scheduled at structured intervals. The general orientation is psychodynamic, but the technique relies on more activity, support, guidance, and disclosure than is common in insight-oriented approaches. To date, no empirical evaluation has been conducted on the model.

Therapeutic Community/Partial Hospital Approaches

Therapeutic communities (TC) have been a mainstay in the rehabilitation of heroin addicts (Platt, Husband, and Taube 1991; De Leon et al. 1991). The "community" arises out of the members' identification with a united peer group. Often the staff consists of former addicts who act as models of successful recovery. The TC usually involves group therapy, loosely defined as time-limited. Members remain in the TC until they are confident of their ability to function outside without resorting to drug use, and may return when relapse is felt to be likely. Dropout rates from TCs range from approximately 25 percent within two weeks to 40 percent within three months of initiating treatment. Favorable outcomes occur in about half of TC clients followed over two years, although rates of abstinence are substantially lower. From 15 to 20 percent of members "graduate" as totally abstinent. For an in-depth presentation of the therapeutic community approach, refer to Chapter 9 (De Leon) in this text.

MATCHING PATIENTS AND TREATMENTS

For some time a strong consensus in the literature has indicated the desirability of matching patients to the most cost-effective treatments (O'Brien, Woody, and McLellan 1983). There are many possible combinations, considering treatments that differ on goals (e.g., abstinence versus moderation) and levels of intensity (e.g., residential versus outpatient) in addition to technique. A few studies of TLGI for substance abuse have identified promising matching variables (Cooney et al. 1991).

Research findings suggest that lower functioning clients benefit more from a structured group therapy, while higher functioning patients may benefit more from an unstructured group therapy. This conclusion is consistent with the findings that social skills training appears to be particularly useful for lower functioning alcoholic patients. Other characteristics identified as potentially important matching variables in treating substance abuse are psychiatric severity, perceived locus of control, family history, life problems, perceived choice of treatment, motivation, and self-image. Matching variables has proven to be one of the most promising areas of inquiry in the field of time-limited group treatments (Piper 1994).

CONCLUSIONS

Interest in TLGI for substance abuse is in keeping with the current priority in health care reform of developing and providing cost-effective treatments. Evidence suggests that less costly treatment approaches, e.g., partial rather than full-time hospitalization, can be effective with many patients and should be utilized. However, substance abuse frequently represents a serious long-term disorder with multiple components. When in an acute form, it requires intensive treatment. Thus, time-limited group therapy for substance abuse is usually only one of a set of coordinated treatments, i.e., only one part of a multimodal program. Its effectiveness may be highly dependent on the presence of other treatments.

Because of their limited time, which is often short term, TLGI require a clear focus. Some objectives involve improvements in substance abuse behaviors and improvements in associated problem areas, such as poor social skills, maladaptive interpersonal patterns, and depression. The objectives cover behavioral, interpersonal, and intrapsychic processes. There is also variety in the theoretical orientations of TLGI including cognitive-behavioral, psychodynamic, and psychoeducational perspectives.

The variability among TLGI appears to correspond with stages in the recovery-treatment process. A three-stage model differentiates an initial, brief detoxification stage, followed by an extended maintenance and treatment stage, which is sometimes called aftercare. Supportive/psychoeducational approaches tend to be offered during all three stages, cognitive-behavioral approaches during the second and third stages, and psychodynamic approaches during the third stage.

TLGI offered at later stages can capitalize on the effects of very different TLGI given at earlier stages or simultaneously. Different TLGI can focus on complementary objectives, e.g., increasing social skills and avoiding maladaptive interpersonal patterns. It is also common for substance abusers to participate in time-unlimited, peer support groups such as Alcoholics Anonymous. To prevent relapse, maintain recovery, and facilitate improvement, it is quite reasonable to regard long-term TLGI as appropriate and time-efficient.

A small but promising research literature suggests optimal matches between types of patients and types of TLGI. The evidence suggests that low functioning patients may benefit more from more structured TLGI, while high functioning patients may benefit more from less structured TLGI. This is an important line of inquiry that merits future research. In general, a lack of methodologically strong clinical trials have investigated TLGI. The fact that TLGI are often only one part of multimodal programs has and will probably continue to impede progress in discovering the unique effects of TLGI. Nevertheless, there are opportunities, e.g., during the aftercare stage, where efficacy and matching questions can be addressed with methodologically strong designs. These opportunities should not be missed.

In conclusion, TLGI for substance abuse are prevalent throughout the treatment process. There is widespread clinical support for their use and limited but promising research support. Continuing pressures from health care initiatives ensure their future presence. Hopefully, the same pressures can be harnessed to learn more about their optimal use in providing cost-effective services to patients with substance abuse problems.

REFERENCES

Alterman AI, O'Brien CP, McLellan AT. Differential therapeutics for substance abuse. In *Clinical Textbook of Addictive Disorders,* edited by Frances RJ, Miller SI. New York: Guilford, 1991, pp. 369-390.

Alterman AI, O'Brien CP, McLellan AT, August DS, Snider EC, Droba M, Cornish JW, Hall CP, Raphaelson AH, Schrade FX. Effectiveness and costs of inpatient versus day hospital cocaine rehabilitation. *Journal of Nervous and Mental Disease* 182(3):157-163, 1994.

Annis HM. Relapse to substance abuse: Empirical findings within a cognitive-social learning approach. *Journal of Psychoactive Drugs* 22:117-124, 1990.

Annis HM, Davis CS. Relapse prevention. In *Handbook of Alcoholism Treatment Approaches,* edited by Hester RK, Miller WR. New York: Pergamon Press, 1989, pp. 170-182.

Bandura A. Self-efficacy: Toward a unifying theory of behavioural change. *Psychological Review* 84:191-215, 1997a.

Bandura A. *Social Learning Theory.* Englewood Cliffs, NJ: Prentice-Hall, 1997b.

Budman SH, Cooley S, Demby A, Koppenaal G, Koslof J, Powers T. A model of time-effective group psychotherapy for patients with personality disorders: The clinical model. *International Journal of Group Psychotherapy* 46:329-355, 1996.

Campbell TC, Brasher B. The pause that refreshes: Opportunities, interventions, and predictions in group therapy with cocaine addicts. *Journal of Systemic Therapies* 13(2):65-73, 1994.

Cooney NL, Kadden RM, Litt MD, Getter H. Matching alcoholics to coping skills or interactional therapies: Two-year follow-up results. *Journal of Consulting and Clinical Psychology* 59(4):598-601, 1991.

De Leon G, Staines GL, Perlis TE, Sacks S, McKendrick K, Hilton R, Brady R. Therapeutic community methods in methadone maintenance: An open clinical trial. *Drug and Alcohol Dependence* 37(1):45-57, 1995.

Dore J. A model of time-limited group therapy for men: Its use with recovering addicts. *Group* 18(4):243-258, 1994.

Duckert F, Amundsen A, Johnson J. What happens to drinking after therapeutic intervention? *British Journal of Addiction* 87:1457-1467, 1992.

Eriksen L, Bjornstad S, Gotestam KG. Social skills training in groups for alcoholics: One-year treatment outcome for groups and individuals. *Addictive Behaviors* 11:309-329, 1986.

Flores PJ. Group psychotherapy with alcoholics, substance abusers, and adult children of alcoholics. In *Comprehensive Group Psychotherapy,* Third Edition, edited by Kaplan HI, Sadock BJ. Baltimore, MD: Williams & Wilkins, 1993, pp. 429-443.

Foy DW, Nunn LB, Rychtarik RG. Broad-spectrum behavioral treatment for chronic alcoholics: Effects of training controlled drinking skills. *Journal of Consulting and Clinical Psychology* 52(2):218-230, 1984.

Fuhriman A, Burlingame GM. Group psychotherapy: Research and practice. In *Handbook of Group Psychotherapy: An Empirical and Clinical Synthesis,* edited by Fuhriman A, Burlingame GM. New York: Wiley, 1994, pp. 3-40.

Gamble EH, Elder ST, Lashley JK. Group behavior therapy: A selective review of the literature. *Medical Psychotherapy: An International Journal* 2:193-204, 1989.

Halliday KS. The efficacy of a modified dynamic group therapy (MDGT) for cocaine abusers: An empirical test of a treatment based on Khantzian's self-medication hypothesis. *Dissertation Abstracts International,* 54(4-B):2201, 1993.

Kadden RM, Cooney NL, Getter H, Litt MD. Matching alcoholics to coping skills or interactional therapies: Posttreatment results. *Journal of Consulting and Clinical Psychology* 57(6):698-704, 1989.

Khantzian EJ, Halliday KS, McAuliffe WE. *Addiction and the Vulnerable Self.* New York: Guilford, 1990.

Mackay PW, Donovan DM, Marlatt GA. Cognitive and behavioral approaches to alcohol abuse. In *Clinical Textbook of Addictive Disorders,* edited by Frances RJ, Miller SI. New York: Guilford, 1991, pp. 452-481.

Marlatt GA, Gordon JR. *Relapse Prevention: Maintenance Strategies in the Treatment of Addictive Behaviors.* New York: Guilford Press, 1985.

Martin S, Privette G. Process model of grief therapy in an alcohol treatment program. *The Journal for Specialists in Group Work* 14(1):46-52, 1989.

Matano RA, Yalom ID. Approaches to chemical dependency: Chemical dependency and interactive group psychotherapy: A synthesis. *International Journal of Group Psychotherapy* 41:269, 1991.

Matulis DJ. An eclectic approach to group work with the alcoholic's "family" system during short-term inpatient treatment. *Social Work with Groups* 8(2):137-139, 1985.

McAuliffe WE. A randomized controlled trial of recovery training and self-help for opioid addicts in New England and Hong Kong. *Journal of Psychoactive Drugs* 22(2):197-209, 1990.

McAuliffe WE, Albert J. *Clean Start: An Outpatient Program for Initiating Cocaine Recovery.* New York: Guilford, 1992.

McKay JR, Alterman AI, McLellan AT, Snider EC, O'Brien CP. Effects of random versus nonrandom assignment in a comparison of inpatient and day hospital rehabilitation for male alcoholics. *Journal of Consulting and Clinical Psychology* 63(1):70-78, 1995.

Monti PM, Abrams DB, Kadden RM, Cooney NL. *Treating Alcohol Dependence: A Coping Skills Training Guide.* New York: Guilford Press, 1989.

O'Brien CP, Woody GE, McLellan AT. Modern treatment of substance abuse. *Drug and Alcohol Dependence* 11(1):95-97, 1983.

Oei TPS, Jackson P. Long-term effects of group and individual social skills training with alcoholics. *Addictive Behaviors* 5:129-136, 1980.

Oei TPS, Jackson PR. Some effective therapeutic factors in group cognitive-behavioural therapy with problem drinkers. *Journal of Studies on Alcohol* 45(2):119-123, 1984.

Piper WE. Client variables. In *Handbook of Group Psychotherapy,* edited by Fuhriman A, Burlingame GM. New York: John Wiley & Sons, 1994, pp. 83-113.

Piper WE, Joyce AS. A consideration of factors influencing the utilization of time-limited, short-term group therapy. *International Journal of Group Psychotherapy* 46:311-328, 1996.

Platt JJ, Husband SD, Taube D. Major psychotherapeutic modalities for heroin addiction: A brief overview. *The International Journal of the Addictions* 25(12A): 1453-1477, 1991.

Prochaska JO, DiClemente CD. Toward a comprehensive model of change. In *Treating Addictive Behaviors: Processes of Change.* New York: Plenum Press, 1986, pp. 3-27.

Rawson RA, Obert JL, McCann MJ, Marinelli-Casey P. Relapse prevention models for substance abuse treatment. *Psychotherapy* 30(2):284-298, 1993.

Rugel RP. Addictions treatment in groups: A review of therapeutic factors. *Small Group Research* 22(4):475-491, 1991.

Sandahl C, Rönnberg S. Brief group psychotherapy in relapse prevention for alcohol-dependent patients. *International Journal of Group Psychotherapy* 40(4): 453-476, 1990.

Spitz HI. Cocaine abuse: Therapeutic group approaches. In *Cocaine Abuse: New Directions in Treatment and Research,* edited by Spitz HI, Rosecan JS. New York: Brunner/Mazel, 1987, pp. 156-201.

Welch BL. Managing managed care: Paradigm I, II, and beyond: Can psychology survive another 100 years? *Practitioner* 5:1-11, 1992.

Chapter 11

Network Therapy

Marc Galanter

INTRODUCTION

Individual therapists in office practice are often considered to have limited effectiveness in treating alcohol and drug dependence. This chapter describes Network Therapy, a group approach designed to assure greater success in such treatment, employing behavioral and psychodynamic therapy, while engaging the patient in a support group composed of a network of family members and peers (Galanter 1993a; 1993b). It was developed over an extended period of time to meet the practical needs of clinical practice, and encompasses group modalities that have been applied in recent years by other clinicians and researchers.

Three key elements are introduced into the Network Therapy technique. First, support from the patient's natural social network is engaged in treatment. Peer support in AA has long been shown to be an effective vehicle for promoting abstinence, and the idea of the therapist's intervening with family and friends in starting treatment was employed as well in one of the early ambulatory techniques specific to addiction (Johnson 1986). The involvement of spouses (McCrady et al. 1991) has since been shown to be effective in enhancing the outcome of professional therapy.

Second, the orchestration of resources to provide community reinforcement gives support for drug-free rehabilitation. In this management role, the "primary care therapist" is conceived as one who functions in direct coordinating and monitoring roles in order to combine psychotherapeutic and self-help elements (Khantzian 1988).

Third, a cognitive-behavioral approach is employed in order to promote relapse prevention. This has been reported to be valuable in addiction treatment, and demonstrated to enhance outcome (Marlatt and Gordon 1985). In Network Therapy, emphasis is placed on identifying triggers to relapse and behavioral techniques for avoiding them, in preference to exploring underlying psychodynamic issues.

Conditioned Abstinence

For many clinicians, the problems of *relapse* and *loss of control* epitomize the pitfalls inherent in addiction treatment. Because addicted patients are typically under pressure to relapse to ingestion of alcohol or drugs, they are seen as poor candidates for stable treatment. Loss of control has been used to describe addicts' inability to reliably limit consumption once an initial dose is taken (Gallant 1987). Although these phenomena are generally described anecdotally, they can be explained mechanistically as well by recourse to the model of conditioned withdrawal, one that relates the pharmacology of dependency-producing drugs to the behaviors they produce. Thus, when an opiate antagonist is administered to addicts maintained on morphine, latent withdrawal phenomena are unmasked. Similar compensatory effects are observed in alcoholics maintained on alcohol, who evidence evoked response patterns characteristic of withdrawal while still clinically intoxicated (Begleiter and Porjesz 1979).

This conception of conditioned withdrawal helps to explain addictive behavior outside the laboratory. A potential addict who has begun to drink or use another drug heavily may be repeatedly exposed to an external stimulus (such as the sight of a liquor bottle) or an internal one (such as a certain mood state) while drinking. Subsequent exposure to these cues may thereby produce conditioned withdrawal symptoms, subjectively experienced as craving.

This model helps to explain why relapse is such a frequent and unanticipated aspect of addiction treatment. Exposure to conditioned cues, ones that were repeatedly associated with drug use, can precipitate reflexive drug craving during the course of therapy, and such cue exposure can also initiate a sequence of conditioned behaviors that leads addicts to lose control and relapse unwittingly into drug use. The sensations associated with the ingestion of an addictive drug, such as the odor of alcohol or the euphoria produced by opiates, are temporally associated with the pharmacologic elicitation of a compensatory response to that drug, and can later produce drug-seeking behavior. For this reason, the "first drink" can serve as a conditioned cue for further drinking. These phenomena yield patients with very limited capacity to control consumption once a single dose of drug has been taken.

Social Supports

Professionals can draw on a network of cohesive relationships to enhance the outcome of treatment. Enhanced outcome was reported when the community reinforcement techniques developed by Hunt and Azrin (1973) were augmented by greater social relatedness in a club-like setting (Mallams et al. 1982). Similarly, higher rates of retention and social recovery result from integrating a peer-led format into a professionally directed alcohol treatment program (Galanter, Castaneda, and Salamon 1987).

Not surprisingly, the cohesiveness and support offered by group and family therapy has been found effective in rehabilitating substance-abusing patients. Yalom et al. (1978) reported on benefits derived when interactional group therapy was used as an adjunct to recovery techniques. Couples' group therapy, as well, has been shown to benefit alcoholics, and to diminish the likelihood of treatment dropout (McCrady et al. 1991).

APPLICATION OF NETWORK THERAPY

The implementation of relapse prevention and engagement of social supports underlie the Network Therapy approach.

Starting a Network

The weight of clinical experience supports the view that abstinence is the most secure goal to propose to most addicted people for their rehabilitation (Helzer et al. 1985; Valliant 1996). For abstinence to be expected, however, the therapist should ensure the provision of a long-term support network, beginning with availability of the therapist and significant others.

The patients should be asked to bring their spouse or a close friend to the first session. Alcoholic patients often dislike certain things they hear when they first come for treatment and may deny or rationalize even if they have voluntarily sought help. Because of their denial of the problem, a significant other is essential to both history taking and to implementing a viable treatment plan. A close relative or spouse can often cut through the denial in a way that an unfamiliar therapist cannot and can therefore be invaluable in setting a standard of realism in dealing with the addiction.

Some patients make clear that they wish to come to the initial session on their own. This is often associated with their desire to preserve the option of continued substance abuse and is born out of the fear that an alliance will be established independently of them to prevent this. Although a delay may be tolerated for a session or two, it should be stated unambiguously at the outset that effective treatment of addiction can be undertaken only on the basis of a therapeutic alliance that includes the support of significant others, and that a network of close friends and/or relatives will be brought in within a session or two at the most.

This begins to undercut one reason for relapse, the patient's sense of being alone and unable to manage the situation. The patient will develop a support network that can handle the majority of problems involved in day-to-day assistance. This generally will leave the therapist to respond only to questions of interpreting the terms of the understanding between himself or herself, the patient, and support network members. If questions arise about the ability of the patient and network to manage the period between the initial sessions, the first few scheduled sessions may be arranged at intervals of only one to three days. In any case, frequent appointments should be scheduled at the outset if a pharmacologic detoxification with benzodiazepines is indicated, so that the patient need never manage more than a few days' dependency-producing medication at a time.

The network must be forged into a cohesive working group to provide necessary support for the patient between the initial sessions. Membership ranges from one to several persons close to the patient. Contacts among network members at this stage may include only telephone calls (at the therapist's or patient's initiative). Dinner arrangements and social encounters can be preplanned to a fair extent during the network sessions. These encounters are most often undertaken at the time when alcohol or drug use is likely to occur. In planning together, however, it should be made clear to network members that relatively little unusual effort will be required for the long-term, and that after the patient is stabilized, their participation will amount to little more than attendance at infrequent meetings with the patient and therapist. This is reassuring to those network members who are unable to make a major time commitment to the patient as well as to those patients who do not want to be placed in a dependent position.

Network Membership

Once the patient has come for an appointment, establishing a network is a task undertaken with active collaboration of patient and therapist. The two, aided by those parties who join the network initially, must search for the right balance of members. The therapist must carefully promote the choice of appropriate network members, as the network will be crucial in determining the balance of the therapy. This process is not without problems, and the therapist must think in a strategic fashion of the interactions that may take place among network members.

Focusing on the Task

As conceived here, the therapist's relationship to the network is like that of a task-oriented team leader, rather than that of a family therapist oriented toward insight. The network is established to implement a straightforward task, that of aiding the therapist in sustaining the patient's abstinence. It must be directed with the same clarity of purpose that a task force is directed in any effective organization. Competing and alternative goals must be suppressed, or at least prevented from interfering with the primary task.

Unlike family members involved in traditional family therapy, network members are not led to expect symptom relief or self-realization for themselves. This prevents the development of competing goals for the network's meetings. It also ensures the members' protection from having their own motives scrutinized, and thereby supports their continuing involvement without the threat of an assault on their psychological defenses. Because network members have kindly volunteered to participate, their motives must not be impugned.

Their constructive behavior should be commended. It is useful to acknowledge appreciation for the contribution they are making to the
therapy. There is often a counterproductive tendency on their part to
minimize the value of their contribution. The network must therefore
be structured as an effective working group with high morale. This is
not always easy:

A forty-five-year-old single woman served as an executive in a large family-
held business—except when her alcohol problem led her into protracted binges.
Her father, brother, and sister were prepared to banish her from the business but
decided first to seek consultation. Because they had initiated the contact, they
were included in the initial network and indeed were very helpful in stabilizing the
patient. Unfortunately, however, the father was a domineering figure who in-
truded in all aspects of the business, evoking angry outbursts from his children.
The children typically reacted with petulance, provoking him in return. The situation came to a head when both of the patient's siblings angrily petitioned me to
exclude the father from the network, two months into the treatment. This presented a problem because the father's control over the business made his involvement important to securing the patient's compliance. The patient's relapse
was still a real possibility. This potentially coercive role, however, was an issue
with which the group could not easily cope. The therapist decided to support the
father's membership in the group, pointing out the constructive role he had
played in getting the therapy started. It seemed necessary to support the ear-
nestness of his concern for his daughter, rather than the children's dismay at
their father's (very real) obstinacy. It was clear to the therapist that the father
could not deal with a situation in which he was not accorded sufficient respect
and that there was no real place in this network for addressing the father's character pathology directly. The hubbub did, in fact, quiet down with time. The children became less provocative themselves, as the group responded to my pleas
for civil behavior.

Use of self-help modalities is also desirable whenever possible.
Some patients are more easily convinced to attend AA meetings. Others may be less compliant. The therapist should mobilize the support
network as appropriate, so as to continue pressure for the patient's involvement with AA for a reasonable trial.

Meeting Arrangements

At the outset of therapy, it is important to see the patient with the
group on a weekly basis, for at least the first month. Unstable circumstances demand more frequent contacts with the network. Sessions
can be tapered off to every two weeks and then monthly intervals af-

ter a few months. Once the patient has stabilized, the meetings tend less to address day-to-day issues.

Sessions begin with the patient's recounting of the drug situation. Reflections on the patient's progress and goals, or sometimes on relations among the network members, may then be discussed. In any case, network members must contact the therapist if they are concerned about the patient's possible use of alcohol or drugs, and the therapist must contact the network members if he or she becomes concerned over a potential relapse.

Pharmacotherapy

For the alcoholic, disulfiram may be of marginal use in ensuring abstinence when used in a traditional counseling context (Fuller et al. 1986) but becomes much more valuable when carefully integrated into work with the patient and network, particularly when the drug is taken under observation. It is a good idea to use the initial telephone contact to engage the patient's agreement to abstain from alcohol for the day immediately prior to the first session. The therapist then has the option of prescribing or administering disulfiram at that time.

The following complex case illustrates the implementation of a regimen of network supports designed to stabilize the patient and secure the use of pharmacotherapy. It also shows how network supports can be used with flexibility.

A twenty-four-year-old college dropout, involved in the arts, came for treatment after she had been using heroin intranasally daily, and drinking heavily for seven days. This was a relapse to her previous long-standing pattern of drug dependence, as she had been hospitalized twice for heroin addiction in the previous two years. Her last hospitalization, six months before, had been followed by episodic heroin insufflation, and bouts of heavy drinking. Her polysubstance abuse as well as her promiscuity and rebellious behavior dated back to her early teens.

One month earlier, while living in a rural area, she had been abducted by a man whom she had befriended at an AA meeting. She managed to escape after being held captive in a motel for a week. She was now living alternately with a friend in the city where she came for treatment, and with her parents who lived 200 miles away; she commuted by train. She had not admitted to her parents that she had relapsed to heroin use. As the patient's history unfolded in her first session, it was clear that she had a long history of social and residential instability, as well as poor judgment since her hospitalization. Nonetheless, she wanted to escape from her self-destructiveness and her pattern of drug use.

The preliminary structure of a network was established in the second session with her and with the friend with whom she was staying some of the time. The patient, however, acknowledged in this session that she was still using heroin intermittently. In the third session, her parents were added by participating via speakerphone from their residence in a remote city. This arrangement allowed for simultaneous planning with other people. Given her previous exposure to addiction treatment and AA, she was willing to accept a concrete plan for achieving abstinence from both alcohol and heroin as an appropriate course of action. She agreed to undergo detoxification from heroin with clonidine while staying in her parents' home, and then to continue with naltrexone and disulfiram treatment. The former was for opiate blockade and for reduction of alcohol craving, and the latter was for securing alcohol abstinence. These medications were to be taken under observation, using the format developed within the Network Therapy regimen described at the end of this case.

The patient was initially concerned that her parents would be upset if she told them that she had relapsed to heroin use after her last hospitalization. The therapist pointed out that they needed to be told so that they could serve as properly informed members of the network. It was agreed in an individual session that this need not be done until the patient's abstinence was stabilized over two weeks of use of the medications. The patient's concern was discussed in light of the judgmental and highly critical attitude of her mother, which had been influential over the course of the patient's adolescence, and had contributed greatly to her rebellious use of drugs. On a few occasions during the initial weeks, the mother became angry when the patient, while staying at home, had not attended AA meetings as planned.

Two more of the patient's friends were added to the network after the initial month of stabilization. This helped dilute the role of her parents in the network, and added additional practical resources, perspective, and support for recovery. The patient herself continued to take the medications under the observation of either her father or her friend, depending on where she was residing.

This patient's circumstances illustrate the value of using the network in combination with the observation of ingestion of a blocking agent or an anti-dipsotropic. (Both were used in this case.) The fact that the patient was taking these two medications on any given day undercut her craving and left her prepared to be compliant with the medication regimen the next day, as well as with the overall treatment plan. In practice, patients experience less craving when such medications are integrated into the treatment regimen because they know that opiates or alcohol are not available to them for the next few days after ingestion of the medication.

Format for Medication Observation by the Network:

1. The patient takes the medication every morning in front of a network member.
2. The patient is observed swallowing the pills.
3. The observer writes down the time of day the pills were taken.
4. The observer brings the list in to the therapist's office at each network session.
5. The observer leaves a message on the therapist's answering machine on any day in which pill ingestion was not clearly observed.

For the sake of the network's stability, the therapist should make clear that the principal role of network members is to participate with the patient and therapist in discussing opportunities for abstinence and stabilization, and not to scrutinize all aspects of the patient's behavior. Problems in compliance with the regimen of medication observation or AA meetings are discussed in network and individual sessions, and not policed by network members. Thus, if the patient misses a pill, the therapist is to be called and the patient not confronted. This removes network members from the role of independent enforcers, although their perspective and assistance may be solicited by mutual agreement with the patient. In this way, the implicit social pressure from members of the network for compliance acts to stabilize the treatment.

Adapting Individual Therapy to the Network Treatment

If network sessions are scheduled on a weekly basis at the outset of treatment, the patient may not be seen individually for a period of time initially. The patient may perceive this as a deprivation unless the individual therapy is presented as an opportunity for further growth predicated on stable abstinence achieved through work with the network.

When the individual therapy begins, the traditional objectives of therapy must be stated so as to accommodate the goals of the substance abuse treatment. For insight-oriented therapy, clarification of unconscious motivations is a primary objective; for supportive therapy, the bolstering of established constructive defenses is primary. In the therapeutic context that is described here, however, the following objectives are given precedence.

The need to address exposure to substances of abuse or to cues that might precipitate alcohol or drug use is of primary importance. Both patient and therapist should be sensitive to this matter and explore these situations as they arise, using cognitively grounded relapse prevention techniques. Second, a stable social life in an appropriate social environment—one conducive to abstinence with minimal disruption of life circumstances—should be supported. Considerations of minor disruptions in place of residence, friends, or job may make the substance abuser highly vulnerable to exacerbations of the addictive illness, and in some respects must be viewed with the considerable caution with which one treats the recently compensated psychotic.

Finally, after these priorities have been attended to, psychological conflicts come to assume a more prominent role in therapy. In the earlier phases, they are likely to reflect directly issues associated with previous drug use. Later, however, as the issue of addiction becomes less compelling from day to day, treatment increasingly will come to resemble the traditional psychotherapy. Given the optimism generated by an initial victory over the addictive process, the patient will be in an excellent position to move forward in therapy with a positive view of the future.

RECENT RESEARCH ON THE NETWORK TECHNIQUE

Pilot Study

A retrospective study was conducted on sixty sequential patients who presented for treatment of alcohol and drug dependence in office practice. The findings demonstrated the mode of operation and the outcome of this approach. Fifty-five of the sixty patients were treated with at least one other network member, and the average network had 2.3 members. Of the fifty-five so treated, sixteen had a parent in the network, thirteen a sibling, twenty-eight a peer, thirty-four a spouse or mate, and four a child of their own. Using DSM criteria, forty-six experienced major or full improvement, and those using disulfiram under observation of a network member showed the best outcome (Galanter 1993c).

Standardization of the Treatment

A Network Therapy Rating Scale was used to rate network-related therapist behavior on videotaped segments of addiction therapy sessions. Half the video segments illustrated the network format, and the remainder were of systemic family therapy. The scale was first applied by medical school teaching faculty who were expert in Network Therapy, and later by psychiatric residents who had received a seminar course on Network Therapy. Responses of both faculty and residents distinguished the two therapy techniques to a highly significant degree, with the faculty distinguishing treatments more effectively than that of the residents (Keller, Galanter, and Weinberg 1997). These scores reflected an acceptable level of integrity and differentiability of Network Therapy, a greater level of expertise among the faculty who would be providing supervision for the trainees, and the ability of both groups to distinguish network therapy techniques from those of nonnetwork approaches.

Study on Training Naive Therapists

A course of training for psychiatric residents naive to addiction and ambulatory treatments was undertaken over a period of two academic years. Before treating patients with this modality, the residents were provided with a structured treatment manual for network therapy and participated in a thirteen-session seminar on application of the Network Therapy technique. Cocaine-abusing patients were eligible to be treated in this study if they could come for evaluation with a friend or family member who could participate in their treatment. In all, twenty-four patients were enrolled. Supervisors' evaluation of videotapes of the network sessions employing a standardized instrument indicated good adherence to the manualized treatment, with effective use of network therapy techniques. The outcome of treatment reflected retention and abstinence rates as good as comparable ambulatory care carried out by therapists experienced in cocaine addiction treatment, and demonstrated the feasibility of teaching the network technique to therapists naive to addiction treatment.

MANUALIZED SUMMARY
OF THE NETWORK TECHNIQUE

The following material is summarized from the treatment manual and defines specific procedures embodied in Network Therapy:

Start a Network As Soon As Possible

1. See the alcohol or drug abuser promptly, as the window of opportunity for entry into treatment is generally brief.
2. If the person is married, engage the spouse early on, preferably at the time of the first phone call. Point out that addiction is a

family problem, and try to enlist the spouse in ensuring that the patient arrives at your office with a day's sobriety.

3. In the initial interview, point out the grave consequences of the patient's addiction before the patient can introduce his or her system of denial; this avoids putting the spouse or other network members in the awkward position of having to contradict the patient.

4. Then make clear that the patient needs to be abstinent, starting now. (A tapered detoxification sometimes may be necessary, as with depressant pills.)

5. When seeing an alcoholic patient for the first time, start him or her on disulfiram treatment as soon as possible, in the office if you can. Have the patient continue taking disulfiram under observation of a network member.

6. During the first session, start arranging for a network to be assembled, generally involving a number of the patient's family or close friends.

7. From the very first meeting, consider how to ensure sobriety until the next meeting, and plan that with the network. Initially, their immediate company, a plan for daily AA attendance, and planned activities may all be necessary.

Manage the Network with Care

1. Include people who are close to the patient, have a long-standing relationship with him or her, and are trusted. Avoid members with substance abuse problems, as they will let you down when you need their unbiased support. Avoid superiors and subordinates at work, as they have an overriding relationship with the patient independent of friendship.

2. Get a balanced group. Avoid a network composed solely of the parental generation, or of younger people, or of people of the opposite sex.

3. Make sure that the mood of meetings is trusting and free of recrimination. Avoid exploring guilt or anger in meetings. Explain issues of conflict in terms of the problems presented by addiction—do not get into personality conflicts.

4. The tone should be directive. Give explicit instructions to support and ensure abstinence. A feeling of teamwork should be

promoted, with no psychologizing or impugning members' motives.

5. Meet as frequently as necessary to ensure abstinence.
6. The network should have no agenda other than to support the patient's abstinence. The members are not there to work on family relations or help other members with their problems, although this may happen indirectly.

Keep the Network's Agenda Focused

1. *Maintaining abstinence:* The patient and the network members should report at the outset of each session any exposure of the patient to alcohol and drugs. They should be instructed on the nature of relapse and plan with the therapist ways to sustain abstinence. Cues to conditioned drug seeking should be examined.
2. *Supporting the network's integrity:* Everyone has a role in this. The patient is expected to make sure that network members keep their meeting appointments and stay involved with the treatment. The therapist sets meeting times and summons the network for any emergency, such as relapse, and secures stability of the membership if the patient is having trouble doing so. Network members' responsibilities are to attend network sessions, although they may be asked to undertake other supportive activity with the patient.
3. *Securing future behavior:* The therapist should support any and all means necessary to ensure the patient's stable abstinence, such as a stable, drug-free residence; the avoidance of substance-abusing friends; attendance at twelve-step meetings; medications such as disulfiram or blocking agents; observed urinalysis; and ancillary psychiatric care. Written agreements may be handy, such as a mutually acceptable contingency contract with penalties for violation of understandings.

REFERENCES

Begleiter H, Porjesz B. Persistence of a subacute withdrawal syndrome following chronic ethanol intake. *Drug and Alcohol Dependence* 4:353-357, 1979.

Fuller R, Branchey L, Brightwell DR, Derman RM, Emrick CD, Iber FL, James KE, Lacoursiere RB, Lee KK, Lowenstam I, et al. Disulfiram treatment of alcoholism. A Veterans Administration cooperative study. *JAMA* 256:1449-1455, 1986.

Galanter M. Network therapy for addiction: A model for office practice. *American Journal of Psychiatry* 150:28-36, 1993a.

Galanter M. *Network Therapy for Alcohol and Drug Abuse: A New Approach in Practice*. New York: Basic Books, 1993b.

Galanter M. Network therapy for substance abuse: A clinical trial. *Psychotherapy* 30:251-258, 1993c.

Galanter M, Castaneda R, Salamon I. *Alcoholism, Clinical and Experimental Research* 11(5):424-429, 1987.

Gallant DM. *Alcoholism: A Guide to Diagnosis, Intervention, and Treatment*. New York: W.W. Norton and Company, 1987.

Helzer JE, Robins LN, Taylor JR, Carey K, Miller RH, Combs-Orme T, Farmer A. The extent of long-term drinking among alcoholics discharged from medical and psychiatric facilities. *New England Journal of Medicine* 312:1678-1682, 1985.

Hunt GM, Azrin NH. A community reinforcement approach to alcoholism. *Behaviour Research and Therapy* 11:91-104, 1973.

Johnson VE. *Intervention: How to Help Someone Who Doesn't Want Help*. Minneapolis: Johnson Institute, 1986.

Keller D, Galanter M, Weinberg S. Validation of a scale for Network Therapy: A technique for systematic use of peer and family support in addiction treatment. *Journal of Drug and Alcohol Abuse* 23:115-127, 1997.

Khantzian EJ. The primary care therapist and patient needs in substance abuse treatment. *American Journal of Drug and Alcohol Abuse* 14(2):159-167, 1988.

Mallams JH, Godley MD, Hall GM, Meyers RJ. A social-systems approach to resocializing alcoholics in the community. *Journal of Studies on Alcohol* 43:1115-1123, 1982.

Marlatt GA, Gordon J. *Relapse Prevention: Maintenance Strategies in the Treatment of Addictive Behaviors*. New York: Guilford Press, 1985.

McCrady BS, Stout R, Noel N, Abrams D, Fisher-Nelson H. Effectiveness of three types of spouse-involved behavioral alcoholism treatment. *British Journal of Addictions* 86:1415-1424, 1991.

Valliant G. A long-term follow-up of male alcohol abuse. *Archives of General Psychiatry* 53:243-249, 1996.

Yalom ID, Bloch S, Bond G, Zimmerman E, Qualls B. Alcoholics in interactional group therapy. *Archives of General Psychiatry* 35:419-425, 1978.

Chapter 12

Self-Help Groups and Substance Abuse: An Examination of Alcoholics Anonymous

Morton A. Lieberman
Keith Humphreys

INTRODUCTION

Self-help groups (SHGs) are ordinarily defined as being composed of members who share a common condition, situation, heritage, symptom, or experience. They are largely self-governing, emphasize self-reliance, and generally offer a face-to-face or phone-to-phone fellowship network, available and accessible without charge. They tend to be self-supporting rather than dependent on external funding.

Development and Origins

Small groups have always served as important healing agents from the beginning of recorded history. Group forces have been used to inspire hope, increase morale, and offer strong emotional support. Religious healers have always relied heavily on group forces, but when healing passed from the priestly to the medical profession, deliberate use of group forces fell into decline until post-World War II.

The most common explanatory model used to account for the current development of SHGs is based upon a functionalist framework, which sees new institutions arising in society when there are mean-

Keith Humphreys' work on this manuscript was supported by a grant from the Rotterdam Addiction Research Institute and by the Department of Veterans Affairs Mental Health Strategic Health Group.

ingful and recognized needs among members of that society that are not being met by existing institutions. The inadequate professional response to problems of alcoholism is proffered as the classic example. In contrast to the functionalist view is the explanation of alternative pathways in which people obtain services already acknowledged in the programs of other institutions in that society. Here the emphasis is not so much on the unmet need as on the incorrectly or inadequately met need; the focus is on the form through which the service is offered. Still another view is that the growth and development of such institutions is best explained by individual needs for affiliation and community with others in similar conditions.

A Brief History of AA

Historical records show that AA was officially founded in 1935. The 1920s and 1930s witnessed the rise of a quasi-religious evangelical movement, characterized by a group known as the Oxford Group. This group attempted to recapture the spirit of early pietist Christianity, and emphasized the importance of confession of and restitution for sins among peers. The Oxford Group counted some alcoholics among its members, including a man named Edwin Thatcher.

Thatcher achieved a period of abstinence with the help of the Oxford Group, particularly from another member who had been treated by the Swiss psychoanalyst Carl Jung, who viewed alcoholism as medically untreatable but perhaps resolved by a spiritual transformation. Thatcher also influenced an alcoholic friend, William Griffith Wilson.

William Wilson (now known as AA cofounder Bill W.) had drinking problems for a number of years. In late 1934 Wilson had a spiritual experience during a detoxification episode. His interpretation of this experience was shaped by what Thatcher had told him, as well as by his own reading of William James' *Varieties of Religious Experiences*. Wilson maintained sobriety until, on a failed business trip to Akron, Ohio, his confidence left him. He got in touch with Dr. Robert Holbrook Smith (now known as AA cofounder Dr. Bob), an Oxford Group member who had also struggled with alcoholism. Their conversation, now recognized as the first AA meeting, had a profound effect on them both. They discovered that they could identify with each other's stories, and provide each other strength and hope. A key lesson they drew from this experience was that the way for alcoholics to recover was for them to help other alcoholics recover.

Over the next few years, alcoholics held mutual support meetings under the auspices of the Oxford Group. However, the religiosity and rigidity of the Oxford Group led the alcoholics to split off into their own organization, which became public in 1939 with their book *Alcoholics Anonymous* (known universally in AA simply as the "Big Book"). The appearance of AA's book was followed by positive media coverage, which helped make the 1940s the decade of AA's fastest growth.

Some aspects of AA, such as the practice of experienced members sponsoring newcomers, were developed specifically to help individual members recover. Others, such as AA's refusal to take any stand on outside issues, were intended to help the organization as a whole survive and function effectively. Much of what AA members learned and decided in both areas was set forth in 1953 in the second most important book in AA, *Twelve Steps and Twelve Traditions*.

AA has continued to grow steadily from the 1950s to the present day. Today, AA's membership survey (which Room and Greenfield, 1993, suggest is a conservative estimate of AA's actual size), records that AA has nearly two million members in over fifty countries. As it has grown in popularity, it has had a substantial impact on the professional treatment system, particularly in the United States. Although consistent with its policy, AA has never taken an organizational stand on professional alcohol treatment service but individual AA members have played key roles in the establishment of the National Institute of Alcohol Abuse and Alcoholism and the National Council on Alcoholism. Further, many treatment programs have adopted parts of AA's approach, have hired AA members as counselors, and refer their patients to AA as aftercare.

SELECTED DEMOGRAPHIC CHARACTERISTICS OF AA

Room and Greenfield (1993) using a 1990 national U.S. adult probability sample [N = 2,058] reported that 9.0 percent of U.S. residents at some point in life attended an AA meeting, 3.6 percent during the past year. However, the proportions reporting AA attendance for problems of their own with alcohol were significantly lower: 3.1 percent lifetime rate, 1.5 percent during the past year.

Capitalizing on the longitudinal design of the Epidemiological Catchment Area program (ECA) survey, Narrow et al. (1993) calculated prevalence rates for use of self-help groups for the year interval between two face-to-face interviews included in the study. About 0.7 percent of the sample reported self-help group use. Among SHG participants, approximately 7.9 percent had substance abuse disorders, 9.7 percent comorbidity marked by substance abuse and mental problems, and 5.1 percent non-substance abuse disorders. Self-help groups' use represented 12.6 percent of the total service use among non-substance abuse diagnosis, and about 20.6 percent among substance abuse disorders; self-help group users attended more sessions than users of every other type of help.

Lieberman and Snowden (1993), in a reanalysis of the ECA sample, reported that the helping resources turned to by respondents diagnosed as suffering from substance abuse problems (DSM-III criteria) were as follows: Current SHG 2.4 percent, current professional 11.1 percent, lifetime SHG 14.2 percent, lifetime professional 38.0 percent.

Meta-analytic research indicates that AA may appeal more to individuals with more severe alcohol problems (Emrick et al. 1993). In part this may be because AA construes alcoholism as an incurable disease and alcoholics as individuals who cannot stop at one or two drinks. To express this conjecture in diagnostic terms, patients who meet DSM-IV criteria for alcohol dependence may find that AA's message resonates better with their experience than do patients whose alcohol problems only meet (or do not even meet) the less restrictive criteria for alcohol abuse. Over the years, AA seems to have expanded its appeal from the stereotypical alcoholic who "hits bottom and loses everything" to less severe problem drinkers.

The best sample for estimating rates of participation can be found in a recent study by Kessler, Mickelson, and Zhao (1997) of self-help group participation in the United States. The sample of 3,032 respondents was recruited from a random digit dial sampling frame of Ss aged 25 to 74. SHGs were defined as, "groups organized and run by people who get together on the basis of a common experience or goal to mutually help or support one another. Groups organized and led by doctors, psychologists, social workers, or other professionals do *not* qualify as SHGs."

Almost 19 percent participated in a self-help group at some time in their life and 7.1 percent did so in the past year. These percentages are equivalent to approximately twenty-five million lifetime participants and ten million participants in the past twelve months. Most participation occurred in groups for substance use problems (6.4 percent lifetime participation, 2.6 percent in past year).

According to *The Self-Help Sourcebook* (White and Madara 1995), over two dozen self-help organizations address alcohol and/or drug abuse. The bulk of this chapter will be devoted to Alcoholics Anonymous (AA), which is by far the largest and most influential. However, because most clinicians would like multiple self-help group referral options, a few alternatives to AA are presented here.

Moderation Management

Founded in 1993, this organization has grown steadily to approximately fifty face-to-face groups in the United States. The organization also operates an electronic listserv group with several hundred members. Moderation Management explicitly states that it does not consider its program appropriate for individuals with more severe and chronic alcohol problems. Moderation Management's program draws heavily from cognitive-behavioral research and theory, and conceptualizes problem drinking as a habit rather than a disease (see Kishline 1994).

Smart Recovery

SMART is an acronym for Self-Management And Recovery Training, a self-help organization that was formed in 1994 and now has approximately 225 groups in the United States. SMART does not label members as "alcoholics" or "addicts," but does recommend lifelong abstinence from drugs and alcohol for members. SMART emphasizes that individual members (rather than God or a "Higher Power") are responsible for bringing about recovery.

Secular Organization for Sobriety

Secular Organization for Sobriety (whose acronym SOS also stands for "Save Our Selves") was founded in 1986 by James Christopher, an AA member who was uncomfortable with the spiritual emphasis of AA and its twelve steps. Christopher created SOS for drug- and alcohol-dependent persons who desire a secular, humanist approach to recovery. With approximately 1,000 groups, SOS is the largest non–twelve-step substance abuse-related self-help organization. Like AA, SOS suggests that members abstain from drugs and alcohol for life.

Women for Sobriety

Like SOS, Women for Sobriety was founded by an alcoholic person (Dr. Jeanne Kirkpatrick) who was dissatisfied with AA. Dr. Kirkpatrick felt that AA was not sensitive to the special needs of alcoholic women, and therefore formed her own self-help organization for them. Women for Sobriety has approximately 300 groups in the United States and Canada, with 1,000 to 2,000 members. They place strong emphasis on restoring self-worth, building self-esteem, and countering stigma, in part through crediting members (rather than a higher power) with attaining abstinence.

HOW SHGs DIFFER
FROM PROFESSIONALLY DIRECTED GROUPS

Aside from some obvious differences, professionally led groups have a designated trained leader, offer services for a fee, and are often marked by a clear beginning and end of service.

The Helping Group As a Social Microcosm

All group psychotherapists view the group as a social microcosm: a small, complete social world, reflecting in miniature all of the dimensions of real social environments. This aspect of the group—its reflection of the intrapersonal issues that confront individuals in a larger society—is most highly prized as a group property linked to an individual's change. Underneath all group activities lies the assumption that change is based on the exploration and reworking of relationships in the group. SHGs develop a rather different stance to the issue of the group as a social microcosm. The interaction among members as a vehicle for change is de-emphasized. AA has a specific negative sanction for this type of behavior. The group is a supportive environment for developing new behavior, not primarily within the group, but outside. The group may become a vehicle for cognitive restructuring, but analysis of the transaction among members is not the basic tool of change.

Psychological Distance/Closeness Between Helper and Helpee

Located at one extreme, many professionals, both through special training and manipulation of symbols and settings attendant to professionalism, increase the psychological distance between themselves and the patient. Of all help systems, SHGs achieve the greatest psychological parity between the helper and those being helped. Not only are helpers frequently similar in social background but, more important, they share the same condition as those seeking help. Client control of the organization also erases psychological distance.

Specificity/Generality of Help Methods

The help provided by nonprofessional therapists and peer counselors tends toward the general. High specificity characterizes self-help groups. Antze's (1976) study of self-help organizations demonstrates how they develop specific ideologies about the nature of the problem and tailor appropriate help methods to the specific afflictions they address.

Differentiation versus Nondifferentiation Among Participants

It is easier for SHGs to stress identity with a common core problem than it is in psychotherapy groups. Although it is typical for a psychotherapeutic group to go through a period of time in which similarities are stressed, this is usually an early developmental phase, and represents an attempt of the group to achieve some form of cohesiveness. It is not the raison d'etre of the group as it may be for a self-help group. In fact, some evidence demonstrates that psychotherapeutic group participants who remain committed to a sense of similarity are less likely to experience positive change. The potency of SHGs, on the other hand, appears to stem from their continued insistence on the possession of a common problem; the members believe themselves to derive support from their identification with a common core issue.

There is a class, however, of group psychotherapy, labeled by Weiner, Williams, and Ozarin (1986) as homogeneous group therapy, whose members are united by their struggle with a common problem. This is a parallel development in group psychotherapy, and represents properties and characteristics shared between more traditional group psychotherapy and self-help groups.

In summary, most SHGs are low on using the group context as a social microcosm, and low on differentiation. They are high on specificity, and low on psychological distance. Traditional dynamic group psychotherapy is high on social microcosm, moderate on specificity, and high on psychological distance and differentiation.

HOW SHGs WORK

Self-help groups are complex entities. They create experiences that are thought to be therapeutic in nature such as inculcation of hope, development of understanding, and the experience of being loved. Self-help groups are also cognitive restructuring systems possessing elaborate ideologies about the core cause and source of difficulty and about the ways individuals can think about their dilemmas in order to get help and cope more effectively. In addition, they are social linkage systems where people form relationships and, in that sense, they provide social support. All types of SHGs are collections of fellow sufferers in high states of personal need, and all require some aspect of the personal and often painful state to be shared in public. Regardless of the type of group, participants uniformly indicated that the abilities of such groups to provide for normalization (universalization) and support were central.

The structural elements provide the basis for how a self-help group delivers its services. They lead to group conditions: characteristics of the group as a social system such as the climate and culture. It is the group culture/conditions that determine the specific types of therapeutic experiences that will take place, which determine the "change mechanisms" that define the efficacy of the self-help group.

Structure

Homogeneity of Problem

SHGs sometimes go through enormous efforts to ensure homogeneity of the central problem. An example of the problem of not ensuring some homogeneity is the repeated failure to organize the elderly into such groups. Without a common base, such as deprived grandparents, or elderly caregivers, or an infinite variety of other common problems of the elderly, perceived similarity with people your own age is a pallid form of identification.

Membership Characteristics

SHGs ideally contain a range of active members, some who have just joined, others who have been members for years. Since SHGs are not conducted by professional leaders, the group must have a mechanism for transmitting the "therapeutic" conditions over time. Without such a mechanism SHGs often fail. In addition, the "helper-therapy principle" (altruism) is a prime process of change; the "senior" SHG members are more likely to experience this.

Cognitive Beliefs, Ideology

All therapeutic systems require an overarching cognitive framework for directing the participants on how to think about their problems, and what needs to be done in the treatment setting in order to get well. Ordinarily, this framework is communicated to the patient in psychotherapy by the therapists.

In SHGs, a similar shared belief system exists, not from the person of the therapist but from the formal and informal communications by the group members. A shared framework about the "cause" and "cure" of their problem or dilemma is apparent among the members. This thesis was shown in an inventive study by Antze (1976) who suggests that each group he studied (AA, Recovery, Inc., and Synanon) has a specific ideology that is closely linked to the underlying associated psychological problem. His analysis of AA ideology suggests that AA provides a specific and thorough antidote to the alcoholic's way of being; its prime therapeutic function is to induce a wide range of contradiction in a member's sense of exaggerated power. To absorb the AA message is to see oneself as less the author of events in life, the active fighter and doer, and more as a person with the wisdom to accept limitations and wait for things to come. Antze's careful analysis of AA and a comparison to Recovery, Inc., which on superficial grounds may appear to function similarly, demonstrates specific and unique characteristics.

Different from "Ordinary" Social Relations

The success of such groups depends, in large respect, on the creation of a tiny society that is separated and marked off from the surrounding culture. In most day-to-day contacts it is widely accepted as a violated norm if one openly criticizes other persons, or reveals one's own feelings about issues culturally defined as private or too personal. SHGs, however, generally create norms that may be counter to those of the larger culture; talking about interpersonal or inner feelings is generally viewed as a decisively good idea, and avoidance of such behavior is ordinarily defined as bad. Similarly, they often support norms that encourage closer relationships than are typical of ordinary social transactions. It is difficult to conceive of an SHG that does not develop norms distinctive from and often opposite to the normative culture of the larger society.

The Purpose of the Twelve Steps

AA believes that alcoholism is rooted in the character problem of self-centeredness, as manifested in egotism and grandiosity. Hence, in AA's view the first challenge for new members is to have the humility to admit that they have a serious problem that they are unable to control.

Step 1 is the only step that mentions alcohol. AA makes a distinction between abstinence (absence of drinking) and "serenity" (a state of emotional and spiritual peace). Because AA believes that alcoholics have characterological problems, it holds that recovery must involve much more than cessation of alcohol consumption. Hence, the other eleven steps focus on the reconstruction of the alcoholics' moral and spiritual character, and the reparation of their relationships with others.

The second key component of the twelve steps, "Surrender to a Higher Power," in AA involves recognizing realistic limits on personal control over some, but not all, of the alcoholic's problems. For example, according to AA, alcoholics cannot change the fact that they are alcoholic. However, alcoholics can choose whether to come to AA and to try to recover, and are held responsible for that decision. Hence, surrender involves making an existentially mature decision to be responsible only for those things over which one can exercise control, and to cease trying to control uncontrollable people, places, and things.

Although in the process of surrender, AA members come to believe that they cannot control their alcoholism, this does not lead them to feel hopeless because of the coupling of the concepts of surrender and Higher Power in AA. In AA's philosophy, a Higher Power can aid the resolution of alcohol problems that the members are helpless to effect on their own (Steps 2 and 3).

Steps 4 through 9 comprise an organized review of members' current and past behavior. In the process of admitting their character flaws and transgressions, AA members relieve their shame and guilt. In some cases, these steps help promote reconciliation with estranged friends and family if those parties are willing to forgive the member and rebuild the relationship that was damaged during the period of active drinking.

AA views alcoholism as a disease that can be arrested but never cured. That is, "once an alcoholic, always an alcoholic." Similarly, AA holds that recovery must also be a lifelong process, such that no one ever really completes the twelve steps. Steps 10 through 12 reflect this viewpoint. These steps are designed to maintain the personal and spiritual changes that members have undergone in their practice of earlier steps. The twelfth step embodies the altruistic spirit of the program by emphasizing that those who have been helped have an obligation to help others who are still suffering.

An Illustration of a "Typical" AA Meeting

Many meetings occur around large tables, and hence are often referred to as "around the tables," "gathering at the tables," etc. AA meetings vary widely in size, with anywhere from a handful to literally over 100 members (in such cases, the group is usually broken down into smaller groups for the main part of the meeting). Each AA meeting develops its own ritual opening. The opening of a meeting is led by the chairperson, who will typically start the meeting by welcoming everyone and introducing himself or herself in AA's traditional format: "My name is (first name only) and I am an alcoholic." Among the openings used, singly or in combination, are reading the steps and/or traditions aloud, reading other AA literature aloud (e.g., the section "How it Works" from the Big Book), and saying a prayer. Opening rituals serve to delimit the AA meeting from the rest of members' lives, to create a "sacred space" with its own norms of conversation and conduct. Further, a meeting's opening ritual provides a sense of comfortable familiarity for AA members who have not attended this particular meeting before. (It is quite common for AA members to go to meetings in other cities when traveling.)

After the opening, the format varies depending on the purpose of the meeting. If it is a speaker's meeting, an experienced member will tell his or her story to the group. In AA's terminology, these stories express "what we were like, what happened, and what we are like now." A typical story will describe how the member began drinking, the problems that ensued, and how life has changed since the speaker joined AA.

If the meeting is not a speaker's meeting, the person chairing the meeting (a rotating responsibility in all AA groups) will usually ask if any newcomers are present. If so, they are welcomed, and in most cases the meeting will then become devoted to discussing the first step of AA. If there are no newcomers, the meeting will usually be devoted to discussing a particular step or topic. Topics are sometimes suggested by the chairperson, and other times by other members of the group.

Although members follow themes in their discussion, they do not as a rule comment directly on a previous speaker's statements or engage other members in conversation during group time (known as "cross-talk" in AA). Most utterances are short (e.g., less than three minutes) in order to allow many speakers to participate.

A Topic Discussion

Ten members sit around a table drinking coffee, smoking cigarettes, or both. After welcoming the group and reading "How it Works" from the Big Book, the chair, Sally, speaks to the group:

SALLY: Before beginning, let us have a moment of silence for the alcoholic who still suffers. [Group members bow their heads for ten seconds.]

SALLY: Thank you. Who has a topic to discuss?

RAY: My name is Ray and I'm an alcoholic. I, uh, I would like to talk about slipping. I got sober here five months ago, but last week things came apart on me and I went and got drunk. [Face flushes.] I can't believe I'm back at square one again. I'd appreciate any experience, strength, and hope on this right now.

ED: My name is Ed, and I'm an alcoholic. I've been there. For me, sobriety has been a process of two steps forward one step back. No pun intended. [Group laughter.] My sponsor has always kept me looking forward, at what I can do today, which is not drink. If I do that today, I am doing all right, even though I've had rough patches and will have more in the future.

CARLOS: I am Carlos and I am an alcoholic. I was a six-month wonder when I first started coming here. And then my wife left me and I went on a real bender. Kicked my ass real good. Most of my sponsors slip sooner or later, too. It's just the way we are.

MARK: I'm Mark. I'm alcoholic. I don't know. I think it's in the Big Book that Bill W. says the desire to drink will return. That's just the way this disease is. I've been sober for seven years, and I still feel the urge sometimes to chuck everything and go back to drinking. That's when I go to a meeting or call someone for help.

LAWANDA: I'm Lawanda. I'm alcoholic. I am grateful to be here and be sober today. Thank you.

ALAN: I'm Alan. I'm an alcoholic. My slip told me I still had work to do, work on the steps. We don't slip by accident. We slip because we haven't accepted our alcoholism and God's will.

ROGER: My name's Roger and I'm alcoholic. It's tough to admit a slip. It takes guts. [Smiles at Ray.] I appreciate that. That's all I've got. Thanks.

RITA: My name is Rita and I'm an alcoholic. The hardest thing for me about slipping was feeling that I had gotten nowhere, that things were just as bad as ever. When I slipped I felt guilty and terrible from the first drink; it just didn't work for me anymore. And I got back to meetings right away and it was a lot easier than I expected, easier than it was to go to my first meeting. So I think my slip didn't ruin everything, even though it seemed that way. I'm grateful that I haven't slipped in three years, grateful to be here today and be sober.

The discussion continued in this fashion until the meeting was over (usually sixty to ninety minutes).

In addition to meetings, many AA members frequently are in contact with one another outside of group, and often talk to their sponsors outside of meetings. A sponsor is an experienced AA member who helps a newer member through the recovery process. In fact, sponsors frequently directly comment on their member's behavior and character (e.g., "You are making progress" or "You are being grandiose") or provide direct advice (e.g., "Just go to a meeting and don't drink, and you'll be fine").

OUTCOMES

Outcomes research on AA is difficult to conduct because of the lack of professional control over the interventions. Efforts to embed AA into the traditional randomized clinical trials evaluation model tend to distort the phenomenon of interest. For example, Brandsma, Maultby, and Welsh (1980) randomized alcohol-dependent individuals court-ordered to treatment to AA (an artificial chapter) or one of three professionally facilitated psychotherapies. Because of the ubiquitous nature of AA, some individuals in every treatment group and the control group attended community-based AA on their own, thereby receiving higher exposure to real-life AA than did individuals assigned to the artificial, researcher-controlled AA group. Along with the study's 60 percent dropout rate, this fact makes the ultimate finding of no differences on alcohol-related measures between conditions at one-year follow-up rather difficult to interpret. In fact, the main contribution of this study may have been to show how hard it is to study AA using traditional research designs.

A more successful randomized study of AA examined blue-collar workers whose alcohol problems had resulted in their coming into contact with an employee assistance program (Walsh et al. 1991). Seventy-three employees were randomly assigned to compulsory inpatient treatment followed by AA, whereas eighty-three others were assigned to attend community-based AA groups only. Attendance, substance use, and job performance were closely monitored throughout the study. Over a two-year period, both groups showed similar and substantial improvement on twelve job-related performance measures. However, the inpatient treatment plus AA condition had better outcomes on several substance abuse measures. Individuals assigned to the AA-only condition improved on substance use measures in absolute terms, but had more frequent relapses over the course of the study than did the inpatient treatment plus AA group. The AA-only group had 10 percent lower health care costs over the course of study ($1,200), so it may have been more cost-effective even though it was somewhat less effective in purely clinical terms.

Project MATCH (1997) was not a study of AA per se, but deserves attention for its methodological rigor, large sample size, and creation of an intervention that allowed quasirandom assignment to self-help groups without corrupting their nature. 1,726 alcohol-dependent patients were randomly assigned to three professionally facilitated psychotherapies, one of which was Twelve-Step Facilitation Counseling. At one year, patients in all three conditions showed comparable and significant sustained reductions in quantity and frequency of alcohol consumption, but twelve-step facilitation was most effective at promoting abstinence for clients with lower psychological problems.

In a naturalistic study, Humphreys and Moos (1996) studied 201 alcohol-abusing individuals who had contacted detoxification units or alcoholism information and referral services. Of these, 135 individuals initially chose to attend AA, and 66 initially chose to seek professional outpatient treatment. Despite the fact that individuals were not randomly assigned to each condition, at baseline there were no significant differences between groups on demographic variables, alcohol problems, or psychopathology. At one- and three-year follow-up, both groups had improved significantly and comparably on measures of alcohol problems and psychopathology. However, alcohol-related health care costs were 45 percent ($1,826 per person) lower in the AA group.

Finally, Emrick and colleagues (1993) conducted a heroic meta-analysis of over fifty years of AA research. They found a consistent pattern of AA attendance being modestly but positively correlated with reductions in drinking and increases in psychological functioning.

Overall, outcome research on AA must be evaluated in the context of the general state of knowledge in alcohol studies. The effectiveness of many professional psychosocial treatments is still very much in doubt, and there is currently no medication of comparable effectiveness to those for other psychiatric disorders, such as depression. Hence, even though some studies find only modest benefits to AA attendance, this is impressive given that AA is free and many highly expensive alcoholism treatment programs can claim no better results.

TREATMENT PLANNING
AND PRETREATMENT ISSUES

Evaluating Whether a Referral to AA Is Appropriate

AA is an extremely decentralized organization. The tradition in AA is for groups to be autonomous, running their meetings as their members please. All AA meetings, of course, are geared to help alcoholics attain sobriety, but their membership composition, style of expression, group process, physical setting, and informal traditions vary enormously. Certain meetings are for particular populations (e.g., all male or all female, couples, gays/lesbians), or have special purposes (e.g., a meeting devoted to a particular step or an invited speaker). AA has also been adapted and changed by different cultural subgroups (Hoffman 1994; Jilek-aal 1981). Therefore the question of referral is more a question of whether referral to a particular type of AA meeting would be appropriate rather than whether any AA meeting would be appropriate. For this reason, there is no substitute for clinicians having visited local AA groups.

Demographics

Given the increasing diversity within AA, there is no good research evidence for making or not making a referral to AA based on demographic variables. National survey data indicate that this is the referral policy adopted by almost all clinicians in the field (Humphreys 1997).

Spiritual Orientation

In a survey of a national sample of substance abuse treatment personnel, Humphreys (1997) found that about one-third of clinicians had reservations about referring atheists to AA and its sister program, Narcotics Anonymous. The twelve steps mention God and a Higher Power repeatedly; spiritual concerns are woven through AA's literature and most of its members' stories; and many meetings open or close with a prayer. Hence, it is certainly possible that a substance abuse patient who was an atheist (or had some animus against God or spirituality) would feel uncomfortable with these aspects of the AA program. As a matter of civil liberties and clinical ethics, no patient should be pressured to accept any spiritual views or to attend AA. At the same time, patients should be made aware of the flexible nature of AA's concept of spirituality. Indeed, some atheists have recovered through AA, as have people of a variety of religious backgrounds.

Psychopathology

Clinicians have reservations about referring dual-diagnosis patients to AA (Humphreys 1997) for two reasons. First, substance abuse patients who also experience florid psychopathology (e.g., hallucinations) may experience social rejection in AA meetings just as they often do in other settings. Second, AA members may stigmatize medication usage and thereby undermine dual-diagnosis patients' medication compliance and therapeutic progress. Some patients may need assistance in adjusting to AA, in continuing to comply with medication, or in finding alternatives (e.g., the self-help organization Double Trouble, which focuses on dual-diagnosis) if AA does not prove helpful.

Preparing Patients for AA

As with any other type of referral, a patient may not follow through on a clinician's suggestion to try AA. Twelve-Step Facilitation Counseling (Nowinski and Baker 1992) has been shown to substantially increase AA attendance (Project Match 1997), and includes several useful techniques for exploring sources of anxiety about going to meetings, such as describing the twelve steps and the general format of AA meetings in advance, and briefly monitoring compliance.

For clinicians who have developed connections with local AA members, an even more intensive form of referral is possible. If an alcoholic client expresses an interest in AA, an in-session telephone call can be made to an experienced AA member who has volunteered to accompany the therapist's clients to their first AA meeting. In a randomized trial of twenty alcohol outpatients, Sisson and Mallams (1981) evaluated the effectiveness of this intensive method of promoting AA involvement and found that it was substantially superior to simply suggesting that a patient attend and providing them with the time and location of local meetings.

Hence, clinicians need not and should not limit themselves to simply suggesting AA attendance. Dealing with initial anxieties, providing some description of AA, monitoring whether the referral was followed, and making a specific connection to an experienced AA member can all maximize the likelihood that a referral to AA will be successful.

REFERENCES

Alcoholics Anonymous. *Twelve Steps and Twelve Traditions.* New York: AA World Services, 1953.

Alcoholics Anonymous. *Alcoholics Anonymous: The Story of How Many Thousands of Men and Women Have Recovered from Alcoholism,* Third Edition. New York: AA World Services, 1976.

Antze P. The role of ideologies in peer psychotherapy organizations: Some theoretical considerations in three case studies. *Journal of Applied Behavioral Sciences* 12:300-310, 1976.

Brandsma JM, Maultby MC, Welsh RJ. *Outpatient Treatment of Alcoholism: A Review and Comparative Study.* Baltimore, MD: University Park Press, 1980.

Emrick CD, Tonigan JS, Montgomery H, Little L. Alcoholics Anonymous: What is currently known? In *Research Alcoholics Anonymous, Opportunities and Alternatives,* edited by McCrady BS, Miller WR. Piscataway, NJ: Rutgers Center of Alcohol Studies, 1993, pp. 41-76.

Hoffman F. Cultural adaptations of Alcoholics Anonymous to serve Hispanic populations. *International Journal of Addictions* 29(4):445-460, 1994.

Humphreys K. Clinicians' referral and matching of patients to self-help groups after substance abuse treatment. *Psychiatric Services* 48(11):1445-1449, 1997.

Humphreys K, Moos R. Reduced substance abuse-related health care costs among voluntary participants in Alcoholics Anonymous. *Psychiatric Services* 47:709-713, 1996.

Jilek-aal L. Acculturation, alcoholism and Indian style Alcoholics Anonymous. *Journal of Studies on Alcohol* 9:143-158, 1981.

Kessler RC, Mickelson KD, Zhao S. Patterns and correlates of self-help group membership in the United States. *Social Policy* 27:27-46, 1997.

Kishline A. *Moderate Drinking: The Moderation Management Guide for People Who Want to Reduce Their Drinking.* New York: Crown, 1994.

Lieberman MA, Snowden L. Problems in assessing prevalence and membership characteristics of self-help group participants. *Journal of Applied Behavioral Science* 29(2):164-178, 1993.

Narrow WE, Regier DA, Rae DS, Manderscheid RW, Locke BZ. Use of services by persons with mental and addictive disorders. Findings from the National Institute of Mental Health Epidemiologic Catchment Area Program. *Archives of General Psychiatry* 50(2):95-197, 1993.

Nowinski J, Baker S. *The Twelve-Step Facilitation Handbook: A Systematic Approach to Early Recovery from Alcoholism and Addiction.* New York: Lexington Books, 1992.

Project MATCH Research Group. Matching alcoholism treatments to client heterogeneity: Project MATCH posttreatment drinking outcomes. *Journal of Studies on Alcohol* 58:7-29, 1997.

Room R, Greenfield T. Alcoholics Anonymous, other 12-step movements and psychotherapy in the U.S. population, 1990. *Addiction* 88:555-562, 1993.

Sisson RW, Mallams JH. The use of systematic encouragement and community access procedures to increase attandance at Alcoholics Anonymous and Al-Anon meetings. *American Journal of Drug and Alcohol Abuse* 8:371-376, 1981.

Walsh DC, Hingson RW, Merrigan DM, Cupples LA, Levenson SM, Coffman GA. A randomized trial of treatment options for alcohol-abusing workers. *New England Journal of Medicine* 325(11):775-782, 1991.

Weiner, Williams RH, Ozarin ID (eds.). *Community Mental Health.* San Francisco, CA: Jossey-Bass, 1986.

White BJ, Madara EJ. *The Self-Help Sourcebook,* Fifth Edition. Denville, NJ: American Self-Help Clearinghouse, 1995.

SECTION III:
SPECIFIC PATIENT POPULATIONS—
DEMOGRAPHIC ISSUES

Chapter 13

Ethnicity and Culture in the Group Therapy of Substance Abuse

David W. Brook

INTRODUCTION AND DEFINITIONS

Definitions of the concepts of culture, race, and ethnicity are infrequently found in the literature on the psychological and psychosocial treatments of substance abuse. The term "race" usually refers to human genetic variation, and is often marked by particular physical characteristics that are common among a specific group with a limited gene pool and a history of common ancestry. Intragroup variation with regard to physical characteristics or phenotypes, as well as genotypes, is often greater than differences between groups, since racial groups rarely live in isolation. In our racially conscious society, political power, the allocation of resources, and socioeconomic discrimination may be based on racially stereotyped characteristics, particularly with regard to stigmatized and misunderstood behavior, such as substance abuse. Substance abuse may occur among all racial, ethnic, or cultural variations of *Homo sapiens*.

Ethnicity denotes membership in a group of people with a sense of relatedness based on common customs, origins, traits, or cultural and social beliefs or activities. Measures related to ethnicity include ethnic identity, acculturative stress, and the psychosociocultural phenomena of acculturation and marginalization (Phinney 1990). Culture is a related broad term that signifies socially transmitted behaviors, customs, values, activities, and groups that characterize a community of people (Sue, Akutsu, and Higashi 1987). Culture acts to channel and shape the expression of biopsychosocial traits, drives, and needs in specific ways. Culture contains subjective and objective aspects. According to Betancourt and Lopez (1993), aspects of subjective culture include social roles (values, norms, and beliefs), familial roles, styles of communication and emotional expression, attitudes, and spirituality and religiosity. Culture also includes the objective aspects of a group's social organization and daily life, such as housing, tools, weapons, food, transportation, and communication methods, as well as types and patterns of substances use and abuse.

It is important to separate "racial" and "cultural" concepts, especially in research studies. The need to control for cultural, social, and environmental variables in order to avoid finding racial correlations with drug use behaviors that do not really exist is noted in a recent study of crack-cocaine abusers. The results of this study initially revealed racial differences in the use of crack-cocaine. However, further analysis showed that these initial results lacked statistical significance when social factors such as neighborhood risk were controlled (Lillie-Blanton, Anthony, and Schuster 1993). There are a number of cultural and racial stereotypes related to various kinds of substance abuse.

Little clinical or empirical research has been conducted in the area of ethnicity and culture and the group psychotherapy of substance abuse. Early papers dealt with cultural issues related to group therapy in general (Brayboy 1971; Kibel 1972; Slavson 1956), including institutionalized racism. Fenster (1996) felt that group therapy could be used to improve relationships among people of different ethnic and racial groups. A number of investigators also have studied the impact of cultural/ethnic factors on drug abuse treatment. An example is seen in the work of Thompson and Cooper (1988), who studied the importance of culturally sensitive substance abuse treatment in African-American adolescents, including self-acceptance and the examination of beliefs, values, and options in the context of an African-American perspective.

This chapter also reviews the significance of ethnicity and culture in the multiracial group therapy of substance abusers. As more therapists treat minority group patients from many ethnic groups, both patients and therapists must have a greater appreciation than ever of cultural variation and potential biases. In groups for substance abusers, a focused and goal-oriented approach to ethnic and cultural differences may be productive in producing cognitive/behavioral changes in relationships and life goals.

ETHNICITY AND SUBSTANCE ABUSE

The societal context is important in substance abuse treatment. For example, the use of drugs sometimes has been thought to be more common among African Americans than among white Americans, Hispanic Americans, or Asian Americans. However, a number of studies have shown that African Americans (and Asian Americans) use most drugs less frequently than white Americans and Hispanic Americans (Newcomb and Bentler 1986; Johnston, Bachman, and O'Malley 1997). Native Americans were found to have the highest frequency of use of most legal and illegal drugs. In a study of alcohol use among adolescents, African Americans were found to have the largest percentage of abstainers among both males and females (Windle 1991), while Hispanic-American adolescents had a higher rate of frequent drinking. It is difficult to generalize from these findings across the broad ethnic and racial spectrum seen in the United States.

Ethnic or cultural factors influence the expression of symptoms of the substance use disorders. The choice of drugs, the way in which drugs are used, the setting of use, and the behavioral effects of drug use are all influenced by ethnic or cultural factors. In some cultures, certain substances of abuse are thought to have religious or medicinal value. For example, some Native American tribal groups use mescaline or peyote in their religious rituals, and smoking various substances other than tobacco is widely accepted in many cultures, similar to the use of alcohol or caffeine in the United States. The use of coca paste (basuco) or coca leaves among rural natives of the Andes is quite common, and is believed to help people to work productively at hard physical labor in an environment of relative oxygen deprivation. Such culturally determined behaviors that may seem aberrant to observers may appear to be within the range of normality to people belonging to a particular cultural or ethnic group.

Despite many cultural variations, there are striking similarities in the developmental pathways leading to substance use and abuse among different ethnic groups. Brook et al. (1992) found similar mechanisms in the development of patterns of substance use among white, African-American, and Hispanic-American adolescents. Risk-taking behavior, lower school achievement, low mutual parent-child attachment, low peer achievement, peer drug use, and a poor school environment were associated with drug use in several different ethnic groups. Among the personality attributes leading to adolescent drug use, three dimensions are of particular importance: unconventionality, intrapersonal distress, and problem behaviors. Difficulty in the mutual parent-child relationship is associated with the development of drug-prone personality attributes, which, in turn, are related to the selection of deviant peers and to an increased risk of adolescent drug use. Such personality-related risk factors for substance use/abuse include sensation seeking, impulsivity, poor emotional control, associating with drug-using peers, low interest in academic or vocational achievement, and conflicted relationships with family members. These risk factors may be influenced by certain ethnic or cultural factors expressed in the parent-child mutual attachment relationship. Longitudinal research, too, has yielded similar findings regarding risk factors for drug use over time (Brook et al. 1997). Rowe, Vazsonyi, and Flannery (1994) concluded, after statistically analyzing six large data sources that had examined developmental processes in African Americans, Hispanic Americans, non-Hispanic whites, and Asian Americans, that such mechanisms did not vary across U.S. racial and ethnic groups.

Culture, Ethnicity, and the Onset and Maintenance of Substance Abuse

The first issue related to culture/ethnicity and adolescent drug use refers to the construct known as "cultural identity," including knowledge about the culture (such as cultural norms), cultural traditions and behaviors, and language preference and proficiency (Phinney 1992).

The second component refers to "ethnic self-identification," which is the degree to which individuals state and feel that they are a member of a particular group, and includes sociocultural aspects of peer relationships and affiliation. Ethnic identification also contains the emotional and intellectual aspects of "a sense of belonging" to a particular group, as well as identification with particular friends, comprising admiration, modeling behavior, and feeling similar to them.

Cheung (1993) has defined ethnic identification as the way people express their psychological attachment to the particular group on the basis of cultural origin or heritage. The presence of protective factors, such as a strong ethnic identification, may serve to offset the adverse affects of risk factors, such as a troubled parent-child relationship, parental substance use, and poverty.

A more culturally specific example of these kinds of issues is seen in the treatment of Puerto Rican patients. According to the work of Singer (1995) and others, a number of economic, cultural, and emotional factors place Puerto Ricans at risk for substance abuse (Centers for Disease Control and Prevention 1995). Puerto Ricans have high rates of birth, school dropout, households headed by women, unemployment, and social and economic difficulties (Deren 1993; Rodriguez 1989; Rodriguez 1984). Some Puerto Ricans have experienced lack of access to mainstream society, as well as discrimination and ethnic hostility (Rodriguez 1989). Peer approval of drug use, peer drug use, and precocious sexuality are also found in Puerto Rican adolescent drug use. Such risk factors interact with certain specific cultural risk or protective factors. Traditional Puerto Rican values include *machismo, marianismo, familismo,* and *respeto.* Although similar factors are seen in other cultures, these values are of particular note among diverse subcultures within the Hispanic-American tradition.

Machismo is defined as a cluster of traits in men that includes aggression, dominance, authority, adherence to strict sex roles, and non-nurturant tendencies or, as noted by Gil (1996, p. 5), "oppressive male supremacy." Marianismo defines a woman's role in society, and includes duty, religiosity, self-sacrifice, caregiving, chastity, and being subordinate to men. Familismo is a close, protective, supportive, and loving connection with one's extended family, putting the family's needs before one's own needs, especially for women. Respeto can be characterized as showing respect for the power of elders and authority figures and receiving respect in return. Particularly for women, it implies deference to male authority and to one's elders of both sexes.

These cultural values often play a role in Puerto Rican substance abuse, and group therapy for these patients very often requires helping them to change their feelings and behaviors related to these cultural values. For example, some evidence supports that machismo is related to male problem behavior, authoritarian and punitive child-rearing, and limited time spent with children, all of which are risk factors for substance abuse in adolescence. Brook et al. (1998) have hypothesized that Puerto Rican young men who score high on measures of both machismo and unconventionality are more likely to engage in drug use and other problem behaviors than those who score high on machismo and low on unconventionality, so that conventionality may act as a protective factor against the risk involved in scoring high on machismo. Brook et al. (1998) also found that one component of respeto, a nonconflictual parent-child relationship, protected the youngster from drug use and buffered psychosocial risk leading to drug use. In addition, a woman who scores higher on marianismo may be at greater risk at the hands of her husband for abusive behavior involving drug use and HIV transmission, than women who score lower.

These culturally defined examples only touch on the ways in which cultural factors can affect the risks for drug use/abuse, or can act as protective buffers against such risks, and also point to goals of treatment. If the group process can focus on ameliorating these risk factors or enhancing such protective factors, then the patient's liability for drug use/abuse or other risk-taking behavior can be lessened or possibly eliminated.

Another component of ethnic identity is ethnic attachment, which includes one's sense of belonging to a particular group, the amount that one identifies oneself as belonging to the group, and one's attitude toward the group. Ethnic identification signifies identification with friends of similar ethnic background, while ethnic affiliation consists of selecting friends from one's own ethnic background. In a recent study of Puerto Rican adolescents, Brook et al. (1998) found that a strong ethnic identity acted as a protective factor against the risk factors leading to drug use. The results of this study also indicate a goal of treatment for group psychotherapy: if the group can help the patients strengthen their ethnic identity, then the patients will be less likely to participate in drug use/abuse. Thus, the group can focus on a specific culturally relevant goal in order to change the cultural risk factors of the patient liable to use or abuse substances.

Research Findings on Ethnicity/Culture and Substance Abuse

Brook et al. (1992) found that the stages of drug use were similar in both white adolescents and African-American and Puerto Rican adolescents. Certain protective factors were common to both groups, but some were specific to each group; both lessened the risks for drug use. In addition, sexual behavior showed a similar developmental sequence in both ethnic groups. In these early adolescents, the degree of their sexual activities was related to their levels of drug use and their delinquent behavior (Brook et al. 1994). The family as a system, with particular reference to the parent-child relationship, has been the focal point of studies utilizing a model suggested by family interactional theory, with an examination of drug use and ethnicity in their relationships to substance use/abuse (Brook, Brook, Whiteman, Gordon, and Cohen 1990). These studies have implications for prevention and treatment, specifically for the group therapy of substance abusers.

ETHNICITY, CULTURE, AND THE GROUP TREATMENT OF SUBSTANCE ABUSERS

With specific reference to substance abuse treatment, culturally determined attitudes may influence such treatment choices as cognitive-behavioral treatment, modified psychoanalytically oriented group therapy, multifamily group therapy, network therapy, or self-help groups. Culturally determined attitudes about sharing feelings and experiences can also affect substance abusers' readiness for change, and their abilities to participate in a group program involving stages of change, culminating in abstinence. Change may be more acceptable for one gender in a culture than for the other, or for one age group as compared with another age cohort. Racism and its adverse effects on personality, including the development and maintenance of trust and self-esteem, may also affect the substance use disorders in different ethnic groups, and the ability to accept change and achieve abstinence. Readiness for treatment, an important consideration in the group treatment of substance abusers, may be evaluated by using the stages of change of Prochaska and DiClemente (1983).

The cultural values of the group therapist may be opposed to the cultural values of the patient. Therapists are often better educated than their patients and, in the United States, often have values emphasizing empathy, individual achievement, emotional independence from parents and family, self-satisfaction (for example, with work), the establishment of a lasting relationship with a significant other, the development of a nuclear family unit, and the maintenance of financial independence. Although such values are often useful elements in the treatment of substance abusers, and indeed may serve as long-term goals for substance abuse treatment, they may not resemble the values of substance abuse patients coming from other cultures, especially those from traditional or non-Western cultures. In those cultures, values may include ties of interdependence rather than independence, extended family ties over peer relationships, financial and emotional dependence on kin, and taking one's place in a defined role in the familial unit or larger society, rather than setting up and maintaining an independent family unit and trying to achieve individual success.

In the past, few facilities have been available for linguistically competent, professional substance abuse treatments for non–English-speaking minorities, and minority groups have been underrepresented in substance abuse treatment. In addition, in some cultures, the existence of a male dominant gender role (i.e., machismo) may serve to discourage men from seeking appropriate treatment, especially for those who are less acculturated and less educated, with the general result that more women than men have sought substance abuse treatment. In order to take these factors into account, substance abuse treatment programs for members of minority groups, especially for those who are less acculturated, should be bilingual and gender and culturally sensitive, showing acceptance and respect for a patient's culture.

Regarding therapist-patient matching with regard to ethnicity, the use of therapists of the same ethnic background, and perhaps other group members as well, may enhance the development of a protective ethnic identification and a better treatment outcome (Sue, Akutsu, and Higashi 1987; Foulks and Pena 1995). Culturally appropriate treatment plans and interventions may offer the most effective and most cost-effective methods of treatment (Campinha-Bacote 1991).

Clinical Implications of Ethnicity and Culture in Transference and Countertransference Issues in the Treatment of Substance Abusers

Differences and similarities in parent-child interactions, the intrapersonal manifestations of ethnicity (i.e., "Black Pride"), and ethnic influences on peer interactions are important in the process of selection for group and in transference and countertransference considerations. The role of relationships and interactions in the extended family, and the part played in a group by "familism" are influenced by ethnicity and culture, and in turn influence the transferences in the interactions among the members of a substance abuse therapy group.

Comas-Diaz and Jacobsen (1991) have examined the common types of transference reactions seen in therapist-patient interethnic dyads: these can include overcompliance and friendliness, or denial of ethnic and cultural differences. Intraethnic transference reactions include idealization of the therapist as omniscient savior, or as a traitor, or the projection of strong negative feelings to the patient's own ethnic group on to the therapist ("orthoracism"). Because of the history of racism and racial tensions in our society, a white patient may experience "pretransference" feelings to an African-American therapist, which are the result not of the patient's past relationships with others, but rather stem from a collection of preconceived ideas and attitudes (Curry 1964). In addition, particularly with an African-American therapist, a patient may have a reaction to the "superior" status of the therapist by becoming resistant to treatment, showing increased defensiveness, or exhibiting massive denial; this is known as "status contradiction" (Griffith 1977).

With reference to countertransference in an interethnic therapy relationship, the therapist may exhibit a number of reactions, including "the clinical anthropologist's syndrome" (Griffith 1977, pp. 396-397), denial of differences, guilt or pity, or aggression. Ambivalence may stem from the therapist's own ambivalence toward her or his own ethnic heritage (Comas-Diaz and Jacobsen 1991). Overidentification, distancing, "cultural myopia," and survivor's guilt, are manifestations of intraethnic countertransference. These authors stress that all such countertransference and transference reactions influence major therapeutic issues such as trust and anger. The therapist's prejudices, feelings, and interventions in group must be seen as dependent also on the therapist's self-knowledge and self-understanding. Substance abusers are particularly sensitive to such matters because of their hypervigilance, low self-esteem, and hypersensitivity to any suggestions of rejection. Many therapists feel uneasy during discussions of race or culture, and believe that group members might feel poorly understood by the group leader, that racial tensions would have a negative impact on the group process and cohesion, and that racist behavior between group members might occur (Davis, Galinsky, and Schopler 1995).

Transference issues in multiethnic/multicultural groups have also been discussed by Hurdle (1990), who stated that communication among group members of different backgrounds was enhanced by role-playing. Although most theoretical work on transference has taken for granted the influence of the nuclear family, many minority patients or those from non-Western cultures have been reared in extended families with a large contribution of other members of the community. Minority members in a multiethnic group for substance abusers may believe that majority group leaders are incapable of understanding or empathy, or may project societal tensions and experiences on to the leaders. Tsui and Schultz (1988) stress the leader's role as a model for identification for group members, which can enhance group cohesion.

The Relationship of Ethnicity to Pregroup Preparation and Group Cohesion

Multicultural therapy groups for substance abusers have the ability to strengthen ethnic identity and to enhance interpersonal and cross-cultural understanding, and help group members cope with prejudice, both in and out of the group setting.

The development of a therapeutic alliance and group cohesion is particularly important in the treatment of substance abusers from diverse cultural or ethnic backgrounds. Without cohesion, the many therapeutic factors that group therapy can offer in substance abuse treatment cannot be utilized effectively, and the group remains relatively less able to deal with the frustrations of group membership and sharing the therapist. Interactions within the group and transferences can more readily become problematic and difficult to resolve. In a multicultural group of substance abusers, ethnic and cultural factors can have a substantial influence on group cohesion, for better or worse.

The group leader can help the group members openly discuss cultural and ethnic diversity as well as substance abuse, which can help increase group cohesion. The establishment of mutual trust via trust in the group leader is especially helpful for substance abusers, who are particularly vulnerable, both in their self-esteem and their ability to trust other people. Over the course of treatment, with shared concern and knowledge of one another, as group cohesion increases, mutual understanding, respect, and tolerance also increase, and the group process becomes increasingly effective. The following example illustrates these processes:

> Mr. W. was one of two African-American patients in an ongoing multiethnic group composed of one other African-American patient, two Hispanic-American patients, and two white patients. Mr. W. was in treatment because of his recurrent alcohol abuse, with a history of long-standing alcohol addiction. Despite the fact that his life had been consumed by his preoccupation with drinking, Mr. W. was still able to work at a part-time job and maintain his relationship with his wife, although their marriage was a difficult one, primarily because of the effects of his drinking. In the group, the other group members quickly focused on Mr. W.'s comorbid depression. There were some derogatory remarks about African Americans, and Mr. W. initially responded defensively and angrily. The therapist intervened in order to promote the group's discussion of these interactions, but with little success. The group members were particularly critical of Mr. W.'s continued drinking and reports of his abusive treatment of his wife. Eventually, Mr. W. was able to discuss his feelings about the derogatory remarks, and the other group members were more able to show empathy and understand the difficulty Mr. W. had in stopping drinking. The topic of AA was discussed, particularly with reference to AA's acceptance of all people who wanted to stop drinking. This discussion led to some shared feelings about the difficulties a number of the other group members had in changing their behaviors.

White (1994) has presented material to show the effectiveness of multiethnic group psychotherapy. In a group, feelings about ethnicity and ethnic identity can be more pronounced than in a therapist-patient dyad, and can be a measure of group cohesion. Fenster (1996) has noted the effect of racial differences in a group on transference, countertransference, and aspects of reality in the interactions among group members.

If group leaders promote discussion of ethnic and cultural differences in the group, the group interaction is enhanced. With substance abusers in particular, because of their generally low self-esteem and vulnerability to criticism, group therapists must be especially alert to the racial or ethnic composition of the group, particularly if there is an ethnic inequality in the group's composition or where there is a single member of an ethnic or racial minority in the group.

Treatment Techniques for Dealing with Culture/Ethnicity in the Group Treatment of Substance Abusers

As with other groups, the leader sets up the group contract, or "ground rules" with each patient, and guides the development of the culture and norms of the group through interventions, modeling, and limit setting. Differences among group members are noted, as are points of similarity. Some North American group leaders tend to use a psychodynamic group approach and techniques that emphasize revealing and discussing feelings, and examining both intrapersonal and interpersonal conflict in the group (Hurdle 1990; Khantzian 1985). When modified for the treatment of some substance abusers, group members from other cultural/ethnic circumstances may feel anxious or resistant to such an approach. For example, disclosure of feelings or discussion of intimate personal matters may be offensive or produce anxiety among Asian or Asian-American group members (Tsui and Schultz 1988). This may be especially true with regard to illegal substance abuse, which may involve shame, embarrassment, and loss of face. The group leader is likely to be viewed as an authority figure by some Asian or Asian-American group members, who may anticipate that the therapist will play a parental role (Tsui and Schultz 1988).

The group must learn norms that acknowledge and respect differences among people, and that foster a willingness to discuss ethnic, cultural, and racial differences. In the absence of such group norms, group members may experience untoward anxiety. Davis, Galinsky, and Schopler (1995) propose a three-step framework to enhance the treatment of multiethnic/multicultural groups, which can be applied to the group treatment of substance abusers:

1. The group leader should assess the ethnic or cultural differences in the group, particularly in relation to the leader's own cultural attitudes.
2. Leaders should be prepared to respond to ethnic or cultural tensions in the group with an appropriate choice of interventions, to foster a group milieu of tolerance and mutual respect.
3. The group leader should respond appropriately with culturally/ethnically relevant and competent interventions.

The group leader must also try to enhance the development of psychosocial protective factors for substance use/abuse in each group member and in the group as a whole. Such protective factors can include a positive parent-child mutual attachment relationship (even in adult children), a supportive mutual attachment relationship with significant others, a positive attitude toward achievement at work or school, the development of a sense of responsibility in relationships with other people, the development and growth of self-esteem, the development of warm and supportive peer relationships outside of the group, and the growth of social skills at work, with peers, and in the family setting. The group may also play a role in enabling members to explore their own ethnic identities and increase their sense of ethnic identification, which may help substance abusers achieve and maintain an abstinent lifestyle, and enhance harm reduction or relapse prevention efforts.

Acculturation and the Treatment of Substance Abusers

Acculturation difficulties can impede attempts to achieve control over substance abuse, and may result in legal and vocational obstacles. They may interfere with the therapeutic work of the group regarding substance abuse as well as the development of a cohesive group. Cultural understanding and tolerance may help smooth out potentially disruptive group interactions.

Acculturative stress arises when there is conflict between a recent immigrant and members of the dominant culture, or when there is conflict among members of different generations in a family that has recently immigrated. Brook et al. (1998) found differences in drug use between adolescents of Puerto Rican descent born in the United States and those born in Puerto Rico and living in the United States. Parents from more traditional cultures often want their children to conform to traditional ethnic customs, while the children want to become more "American" in their attitudes and behaviors and may have serious clashes with their parents or grandparents about this issue. There may be open conflict among group members about the appropriate attitudes toward substance use/abuse, and group cohesion may suffer unless the group leader helps the group members explore and better understand these cultural differences.

A Chinese-American group member had discussed her family relationships in the group. Although her parents immigrated to this country many years ago from China, they still primarily spoke Chinese and maintained traditional Chinese customs and beliefs. Their daughter, the group member, was born in this country, had attended an elite college, and worked in the travel business. Her adolescent son attended high school, was totally assimilated, and had many "American" friends and interests. Despite the family's attempts to inculcate in him the components of traditional Chinese culture, language, and beliefs, he understood and spoke very little Chinese, but instead spoke idiomatic English without an accent and had some common American adolescent interests. These included experimentation with drugs, which was met with shock and disapproval by his upper middle-class family. Mrs. L. brought up the hurt feelings and distress felt by the family members in the group, with the support of the group leader. She felt confused, anxious, and depressed about her role as the member of the family who was responsible for the communications among the other family members. She was uncertain as to how to deal with her son's drug use, and felt vulnerable to his criticisms of her parents. In the group, she received support, compassion, and understanding, as other group members explored with her their own reactions to drug use in their families. After these revelations, she became more effective in addressing the acculturative stress and conflicts around acculturation in her family and in approaching her son about his drug use.

Similar examples cannot be explored here because of space limitations, but include the high rates of alcoholism and drug abuse, mental illness, dysfunctional families, poverty, and childhood neglect all too frequently seen in the lives of many Native Americans.

CLINICAL RECOMMENDATIONS

The following conclusions concerning the influences of ethnic and cultural issues on the group treatment of substance abusers are based on the results of both research studies and clinical experiences.

1. Early life experiences and development have been influenced by specific ethnic/cultural events and experiences.
2. All of the psychosocial domains that have an impact on substance abuse interact with a number of such ethnic/cultural factors.
3. Different ethnic/cultural groups may have different kinds (and sets) of risk factors for substance abuse, especially in the domains of personality and behavior, child-rearing techniques, and the parent-child mutual attachment relationship.

4. Therefore, different ethnic/cultural groups require different kinds of culturally specific and culturally relevant interventions to bring about change in substance use behavior.
5. The influences of ethnicity and culture on substance abuse occur as group phenomena, through participation and involvement in one or more groups, and so they are especially significant for group psychotherapy.
6. Ethnic and cultural experiences around substance use/abuse are transferred from a culture to an individual through involvement in a variety of kinds of groups.
7. An assessment of such cultural and ethnic influences concerning substance use should be made a part of each patient's treatment plan.

These considerations lead us to specific recommendations for culturally aware treatment:

1. A culturally relevant, biopsychosocial approach is necessary for appropriate assessment and evaluation for group therapy of patients who are substance abusers.
2. Group therapists must consider the interplay between ethnic and psychodynamic factors and the role of culture in channeling biopsychological drives.
3. Cross-cultural conflicts may influence the substance-related behavior of group members.
4. In a multicultural group for the treatment of substance abuse, the therapist should understand the influences of ethnicity/culture on the interactions in the group and on group cohesion, as well as on the development and maintenance of substance abuse.
5. Ethnicity/culture and substance abuse can be addressed in many contexts, both in time-limited and long-term groups, and in a variety of treatment settings.
6. Ethnic and cultural issues have profound effects on such group dynamic factors as transference, countertransference, and resistance. If these ethnic influences are not discussed openly in the group or by the group therapist, especially if they involve substance abuse directly, the group's cohesion can be adversely af-

fected, with the loss of the therapeutic effectiveness of the group.

7. The therapists must be knowledgeable about and comfortable with their own feelings and attitudes about their ethnicity and culture, as well as the ethnicity and cultural beliefs of the group members, particularly with regard to issues of substance abuse and ethnic identification. Countertransference reactions and negative or hostile feelings influence the therapeutic effects of the group.

CONCLUSIONS

Ethnic and cultural factors play a significant role in the practice of group psychotherapy and in the group treatment of substance abusers. Since we live in a social milieu in which ethnic and cultural diversity are increasingly common, group therapists must pay attention to the influences of such factors to enhance therapeutic effectiveness in the group treatment of substance abusers.

REFERENCES

Betancourt H, Lopez SR. The study of culture, ethnicity, and race in American psychology. *American Psychologist* 48:629-637, 1993.

Brayboy T. The black patient in group therapy. *International Journal of Group Psychotherapy* 21:288-293, 1971.

Brook JS, Balka EB, Abernathy T, Hamburg BA. Sequences of sexual behavior in African-American and Puerto Rican adolescents. *Journal of Genetic Psychology* 155(2):147-149, 1994.

Brook JS, Brook DW, Whiteman M, Gordon AS, Cohen P. The psychosocial etiology of adolescent drug use and abuse. *Genetic Social and General Psychology Monographs* 116(2):111-267, 1990.

Brook JS, Whiteman M, Balka EB, Hamburg BA. African-American and Puerto Rican drug use: Personality, familial, and other environmental risk factors. *Genetic Social and General Psychology Monographs,* 118:417-438, 1992.

Brook JS, Whiteman M, Balka EB, Win PT, Gursen MD. African-American and Puerto Rican drug use: A longitudinal study. *Journal of the American Academy of Child and Adolescent Psychiatry* 36:1260-1268, 1997.

Brook JS, Whiteman M, Balka EB, Win PT, Gursen MD. Drug use among Puerto Ricans: Ethnic identity as a protective factor. *Hispanic Journal of Behavioral Science* 20(2):241-254, 1998.

Campinha-Bacote J. Community mental health services for the under-served: A culturally specific model. *Archives of Psychiatric Nursing* 5:229-235,1991.

Centers for Disease Control and Prevention. *HIV/AIDS Surveillance Report* 7(2): 5-39, 1995.

Cheung YW. Approaches to ethnicity: Clearing roadblocks in the study of ethnicity and substance use. *International Journal of Addictions* 28:1209-1226, 1993.

Comas-Diaz L, Jacobsen FM. Ethnocultural transference and countertransference in the therapeutic dyad. *American Journal of Orthopsychiatry* 61:392-402, 1991.

Curry AE. Myth, transference and the black psychotherapist. *Psychoanalytic Review* 51:7-14, 1964.

Davis LE, Galinsky MJ, Schopler JH. RAP: A framework for leadership of multi-racial groups. *Social Work* 40:155-165, 1995.

Deren S, Beardsley M, Tortu S, Davis R, Clatts M. Behavior change strategies for women at high risk for HIV. *Drugs & Society* 7:119-128, 1993.

Fenster A. Group therapy as an effective treatment modality for people of color. *International Journal of Group Psychotherapy* 46:399-416, 1996.

Foulks EF, Pena JM. Ethnicity and psychotherapy: A component in the treatment of cocaine addiction in African Americans. *Psychiatric Clinics of North America: Cultural Psychiatry* 18:607-620, 1995.

Gil RM, Vazquez CI. *The Maria Paradox*. New York: GP Putnam's Sons, Inc., 1996.

Griffith MW. The influences of race on the psychotherapeutic relationship. *Psychiatry* 40:27-40, 1977.

Hurdle DE. The ethnic group experience. *Social Work with Groups* 13:59-69, 1990.

Johnston LD, Bachman JG, O'Malley PM. *Monitoring the Future: Questionnaire Responses from the Nation's High School Seniors, 1995*. Ann Arbor, MI: University of Michigan, Institute for Social Research, 1997.

Khantzian EJ. Psychotherapeutic interventions with substance abusers—the clinical context. *Journal of Substance Abuse Treatment* 2(2):83-88.

Kibel HD. Interracial conflicts as resistance in group psychotherapy. *American Journal of Psychotherapy* 26:555-562, 1972.

Lillie-Blanton M, Anthony JC, Schuster CR. Probing the meaning of racial/ethnic group comparisons in crack cocaine smoking. *JAMA* 269:993-997, 1993.

Newcomb MD, Bentler PM. Substance use and ethnicity: Differential impact of peer and adult models. *Journal of Psychology* 120(1):83-95, 1986.

Phinney JS. Ethnic identity in adolescents, and adults: Review of research. *Psychological Bulletin* 108:499-514, 1990.

Phinney JS. The multigroup ethnic identity measure: A new scale for use with diverse groups. *Journal of Adolescent Research* 7(2):156-176, 1992.

Prochaska JO, DiClemente CC. Stages and processes of self-change of smoking: Toward an integrative model of change. *Journal of Consulting and Clinical Psychology* 51(3):390-395, 1983.

Rodriguez C. *Puerto Ricans Born in the USA.* Boston, MA: Unwin Hyman, 1989.

Rodriguez O, Burger W, Banks L. *Crime Rates Among Hispanics, Blacks, and Whites in New York City.* Research Bulletin 71(2), Hispanic Research Center, Fordham University, 1984.

Rowe DC, Vazsonyi AT, Flannery DJ. No more than skin deep: Ethnic and racial similarity in developmental processes. *Psychological Review* 101:396-413, 1994.

Singer M. Providing substance abuse treatment to Puerto Rican clients living in the continental United States. In *Substance Abuse Treatment in the Era of AIDS,* edited by Amulezu-Marshall O. Rockville, MD: Center for Substance Abuse Treatment, 1995, pp. 93-140.

Slavson SR. Racial and cultural factors in group psychotherapy. *International Journal of Group Psychotherapy* 2:152-165, 1956.

Sue S, Akutsu PD, Higashi C. Training issues in conducting therapy with ethnic-minority-group clients. In *Handbook of Cross-Cultural Counseling and Therapy,* edited by Pedersen P. New York: Praeger, 1987, pp. 275-280.

Thompson T, Cooper C. Chemical dependency treatment and black adolescents. *Journal of Drug Issues* 18(1):21-31, 1988.

Tsui P, Schultz GL. Ethnic factors in group process: Cultural dynamics in multi-ethnic therapy groups. *American Journal of Orthopsychiatry* 58:136-142, 1988.

White JC. The impact of race and ethnicity on transference and countertransference in combined individual/group therapy. *Group* 18:89-99, 1994.

Windle M. Alcohol use and abuse: Some findings from the National Adolescent Student Health Survey. *Alcohol Health and Research World* 15(1):5-10, 1991.

Chapter 14

Group Treatment
for Women Substance Abusers

Valerie Gibbs

INTRODUCTION

Traditionally, diagnostic criteria for alcoholism have been based upon familiar male behavioral characteristics, yet women diagnosed with alcoholism have been seen as evidencing greater pathology and poorer outcome when compared to their male counterparts (Vannicelli 1989; Wilsnack et al. 1991). For example, the focus when treating women with alcoholic behavior changes (i.e., excessive acting out, anger, or stubbornness and moodiness) was to help to establish "sober attitudes," such as acting more "mature," like the "good girl," the young lady, the devoted wife, and unconditionally loving mother and homemaker.

Despite various research studies concerning behavioral variables and substance abuse (i.e., treatment and outcome), little empirical data concerning the complex roles of gender differences within and across cultural behaviors have been applied to substance abuse treatment (Miller and Hester 1986; Nelson-Zlupko, Kauffman, and Dore 1995).

HISTORICAL PERSPECTIVE

The women's movement in the 1960s fostered an environment in which early feminist practitioners challenged the underlying assumptions of the prevailing women's treatment model (i.e., to allow for the exclusive, expected role of being in the home and mothering children). Feminists retaliated strongly against the chauvinistic model, stating their own views. For example, although men saw women as subjects of utility, these feminists felt they could develop themselves independently by repudiating the usual feminine roles, such as maternity.

Theories of feminist therapy first began to appear in the literature in the 1960s and 1970s (Reed and Garvin 1996). A number of early theorists believed that all-women groups were necessary for women (Sturdivant 1980). Many authors documented the influence of pervasive sex-role stereotypes in therapy, and their influences on definitions of mental health, which played a role in the goals of treatment, diagnosis, and hospitalization. Freud's assumptions about the psychology of women were questioned, and the fallacy of blaming women for acts of violence against them was explored (Brownmiller 1975). Some of the limitations of therapy for women based on theory and data were delineated, as were differences in function and outcome in treatment groups composed of men, women, and mixed gender groups.

With reference to the development of substance abuse, correlations were noted between sexual and physical abuse and the later development of substance abuse. The high level of sexual abuse of female children was shown to be real (Rush 1980), and its consequences for the later development of substance use disorders and their treatments were elaborated. A number of theorists developed feminist therapy interventions, and some authors focused on such interventions in groups (Reed and Garvin 1983; Brody 1987; Butler and Wintram 1991). The application of a feminist or gender-sensitive approach to psychodynamic group practice in general was recently the focus of an excellent chapter by Reed and Garvin (1996), and a number of important concepts and suggested types of approach were examined in DeChant's excellent collection of papers on the topic (DeChant 1996).

Over the past decade, a clearer, more balanced definition of women's roles in society has emerged (Blume 1994; Chodorow 1989). Gender role changes, however, have been slow even in comparison to the gradual accretion of various changes within the legal system and government, politics, economics, and culture. The vast majority of national mental health treatment models that focus on family support systems still rely on traditional role patterns; the father's role is depicted as a desirable position of independence, whereas the mother's role is depicted as a dangerous symbol of regressive merger and unwanted dependence. Many of these polarized views are the result of society's difficulty in giving value to dependent and affectionate behaviors, which are traditionally associated with females. Valian (1998) has discussed thoroughly some of the internalized changes within women and men that may have hindered the emergence of gender role equality, both intrapsychically and within relationships and societal institutions.

Unfortunately, many of the traditional, chauvinistic assumptions and expectations about women are still alive, especially those concerning female substance abusers. The argument against such stereotyped limitations is that the context in which people live mediates the association between gender and alcohol-related problems. Concerning gender risks for substance abuse, in general, more successful developmental guidelines for recovery for women, as well as men, can be established with greater specificity. "Modernity" versus "traditionality," with respect to women's place in society, allows for a reworking of gender risks and gender differences in the process of recovery from substance abuse problems. In substance abuse treatment settings, it is well recognized that women who appear to behave too emotionally (i.e., too angry, too "hysterical," too dependent, or too passive), may be quickly diagnosed as depressed, or worse, character disordered. A primary or secondary diagnosis for these women is often purely psychiatric, with substance abuse or dependence taking a distant back seat.

Unfortunately, disagreement still exists with respect to women's alcohol dependence problems. With regard to comorbid diagnoses, even though research and case-study literature advocates the success of treating substance abuse first, especially with the diagnosis of depression, there is disagreement over treatment. If women continue to be diagnosed using a combination of male-oriented diagnostic criteria and negative female stereotyping, there will continue to be underdetection of alcohol-related problems in women, stigmatization of women alcoholics, and underutilization of alcohol treatment services by women (Wilsnack and Wilsnack 1995).

Many treatment settings have begun to challenge traditional beliefs by integrating feminist principles into contemporary cognitive-behavioral models. With respect to cognitive-behavioral concerns, treatment of substance-abusing women is concerned primarily with maladaptive thinking patterns. It should be noted that 40 to 50 percent of substance abuse patients have mild to moderate cognitive problems while using drugs; these problems usually remit with abstinence (Zerbe 1999). A number of maladaptive thinking patterns are commonly found in substance abuse with respect to assertiveness or sexuality, which lend themselves to social immaturity and negative symptoms. Such negative outlooks or dichotomous "black and white" thoughts need to be modified to assist recovery.

Other targets for treatment include low self-esteem, "all or none" assessments of self and others, feelings of anger and jealousy regarding other women caused by oppression or by forms of institutionalized discrimination (i.e., the "glass ceiling" noted by women in many work settings), mother-daughter issues at work, and fear of male hostility or repression. These issues are of special relevance for women substance abusers because of their effects on self-image and achievement orientation, which are so important as protective and curative factors for such women. Overcoming societal limitations and expectations regarding the abilities and achievements of women can have important therapeutic effects, and group treatment can be a useful method of helping women substance abusers achieve these goals and substitute positive achievements and successful relationships for self-destructive connections with substances of abuse.

PRETREATMENT ISSUES: GENDER AND GROUPS

Although many substance abuse treatment and training group models do not actively explore how and to what extent group process factors should be fostered, social skills training and treatment models should actively include interpersonal group process strategies. Such strategies can encourage motivation for learning and can facilitate the creation of interpersonal relationships among group members.

Controversy exists as to whether men and women should be treated in single-sex or mixed group settings. Levine (Levine and Moreland 1990) believes mixed-gender groups are most successful for treating substance abuse clients because mixed groups remind people of their conventional and expected gender roles which, in turn, lead them to redefine their roles, either through personal choice or through group persuasion. Other advocates of heterogeneous groups state that this awareness of traditional stereotypes can help examine, enlighten, and moderate the impact of group functioning. For example, mixed-gender groups offer the opportunity to examine the adverse qualities of female nurturing and the destructive nature of male separateness and dominance. Ideally, men and women can be mutually supportive in mixed-gender groups, particularly with regard to examining and dealing with societal sexist attitudes and restrictions on women's roles. This can occur both in the context of the group, as noted above, and with respect to giving each other mutual support for coping with such issues in the real world. It is important to keep in mind that women substance abusers may face numerous difficulties, both overt and covert, with regard to their participation as active group members. Women often incorporate sex-role stereotypes and culturally imposed behavioral restrictions into their intrapsychic and interpersonal mental representations and interactions beginning in early childhood. If an examination of gender roles does not permit dependable, consistent, and confident self-assessment, women need to decide for themselves which nurturing behaviors they enjoy and which they believe may be harmful.

With regard to dynamic and developmental gender differences, unlike boys, girls do not completely separate from their mothers when they reach adulthood. Significantly most girls utilize internalization and involvement in relationships in the resolution of identity issues, while boys seek their identity by utilizing externalizing roles to build self-confidence and clarify identity issues (Benjamin 1993).

This difference may be a rationale for the use of homogeneous groups for women. For long-term groups, investigation into how female development may be derailed by both social and psychological forces in childhood, adolescence, and/or early adulthood may be useful for sustained recovery from substance abuse. Of particular relevance is the connection between early sexual abuse and later substance abuse (Brook 1996). Sexual abuse is experienced by about one-third of women in childhood (Gordon and Riger 1989), and the ramifications of this common experience, as well as later sexual harassment and discrimination, should be a focus of examination in a group for female substance abusers. This issue and the traumatic fears that result should be addressed both as intrapsychic representations and as real events in the lives of these women. Women substance abusers are frequently exploited sexually, or trade sex for drugs out of despair, depression, poverty, and feelings of low self-esteem and helplessness. This is now a major reason why HIV infection is increasing so rapidly among these women, especially in marginalized minority groups (Brook et al. 1999).

In dynamic terms, in order to recognize, validate, and affirm their individual insights and to accomplish the necessary identification with other group members, women benefit from being with other women in a homogeneous group. This ideology clearly contradicts the idea that women depend upon and need validation of self-worth from men. In a homogeneous group, women are able to relate to others quickly, which facilitates group cohesion and enhances support and validation among group members. Together, women's perceptions of their roles in group and their roles as models are strengthened. Moreover, the homogeneous collective identification and support is essential for exploring alternate responses to situational difficulties. A particular situational difficulty for women substance abusers is the occurrence of pregnancy. A group for women substance abusers may be a particularly useful setting for such women to explore sensitive issues including the higher risk of fetal abnormalities, such as fetal alcohol syndrome or "crack babies," in pregnant substance abusers. In addition, risks for relapse associated with the postpartum period may be usefully explored in a women's group.

This chapter presents a description and assessment of the importance of an interpersonal cognitive-behavioral model in the treatment of substance-abusing women. Cognitive-behavioral techniques for instruction, modeling of various roles, and group process strategies will be described within three group stages: Early, Middle, and Later. Such interventions increase motivation for learning, improve acquisition of social skills, and enhance overall social competence, as the therapeutic group process itself appears to reduce negative symptoms by increasing motivation for social learning. Group members learn to participate fully in the social world and act as vehicles of social learning without the sustained use of chemical substances. Patients manage affect and test reality using interpersonal behavioral and problem-solving techniques. In fact, the use of cognitive-behavioral and interpersonal group process strategies may offer the most comprehensive and dynamic social skills treatment package for women substance abusers.

The application of cognitive-behavioral social skills techniques combined with group process strategies may, in the future, fill the gap between outcome research on social skills and research on social competence in the substance abuse population. Preliminary data collected in the past five years, with a regimented follow-up (six and twelve months; 79.5 percent retrieval of subjects by telephone contacts, yield of 68 percent abstinence), compares the efficacy of these groups with other women's abstinent treatment groups and suggests more positive changes in social functioning for significant lengths of time during recovery. The research tested the following hypotheses:

1. Women's Substance Abuse Groups-Interpersonal Cognitive-Behavioral Model of Treatment (WSAG-ICBMT) will increase the overall social competence of substance-abusing women who exhibit sustained abstinence.
2. WSAG-ICBMT will improve the negative symptoms often associated with poor treatment for women diagnosed with substance abuse disorders.
3. WSAG-ICBMT will facilitate the emergence of those therapeutic group process factors found to enhance social competence in women with substance abuse.

TREATMENT AND TECHNIQUE

Patients engaged in this study were referred from two large metropolitan medical teaching hospitals (i.e., the Ambulatory Outpatient Clinic and the Adult Continuing Day Treatment Program). These sites were selected because they were frequently chosen by patients in recovery from substance abuse who, in many instances, exhibited comorbid depression. All willing patients who met the DSM-IV (American Psychiatric Association 1994) diagnostic criteria for substance abuse or substance dependence disorder were screened and evaluated by a doctoral-level clinician and an experienced diagnostician. Patients who currently were noncompliant with medication, or who had a history of schizophrenia or a schizoaffective disorder within the last year, were excluded from the study. Those with a history of moderate to severe neurological impairment or mental retardation, or those who were considered psychiatrically unstable as defined by scores of 5+ (maximum score per item = 7) in adaptation to substance abuse or in the Positive and Negative Syndrome Scale domains (i.e., conceptual disorganization, pseudohallucinatory behavior, or unusual content of thought), were also excluded (Kay, Fiszbein, and Opler 1987).

After being screened and giving informed consent, forty subjects (mean age = 33.7 years, age range 19-61), over the course of several years, were included in this treatment.

Subjects were not randomly assigned to group treatment, but were assigned upon finishing intake and preparation procedures when the appropriate number of group members (n = 10) were available. Groups followed a fifteen-session format meeting of fifty minutes per session. Each group met once a week and had two leaders. Group leaders were required to have a minimum of three years' Interpersonal Cognitive-Behavioral Group Treatment (ICBGT) supervision experience. The coleader was required to have a minimum of one year of supervisory experience and two years of experience working with substance abuse populations.

The Role of the Leader

The tasks of the leaders included offering and facilitating the use of cognitive-behavioral techniques by the group members. Leaders were also available for support and modeling, teaching social skills, acting to help group members test reality, and helping group members learn to avoid using self-destructive patterns of thought and behavior. Moreover, leaders collected data, actively facilitated interactions between group members, and utilized modified interpersonal group process techniques. They assisted the group members in setting group goals, making effective use of feedback, and actively helping the group members during the termination phase.

Treatment Stages and Phases of Group Development

Each Interpersonal Cognitive-Behavioral Treatment (ICBT) session was divided into four phases: Orientation and Cognitive Networking Phase, Warm-up and Sharing Phase, Enactment Phase, and Affirmation and Termination Phase. There were fifteen group sessions evenly subdivided into stages: Early (five sessions), Middle (five sessions), and Later (five sessions).

(1) Orientation and Networking Phase (Fifteen . . . Three to Five Minutes)

In the Orientation and Cognitive Networking Phase, leaders encouraged and facilitated social interactions among group members. For instance, the leader would make the following statement: "Evelyn, your comments seem to suggest that you understand the issue Joanne is raising. What might Joanne be feeling about the issue?" This phase began as a ten- to fifteen-minute segment but, with the introduction of group process factors (altruism and self-disclosure), its duration was changed to an average of three to five minutes by session eight.

(2) Warm-up and Sharing Phase (Fifteen Minutes)

During the Warm-up and Sharing Phase, the second phase of the treatment model, a strong emphasis was placed on self-disclosure. Members were encouraged to share concerns or personal issues with other group participants:

At the ninth session, Sally, a thirty-eight-year-old single professional accountant with a twelve-year history of substance abuse, reflected how strange she felt having finally divulged so many intricacies surrounding her alcohol abuse with someone other than her long-term individual therapist. Although she had read a lot of material on substance abuse disorders and could relate to many of the cited personal accounts, she had always believed that these afflicted individuals would somehow look and act totally different than she. It surprised her that some of the other members had similar lengthy substance abuse histories and that they too had become masters in deception, hiding from view their intense feelings of loneliness and low self-esteem.

Having worked predominantly with males, she was not accustomed to relating to females. In fact, she regarded herself as superior to other women and had always held the general belief that females were 'flighty, catty, and mistrustful.' These revelations triggered other members to reflect both on their initial personal disclosures and on their perceptions of the women's group. Moreover, throughout this brief discussion, many members interjected their relief that members were understanding and accepting; they expressed the notion that the group was beginning to feel safe for them.

(3) The Enactment Phase (Twenty Minutes)

During the twenty-minute Enactment Phase, an interpersonal situation was created by each patient, which included group members as active participants. This phase involved certain basic elements: (1) using an interpersonal group process technique, (2) directing an encounter, and (3) using cognitive-behavioral strategies. An average of three enactments per group session was typical over the course of treatment.

To foster therapeutic group process factors typically associated with positive treatment outcome (i.e., cohesion, universality, and learning/modeling), we included the following modified interpersonal group process techniques: doubling, role reversal, and future projection (i.e., relapse issues).

Doubling. With doubling, the protagonist (participant) was encouraged to express feelings evoked by an interpersonal situation. Another group member was then asked to represent and establish identity with the protagonist by verbalizing what the group member thought the protagonist was feeling. The group member, in effect, confirmed the accuracy of her own feelings by "checking in" with the protagonist. In multiple doubling, more than one group participant was asked to identify with the protagonist. This created multiple perspectives for both the protagonist and other group members, and provided the protagonist with a feeling of being understood and supported. The following is an example of such doubling:

Alice, a twenty-seven-year-old who complained of depression, loneliness, and a lack of direction in life, typically presented herself as passive, calculating, accommodating, and self-deprecating. Anything she vocalized was predictably preceded by a scanning of the faces of leaders and members so to receive clues as to what they would want to hear. She eventually began to challenge this defense and to show herself as more uninhibited and opinionated. She appointed someone in group to assist her in this effort. She also began to notice that other group members were more interested in her opinions. Group members told her that her former meekness was often boring and that the more she expressed her own desires and feelings, the more they were attracted to her. Thereafter she was able to gain insight into her fears of abandonment and rejection and her subsequent need to play it "safe." She eventually became very popular and well liked in the group, which helped bolster her self-esteem and provide her with the needed encouragement to begin taking more risks in her personal life.

Role Reversal. Although doubling proves helpful, the "role reversal" technique provides both role clarification and reality testing, for the protagonist is asked to "step into the other's shoes." During the Enactment Phase within the Middle Stage (ninth session), role reversal members took the opportunity to focus on the roles they assumed in group, which often mirrored those assumed in outside relationships. Considerable interpersonal learning took place as members experimented with new and modified roles. The following is an example of role reversal:

> Mary, a thirty-three-year-old, became aware of her tendency to adopt a very sociable, mediating, and cotherapeutic role within the group that paralleled the role she assumed in her family and among her friends. She was very supportive of other members, attempting to ensure that everyone had an opportunity to participate. She filled silences in the discussions, endeavored to keep the group on a positive emotional tone, and assumed a peacekeeping position whenever she sensed friction between members. Although helpful to the group in its formative stage, Mary's rigidity within this role began to restrict the group's progression into different phases. With the assistance and encouragement of the group to relinquish this role, Mary gradually began to experiment with new roles despite her extreme anxiety and fear that things would fall apart if she were not "on hand to glue them back together."
>
> By "putting on others' shoes," Mary was able to demonstrate more role flexibility within the group, which would allow more flexibility in her outside roles. Thus she was able to confront the "parentified" position she had adopted as a preteen In response to the distress of her parents and their helplessness surrounding the rebelliousness and acting-out behavior of her older teenage sister. She gained insight into how her development of excessive drinking and drug abuse paradoxically helped her to maintain some semblance of self-control and coping.

Future Projection. With "future projection," during the Middle or Later Stage of group and specifically with relapse issues, the protagonist acted out how she wanted her future to shape itself by selecting a point in time, a place, and the people with whom she expected to be involved. Relapse targets, as future projections during the Enactment Phase, also were incorporated. For example, when a group member or members were interacting with strong affects of anger or sadness with others in the group, members were trained to interrupt the interactions at sensitive points to illustrate the group's experience of tension and high emotion, reactions that were likely to occur outside of the group. Simultaneously, the group identified with the individual group member's experience, thereby providing the benefits of living through "the pressure" of an intense interaction. The group gave support to the individual member(s) in adopting momentarily the role of witness, separating emotionality from impulsive responses.

These experiences within the supportive environment helped the individual group member to entertain the idea of replacing impulse with reasoned response. Once this skill was practiced, it provided each member with a clear and integrated experiential approach to behavior changes emerging from a newly evolving sense of self. Moreover, reinforcing these behavior changes demonstrated that one had achieved a level of mastery over areas that formerly produced overwhelming anxiety, failure, and unrealistic fears.

Following the use of group process techniques, the individual was given affective, behavioral, and cognitive feedback. She, along with other group participants, gained practice in cognitive-behavioral strategies including modeling and behavioral rehearsal. The group also offered alternative solutions to the interpersonal problems presented, allowing the individual to role-play or enact a new response.

(4) Affirmation and Termination Phase

Nearing the end of group treatment, specifically at the Later Stage of group treatment with approximately three group meetings left, the Affirmation and Termination Phase became lengthened to ten to fifteen minutes. During this important period, group development, including the termination of group treatment, was critical to the group developmental process and served as an important force in promoting the continuation of change. The group task entailed the disengagement of members in such a manner so that they could function without feeling a sense of demoralization or hopelessness. Group members gave up the safe, containing environment of the group. This crucial development and its threatened loss might have precipitated all the original self-definition issues.

Here too, the focus of cognitive-behavioral attention was centered on events and issues external to the group. Future plans and ambitions were compared and contrasted with events that had occurred in the group and the progress of individual members. This assisted the group members in assimilating the group as a personally significant and enduring experience. Each member's task was to accept personal responsibility for her behavior without the presence or support of the group. The leaders also personally participated in the termination process.

In the last session, emphasis was placed on the reality of termination. To say good-bye to one another was an emotionally laden experience for members who knew they might never see one another again due to life circumstances. The termination of group at the end of the fifteenth session allowed positive emotional closure, which further enhanced the group process and future relationships by fostering universality, cohesiveness, and increased motivation.

SUMMARY

In general, the preliminary observational data supported all three hypotheses: (1) the WSAG-ICBMT leads to an increase in overall social competence for individuals diagnosed with substance abuse; (2) the effects of ICBMT lead to a reduction of negative symptoms, which increases overall psychosocial functioning; (3) the possible emergence of therapeutic group process factors suggested that ICBMT was a salient facilitator of many of the therapeutic group process factors found by researchers to be instrumental in enhancing overall social functioning (Yalom 1995).

Women's Substance Abuse Groups-Interpersonal Cognitive-Behavioral Model of Treatment offers women an important modality of treatment. The holding environment and social microcosm created in the women's group provides an effective means for addressing the cognitive skills to deal with distortions and self-deficits that typify substance abuse. Resolution of these issues allows the individual to mature toward improved social skills, self-regulation, integration, and the experience of greater autonomy and improved self-esteem. The peer interaction available in the group modality offers the unique advantage of identifying overall social function and competence. The group also offers an inclusive approach to the reduction of negative symptoms.

REFERENCES

American Psychiatric Association. *Diagnostic and Statistical Manual of Mental Disorders,* Fourth Edition. Washington, DC: American Psychiatric Association, 1994.

Benjamin LS. *Interpersonal Diagnosis and Treatment of Personality Disorders.* New York: Guilford Press, 1993.

Blume SB. Gender differences in alcohol-related disorders. *Harvard Review of Psychiatry* 2(1):7-14, 1994.

Brody CM (ed.). *Women's Therapy Groups: Paradigms of Feminist Treatment.* New York: Springer, 1987.

Brook DW. Adolescents who abuse substances. In *Group Therapy with Children and Adolescents,* edited by Kymissis P, Halperin D. Washington, DC: American Psychiatric Press, Inc., 1996, p. 248.

Brook DW, Brook JS, Richter L, Whiteman M, Win PT, Masci JR, Roberto J. Coping strategies of HIV-positive and HIV-negative female injection drug users: A longitudinal study. *AIDS Education and Prevention* 11(5), 373-388, 1999.

Brownmiller S. *Against Our Will: Men, Women, and Rape.* New York: Simon & Schuster, 1975.

Butler S, Wintram C. *Feminist Groupwork.* Newbury Park, CA: Sage, 1991.

Chodorow N. *Feminism and Psychoanalytic Theory.* New Haven, CT: Yale University Press, 1989.

DeChant B. *Women and Group Psychotherapy: Theory and Practice.* New York: The Guilford Press, 1996.

Gordon MT, Riger S. *The Female Fear.* New York: Free Press, 1989.

Kay SR, Fiszbein A, Opler LA. The positive and negative syndrome scale (PANSS) for schizophrenia. *Schizophrenia Bulletin* 13:261-276, 1987.

Levine JM, Moreland RL. Progress in small group research. In *The Annual Review of Psychology,* edited by Rosenzweig MR, Porter LW. Palo Alto, CA: Annual Reviews, 1990, pp. 585-634.

Miller WR, Hester RK (eds.). *The effectiveness of alcoholism treatment: What research reveals.* New York: Plenum Press, 1986.

Nelson-Zlupko L, Kauffman E, Dore M. Gender differences in drug addiction and treatment: Implications for social work intervention with substance-abusing women. *Social Work* 40:45-54, 1995.

Reed BG, Garvin CD (eds.). *Groupwork with Women/Groupwork with Men.* Binghamton, NY: The Haworth Press, 1983.

Reed BG, Garvin CD. Feminist psychodynamic group psychotherapy: The application of principles. In *Women and Group Psychotherapy: Theory and Practice,* edited by DeChant B. New York: Guilford Press, 1996, pp. 127-154.

Rush F. *Best Kept Secret: Sexual Abuse of Children.* Englewood Cliffs, NJ: Prentice-Hall, 1980.

Sturdivant S. *Therapy with Women.* New York: Springer, 1980.

Valian V. *Why So Slow? The Advancement of Women.* Cambridge, MA: MIT Press, 1998.

Vannicelli M. *Group Psychotherapy: Adult Children of Alcoholics.* New York: Guilford Press, 1989.

Wilsnack SC, Klassen AD, Schur BE, Wilsnack RW. Predicting onset and chronicity of women's problem drinking: A five-year longitudinal analysis. *American Journal of Public Health,* 81:305-318, 1991.

Wilsnack SC, Wilsnack RW. Drinking and problem drinking in U.S. women. Patterns and recent trends. *Recent Developments in Alcoholism* 12:29-60, 1995.

Yalom ID. *The Theory and Practice of Group Psychotherapy,* Fourth Edition. New York: Basic Books, 1995.

Zerbe KJ. *Women's Mental Health in Primary Care.* Philadelphia, PA: WB Saunders & Co., 1999.

Chapter 15

Group Therapy for Substance Abuse with Gay Men and Lesbians

David M. McDowell

INTRODUCTION

The variety of sexual expression is as varied as humans are themselves; consequently, sexuality should be understood as complex and nuanced. Throughout history, individuals have loved and have had sexual relationships with members of their own sex. Sometimes, like-gender relations were the norm, while at other times homosexuality was considered extremely aberrant and even criminal (Bayer 1987). This century has seen different cycles of popular opinion in terms of tolerance and intolerance. In recent years, homosexual individuals have more commonly referred to themselves as gay (for men) or lesbians (for women). These terms differ from the term homosexual for they refer to a larger identification with an internal identity and lifestyle. Homosexual behavior is different from a homosexual identity. That is, a person who does not identify as being homosexual may have and enjoy sex with someone of the same sex.

Substance use and abuse is an enormously important problem in the gay "community." The clinician interested in substance abuse is likely to encounter gay individuals. Group therapy is often the treatment of choice if substance dependence has developed. This chapter will serve as an introduction to issues concerning the lives of gay men and women, particularly issues that must be acknowledged and addressed before treating this group of people. This chapter is geared to familiarize the clinician with issues important to gay/lesbian patients who use or abuse substances.

Definitions and Terms

Homosexuality, as a term, was first used by Krafft-Ebing to imply a clinical, pathological condition (Krafft-Ebing 1898). Although the term *gay* has for a long time been associated with homosexual men alone, it is now used intermittently for women also and has been for several hundred years (Boswell 1980). The term *lesbian,* which refers to a homosexual woman, is derived from the name of the Greek island Lesbos, home of the ancient world's great female poet, Sappho. The term *bisexual* refers to those individuals who are sexually attracted to both sexes. These individuals are able to carry on sexual relations with either gender, but often they prefer one over the other. Even individuals who identify themselves as heterosexual can have fleeting homosexual thoughts and attractions, and it is quite normative during adolescence to have sexual feelings for others of the same sex.

The term *sexual identity* refers to the internal identification of one's self as either male or female. The term *sexual object choice* refers to the sex that serves as the primary focus of an individual's erotic life, dreams, and fantasies. For our purposes, the terms *gay* and *lesbian* refer to those individuals who have a predominant sexual attraction to males and females, respectively. Their sexual fantasies are either entirely or almost entirely directed at others of the same gender, and have been since childhood (Isay 1989). Because of societal pressure and other factors, such individuals may never have had sex with someone of their same sex. Nonetheless, their internal identity is homosexual.

THE CASE FOR "GAY SUBSTANCE ABUSE GROUPS"

It is generally understood that although there is no pat formula for choosing the best mixture of patients, there should be a principle of "maximum tolerable heterogeneity" in selecting group members (Vannicelli 1990). This flexibility, however, may not apply for gay and lesbian substance abusers. Gay men and lesbians often feel that specific developmental and social issues confront them, of which most dynamically oriented therapists have little knowledge. Yet, there are numerous other reasons for recommending substance-abusing gay men and lesbians to groups composed exclusively of gay men and women. A great deal of prejudice exists in the outside world concerning gays and lesbians although recent strides have helped them feel more integrated in society. Moreover, it is often quite difficult to have intimate discussions about gay sexuality and substance abuse in a context in which group members may legitimately believe they are being judged.

Numerous behaviors that are considered normal in the gay "world" can be viewed as unusual and provoke judgment and rebuke. These issues support the argument in favor of creating separate gay and lesbian groups to deal with gay topics, including substance abuse. The following example illustrates several important points about treating gays and lesbians, as well as treating substance abuse in general:

> Ted is a thirty-three-year-old single banker living in a midwestern city. He first used cocaine in social settings, especially on Saturday nights when he went dancing at the local gay disco. He also used numerous other drugs such as "Ecstasy," (MDMA), "Special K," (ketamine), and "Crystal" (methamphetamine). In a random drug test at work, his urine tested positive for drug use. Ted was surprised that his employer used random drug testing, and because it happened after one of his rare "circuit party weekends," he felt unlucky. His employer insisted that he be sent to a drug counselor. The drug counselor, who had not heard of many of the drugs Ted had used, said that anyone who used drugs like that was an addict. He made Ted join his twelve-step–based group. This group included many older men, most of them members of the Teamsters' Union. In the first meeting, several of the members made homophobic remarks, which went unchallenged by the group leader and seemed to promote solidarity among the other members. Ted attended the group for a few weeks, but then stopped. His employer was informed of his absence, and Ted was terminated.

The counselor made several mistakes in Ted's treatment. Some gay men and women do use drugs recreationally and, although not healthy, it is the cultural norm. Based on his history of drug use, whether Ted has a particular problem with drug abuse or addiction is unclear. Moreover, Ted was placed in a group with whose members he had little in common, and he was likely to be met with scorn and prejudice. In Ted's case, there were numerous reasons, other than a possible addiction, not to be self-revealing. The counselor was neither sensitive, nor even aware, of the special problems Ted was facing. Groups act as a cornerstone of substance abuse treatment, but they are not the only means for treating gay men and women. In Ted's case, either a more sensitive group or a different form of treatment may have proven successful.

In recent years, recognition of substance abuse in the gay and lesbian community has increased. Several treatment programs have special tracks for gays and lesbians. Furthermore, various twelve-step meetings have been developed that are more "gay friendly" than others. In fact, a number of programs cater especially to gays and lesbians.

COMMON THEMES OF BEING GAY

A number of issues concerning gay men and lesbians need to be understood by the clinician working with this population. Many gays share similar common experiences, although these experiences do not necessarily occur universally. The following are examples of typical shared events.

Coming Out

"Coming out" or "coming out of the closet" is a process experienced by all individuals who identify themselves as homosexual and refers to acknowledging and dealing with one's identity as a gay man or lesbian. This process is divided into the internal and the external. The internal part of "coming out" involves the intrapsychic realization that one is attracted to members of the same sex. The internal aspect of the process is usually referred to as "coming out to oneself." The external part of the "coming out" process involves the gay individual's public identification as a gay man or woman. This public "coming out" may be limited to one or a few friends, to family members, or it may be universal.

"Coming out" is different for each individual. There is, in fact, an extreme amount of variation in the process. In some cases, patients will report that they have always known they were homosexual and have readily accepted it and admitted it to others. These individuals are rare, but they do exist. Such an individual would be said to have "always been out." When individuals' sexual orientation is exposed in a way not intended, however, the resulting humiliation may lead them back into denying their identity.

Most gay men and women report that they were aware of feelings of attraction to the same sex from a very early age. Often there are consequences for revealing gay feelings at an early age; that is, they are met by the family with disappointment, consternation, or worse. Subsequently, the typical homosexual child enters a phase of latency during which sexual feelings are not so prominent. During adolescence, sexuality awakens and the gay or lesbian adolescents realize their feelings, which may be intensely erotic, are different from the majority of their peers. This difference leads to feelings of isolation and confusion. Often the gay individuals try to convince themselves that they are undergoing a "phase" that will soon pass. Eventually, if it occurs at all, the gay individuals come to finally and completely accept themselves as gay. This self-acknowledgment may take place long before engaging in actual gay sex, or it may take place after years of having sex with homosexual partners. The public phase is the last stage of "coming out." It includes "coming out" to friends, family, and co-workers. While many gay people are "out to everyone," it is common for homosexuals to have compartmentalized lives in which one segment of people in their world knows they are gay, while another does not.

Prejudice

Although much improved, prejudice is rampant in the public's perception of gays and lesbians. The stereotypes that gays and lesbians are more promiscuous than heterosexuals, cannot form relationships, and are more likely to be child molesters are still common concerns for many members of the general public despite the fact that they are not true (Cabaj 1995). Prejudices continue to influence policy at every level of society. Although every responsible, scientific study has indicated that gays and lesbians can serve equally well as can their heterosexual counterparts, being homosexual is cause for dismissal from the American armed forces. In addition, the majority of states continue to have laws against sodomy, making consensual homosexual sex among adults a crime.

The clinician must be aware that although prejudice is no excuse for substance abuse, antigay prejudice is real. Similarly, violence against gay people is all too common. The term "gay bashing" refers to violence against individuals solely because they are, or are perceived to be, gay.

Homophobia

Homophobia refers to the fear of homosexuality, in general, and the homosexual person, in particular. It exists in two forms, internal and external. External homophobia is the root cause of the prejudice discussed previously and has a variety of complex societal and psychological origins. It exists on a spectrum; it may be overt, violent (as in the case of individuals who promote and defend gay bashing), or extremely subtle (in the case of heterosexuals who believe they have no prejudice but, in fact, harbor some hidden beliefs that gays are inferior).

Internalized homophobia refers to prejudice and negative feelings gay people have about themselves and other gay people. This homophobia is very real and common among gays and lesbians and is enormously destructive to self-esteem.

Growing Up and Adolescence

Growing up with the confusing feelings involved with being gay is extremely difficult for most people. Many gay people describe feelings of isolation, loneliness, and fears of exposure and ostracism. These are not simply neurotic fears; in many cases, they are real. Gay youth are much more likely to be thrown out of their homes, become homeless, and be subject to violence. Moreover, gay youth are four times more likely to commit suicide than heterosexuals. Thus, while feelings of isolation, loneliness, and thoughts of suicide are common among adolescents, they are more common among gays and lesbians. As such, they often become the topic of conversation in group therapy. These feelings and experiences form part of the initial motivation to begin the use and abuse of substances.

CURRENT THEORY OF HOMOSEXUALITY

Current views indicate that the formation of a gay identity is the result of a complex interaction of genetic, environmental, and psychological factors. Although controversial, there is little doubt that a strong genetic component is involved in sexual persuasion (Byne 1996), and there may be some hormonal and neurological cerebral differences in gay people. The fact that identical twins have a 50 percent concordance rate for homosexuality clearly demonstrates that homosexuality is not entirely biological. Although there is no one consensus on the psychological issues that contribute to a gay identity, there is no such thing as a stereotypical family dynamic that produces a gay child (Cabaj 1995). What is clear, however, is that the formation of sexual orientation occurs early in development, probably before the end of the second year, and is extremely difficult to change (Isay 1989).

THE NORMATIVE ROLE OF SUBSTANCES IN GAY LIFE

Most studies report that the incidence of substance abuse is higher in the gay and lesbian population than in the general population (Cabaj 1995). Clinicians who work with the homosexual population also indicate that gays and lesbians seem to drink and use substances more often than the general public (Finnegan and McNally 1987).

To distinguish between substance use, abuse, and dependence, one needs to take into account the social milieu of the particular patient. Substance ingestion may be said to go from use to abuse when it impairs some functioning in the person's life. For many gays and lesbians, the use of recreational drugs is quite common and socially acceptable and is, therefore, in some sense "normal." That is, certain types of alcohol and drug use may be more common and typical than in some other subcultures.

Heavier drinking also occurs more commonly in gay and lesbian populations than in heterosexual populations. Moreover, this tendency continues further into the life cycle than it does in heterosexual circles, where heavy and binge drinking are quite common during late adolescence (McKirman 1989). This pattern often begins in high school and continues through college. After college, most people begin to moderate their patterns (Goodwin and Gabrielli 1995), while only a minority continue to drink heavily. The minority, therefore, is more likely to become alcoholic. In the case of gays and lesbians, most clinicians agree that the pattern of heavy and binge drinking is prolonged.

One of the reasons why alcohol proves so influential to gay men and lesbians is because the "gay bar" is an important part of their lives. These bars have a clientele that is either strictly or primarily gay, and is often the center of gay social life. They allow readily available and easy access to alcohol and drugs and undoubtedly facilitate the use and potential abuse of these substances.

For many gay men, sex and intimacy are often completely separated. This is, of course, not exclusive to the gay population. Subculturally sanctioned outlets for sex without intimacy are more readily available to gays than to some other parts of society. Gay men, at least in urban areas, can find anonymous partners rather readily.

Substance use helps many gay people brace themselves for the trauma associated with experiencing themselves as gay men and women. The use of substances to medicate anxiety is a tremendous temptation. Moreover, substances can provide a convenient excuse for the sexual behavior about which many gay men and lesbians feel deeply conflicted, thereby making denial and dissociation easier. A common line heard by clinicians is, "I was so drunk (or stoned, or high), I didn't know what I was doing last night." This allows the gay individuals to disavow the powerful and deeply disturbing sexual feelings they have experienced and the actions they have taken on account of them.

SUBSTANCES OF ABUSE CHARACTERISTIC OF THE GAY AND LESBIAN COMMUNITY

Gays and lesbians experience problems with numerous substances. A number of drugs used by gay men and women are not nearly as common in any other population, except perhaps for certain adolescent groups. The so-called "club drugs" commonly found in gay social settings include, but are not limited to, methamphetamine (crystal meth), methylenedioxymethamphetamine (MDMA or Ecstasy), ketamine (Special K), and gamma hydroxybutyrate (GHB or liquid x). These substances are unique compounds, differing in terms of their pharmacological properties and their phenomenological effects. The clinician working with a gay or lesbian population is urged to learn about the nature and effects of these drugs (McDowell and Kleber 1994; Vickers 1969).

GROUP PSYCHOTHERAPY

Group psychotherapy is often the center of psychotherapeutic management for gays struggling with substance abuse issues. There has been a proliferation of such groups for gay men and lesbians. Group therapy for substance abusers, and for those who are gay and lesbian, often blends the two most frequently employed group models: the self-help group and the psychotherapy group.

Psychotherapy and Self-Help Groups

Very often, self-help groups and psychotherapy groups are simultaneously used in treatment plans. While mutual-help groups advocate "sharing" of experiences and feelings, allowing participants to gain insight into their own experiences, they also provide a basis for understanding that experiences are not necessarily unique. Such experiential learning can be enormously therapeutic (Flores 1997). Psychotherapy groups, on the other hand, tend to emphasize interaction/confrontation with the leader or with other members, using traditional psychodynamic constructs. Patients are encouraged to deal with problems "in the group"; interactions outside are usually discouraged. Such a structure promotes the psychodynamic work of the group and minimizes pathological behavior from being "acted out."

The self-help group is any group that includes twelve-step meetings. Many areas have twelve-step meetings that are designed for gay and lesbian membership. Participation in these groups, however, is not strictly forbidden to others, as such "exclusion" would go against the general philosophy of the twelve-step tradition (Kurtz 1979). These groups are open, free, and readily available. On the contrary, psychotherapy groups are usually held in a clinical or private setting, have a leader, and require a fee.

Pregroup Issues

The purpose of the pregroup phase is to thoughtfully select and prepare prospective group members. Members who are well oriented come into group with realistic goals and expectations.

The group leader in the pregroup phase selects appropriate members and then sets the ground rules and policies that will prevail during the group process. Examples of ground rules include whether the group will be open or closed, and whether the group will be time-limited or open-ended. The ground rules for a gay/lesbian group do not substantially differ from those of any other substance-abusing group.

Policies relating to contact outside of the group, however, are perhaps more fraught with difficulty for gays and lesbians. Because many gays and lesbians choose predominantly gay social lives, restricting contact outside a group is very complex and almost unrealistic. The group leader should be aware of the difficulties involved in separating social worlds in the various spheres of community interaction. Another reason for leniency regarding contact outside of the group is that since so much of "gay life" centers around a culture where drugs and alcohol are available, there may not be as many sober social outlets as are available for nongay populations. In the early stages of recovery, when individuals break their ties with drug- and alcohol-using gay and lesbian subcultures to achieve sobriety, they often simultaneously cut their interpersonal attachment bonds. Group membership helps to anchor the member during this time of great change and turmoil. The group helps counter feelings of loneliness, isolation, and alienation. If contact outside the group is healthy and is in the interest of maintaining sobriety, it should be allowed. However, care should be taken to observe that this outside contact does not sabotage the group's goals (Zweben 1986).

Group Goals

Once detoxification and early sobriety have been attained, the central goal of the group becomes helping the participant to maintain sobriety and emotional health. Emotional health, in this context, is defined as the state and ability to cope with the world and uncomfortable feelings in a productive manner without the use of drugs or alcohol. Gay/lesbian group members will have many common experiences that can serve as a basis for relationships, bonds, and group cohesion. Issues of relevance may include dealing with strong feelings, problems with self-esteem, and feelings of isolation and loneliness. The leader must be aware that many of these feelings that gays and lesbians experience are the result of real and persistent homophobia, not neurotic paranoia (Wolfe 1998). Goals should therefore include how to incorporate fulfillment and meaning into one's life without resorting to drug use.

Another goal of any substance abuse group is to teach the psychological and practical mechanisms for monitoring one's behavior and avoiding relapse. These techniques, covered in other chapters of this volume, are no different for gays and lesbians. Through the group process, the members learn new drug-free methods of dealing with painful affects, practical problems, and the difficulties of negotiating between life and relationships.

LEADING A GAY AND LESBIAN SUBSTANCE ABUSE GROUP

Leaders of drug and alcohol groups begin with an emphasis on support and cohesion. Differences and conflicts at the beginning should be minimized. This sets the stage for repairing ruptured attachment bonds. A strong initial alliance among members and the leader helps deal with the eventual conflicts and difficulties that may occur during later stages of the group.

Unlike some psychodynamic groups, the support offered in a substance abuse group is not unconditional. The primary goal of the group is to attain and maintain sobriety, teaching the mechanisms that foster that goal. Group members who undermine these goals are confronted, in order to avoid subverting the goals of the group. Examples of such behavior are irregular attendance, incomplete disclosure about drug use, and romanticizing drug life. Although this is a complex matter, homosexual individuals may encounter more difficulty and discrimination than do their straight counterparts. Nevertheless, this cannot be used to intellectualize or rationalize relapse and drug use.

As in other substance abuse groups, confrontation is an integral and invaluable tool. The leader must scrupulously avoid subtle homophobia among members leading to scapegoating of a group member. It is quite common since many gay men and women continue to foster hostile feelings toward their own sexuality (Isay 1991).

Much learning takes place during the early stages of substance abuse groups. Often one learns how to deal with powerful affects that have been anesthetized for years. The leader needs to assume that drugs have served, at least in part, as a means to avoid the powerful and uncomfortable feelings associated with such issues as intimacy, attachment, dependency, and loneliness. Because these feelings may possibly flood a member in the group setting, one of the leader's primary goals is to monitor and prevent these feelings from taking a destructive path.

The most effective substance abuse groups for gays and lesbians provide a mixture of cognitive education about substance abuse itself, techniques to avoid relapse, and psychodynamic work. Members are taught to understand the meaning behind their substance use, as well as to understand themselves in a deeper, more complete manner. Although the focus of the group is usually the "here and now," past experiences and developmental and family issues must be explored. Intensive dynamic work should only be used when group cohesion is firmly established and sobriety is achieved.

Membership in a substance abuse group provides gays and lesbians with a positive environment of acceptance, exploration, and mutuality. Such sanctuary is a radical change from the more common life experience of these individuals. Continued membership in a gay group is therapeutic because it provides a corrective emotional experience for common issues experienced by group members.

Leadership Considerations in Substance Abuse Groups

Identity Issues for the Leader

Self-disclosure concerning the sexual orientation of the group leader is a vital question. Whether the leader is gay, lesbian, or "straight" will have a profound impact on the process of the group. Members will likely feel a more immediate connection and identification with gay or lesbian leaders. Issues of rivalry, competition, and envy, however, will also be more likely to surface earlier. A heterosexual leader will likely be met with complaints concerning his or her not being able to empathize with or relate to the group. Although these fears may be valid, they can also be used to create a powerful resistance to treatment. In general, it is probably preferable for the group leader to be gay or lesbian because he or she can serve as a powerful role model. If a leader is heterosexual, it is usually, but not always, wise to reveal his or her sexual orientation. Not to do so would likely cause tension that would lead to subversion as the group evolves. The leader must also keep in mind that the purpose of the group is to promote and enable sobriety, and that goal has no sexuality.

It is all too common for gays and lesbians to use their differences and the real homophobia of society as tools of resistance. The leader, gay or straight, must be very careful about this type of evasion.

Leading the Group

In all substance abuse groups, structure and firmness are essential. The group norm must be total abstinence from all drugs and alcohol, and this is nonnegotiable (Spitz and Spitz 1998). To adopt any other policy would be to invite subterfuge and disaster. Many gays and lesbians, however, will likely be advocates of "harm reduction." Although harm reductionists have many valid points, once individuals have presented themselves for treatment they have demonstrated an inability to regulate the use of substances. In group, arguments for a harm reduction approach should be interpreted as resistance, an elaborate form of intellectualized enabling that, in fact, is harm producing (Kleber 1997).

Group Composition

Many factors have to be taken into account in composing a therapeutic group experience for gay and lesbian addicted members. Gay men and lesbians are as diverse as their heterosexual counterparts and the same considerations for their treatment need to be maintained (Spitz and Spitz 1998).

Age is often a consideration in creating substance abuse groups. In general, although groups of similar age will be more cohesive and have more in common, a spectrum of ages can also have benefits in providing role models for longer-term sobriety (Richardson 1995). The adolescent substance abuse group is a prototype of age-specific group composition. An adolescent group dealing with issues of acceptance and coming out may be more likely to address such issues in a healthy manner. Groups are helpful for ego and identity formation, especially for gay and lesbian teens, whose ego and identity issues may be even more confused and pained.

Gender considerations are vital. Forming and maintaining intimate relationships is a critical issue for almost anyone with a substance abuse problem. Same sex groups allow for more commonalities. In order to concentrate on achieving a stable state of sobriety, it may be advantageous to place substance abusers with high levels of relationship anxiety in a same gender group (McDowell and Spitz 1999). Common issues of gays and lesbians may be enough to provide the cohesion necessary for a group to work. In coed groups, if possible, having two leaders, a gay man and a lesbian, may work out best.

Group therapists must be aware of the family circumstances of every group member. Families are crucial to the recovery process and their participation must be considered. With gay and lesbian patients, however, "family" may not always be family of origin. Although a large number of individuals have good relations with their biological families, many gays and lesbians consider their "families" to be a network of other gay men and women with whom they share feelings of intimacy. Such networks often have the same flavor, as well as the same pathology, of more traditional family units.

The issue of contact outside of the group is a complex one. Traditional psychodynamic psychotherapy prohibits such contact so as to keep analysis and observation within the group alone. Early on in sobriety, however, it may be very useful for group members to be able to contact one another, either by telephone or socially, as long as such contact is discussed at the next meeting. Contact may help to promote the establishment of healthy and non-drug-focused social interaction. Moreover, if extra group contact and the resulting discussion are based on honesty, trust, and caring, then such an interaction may, in fact, be quite beneficial and therapeutic.

Confidentiality is especially important in a gay and lesbian substance abuse group because some members may not be "out" about their drug use or their sexuality. In addition, some members may be HIV positive, an issue that most do not want discussed. An atmosphere must therefore be created where individuals feel comfortable in discussing even the most delicate problems. In addiction groups, failure to adhere to the group contract regarding confidentiality is grounds for dismissal from the group. It is the group leader's responsibility to make clear the importance of maintaining confidentiality.

Case Studies

Several cases are illustrative of different group compositions and structures.

Leslie is a thirty-eight-year-old single lesbian who lives in a small northeastern town. She began using drugs, mostly marijuana and cocaine, at the age of fourteen. By sixteen, she was using cocaine regularly as well as drinking and sniffing glue. Except for several brief periods, she was never sober. After her last arrest, she was offered the choice of jail or a special program in a therapeutic community for women with a special track for lesbian issues. She chose the latter. The main form of treatment there was group treatment. Leslie said that she did not like groups, but agreed to attend. Although she participated in an almost automatic manner, she blamed all of her problems on the homophobia of her hometown. The group leaders and members were sensitive to these issues and at times agreed that her feelings were justified, but said that her coping mechanisms were not healthy. When confronted with the opinion of the other group members that she was using the putative homophobia of others as a resistance to accepting the seriousness of her problem, she became furious.

This case illustrates the important point that although homophobia does exist, and the group members and the group leader must be sensitive to it, it cannot be used as an excuse for addictive behavior. Addicts typically blame their condition on outside factors and stresses, but homophobia, as real as it is, is no excuse for continued drug use and the self-destructive addictive behavior associated with it.

John is a twenty-eight-year-old gay graduate student studying psychology in a midwestern city. He has long been interested in gay issues and proposed a project to set up a gay group for dealing with issues concerning substance abuse. He searched high and low and finally created a group whose composition, on the first night, included Jack (a wealthy lawyer and periodic user of cocaine), Linda (a seventy-four-year-old lesbian who had been in recovery, through AA, for over thirty years), Fred (a seventeen-year-old adolescent who had been sent to the local clinic for his marijuana use and thought he might be gay), Karen (a thirty-eight-year-old lesbian in a stable relationship, with a long history of alcohol use exacerbated by periodic depression), and Jackie (a transsexual, transgendered lesbian with a long history of chaotic relationships and heavy use of methamphetamine).

In the first meeting, a nervous John introduced himself, but said that because of anonymity issues he would not identify himself as either gay or straight. As the conversation sputtered around, it was marked by awkward silences and a search for commonalities, of which there were few. In the second session, only two of the group's members returned; it was concluded that the others were in "resistance" to their addictions. There were no subsequent meetings.

The previous case illustrates several potential pitfalls in gay groups. Attempting to put this group together with many disparate age, sex, socioeconomic, and lifestyle differences was a recipe for, if not disaster, disunity. Furthermore, John, an inexperienced therapist, chose not to self-disclose and set an inhibiting tone for the group. In addition, each member was involved with a different drug, so there were different issues surrounding each member's drug use, and each may be at a very different stage in recovery. For at least two of the members, it was unclear if they were addicted or merely using problematically. Although well-intentioned, this group had very little chance of succeeding due to the noted leadership errors.

Linda is a twenty-four-year-old junior executive who has had problems with alcohol since her early teens. She was referred to group by her psychotherapist who believed that her issues with alcohol were becoming serious and that they were interfering with psychotherapy. Linda had recently "come out" as a lesbian. She blamed many of the issues she had with alcohol on the stress of being a lesbian. Her therapist referred her to a lesbian group, consisting of women from their early twenties to late forties. It was run by a well-trained lesbian therapist with a particular interest in substance abuse. Linda felt a growing kinship with the members of the group. She was able to explore her issues of isolation and rejection and felt that she was understood. After six months she felt comfortable enough to discuss some issues of abuse she had experienced in the past. The group was supportive and several members revealed that they had had similar experiences. Linda began to appreciate the gentle confrontations she experienced when she blamed her drinking on homophobia or on her previous abuse. She also began to understand the role she played in her own personal and social isolation. She continues to go to the group, after three years of attendance, and finds it a source of comfort and knowledge.

This is an example of a successful group experience in which the patient was able to deal with a variety of psychological and addictive behaviors. Combining people with much in common, along with a practical and well-trained leader, is often a recipe for success. Not only are psychological insights discovered and confirmed, the tools to remain sober and to deal with the world in a healthy way are learned and reinforced.

SUMMARY

For many reasons groups have become the most important part of the comprehensive treatment of substance abuse. The principles imparted through peer education, support, and shared common experiences with painful feelings and difficult problems are enormously therapeutic. Given the problems and isolation that many gays feel and the significance of substance use and abuse in the gay world, substance abuse groups for gay men and lesbians enjoy a position of prominence in the treatment field. Every indication exists that these groups are beneficial and will continue to play an even greater role in recovery.

REFERENCES

Bayer R. *Homosexuality and American Psychiatry*. Princeton, NJ: Princeton University Press, 1987.

Boswell J. *Christianity, Social Tolerance and Homosexuality*. Chicago: Chicago University Press, 1980.

Byne W. Biology and homosexuality: Implications of neuroendocrinological and neuroanatomic studies. In *Homosexuality and Mental Health: A Comprehensive Review,* edited by Cabaj RP, Stein T. Washington, DC: American Psychiatric Press, 1996, pp. 115-128.

Cabaj R. Gays, lesbians, and bisexuals. In *Substance Abuse: A Comprehensive Textbook,* edited by Lowinson JH, Ruiz P, Millman RB, Langrod JG. Baltimore, MD: Williams and Wilkins, 1997, pp. 725-733.

Finnegan D, McNally E. *Dual Identities: Counseling Chemically Dependent Gay Men and Lesbians*. Center City, MN: Hazelden, 1987.

Flores P. *Group Psychotherapy with Addicted Populations*. Binghamton, NY: The Haworth Press, 1997.

Goodwin DW, Gabrielli WF Jr. Alcohol: Clinical aspects. In *Substance Abuse: A Comprehensive Textbook,* edited by Lowinson JH, Ruiz P, Millman RB, Langrod JG. Baltimore, MD: Williams and Wilkins, 1997, pp. 142-148.

Hooker E. The adjustment of the male overt homosexual. *Journal of Projective Techniques and Personality Assessment* 21(1):18-31, 1957.

Isay R. *Being Homosexual: Gay Men and Their Development*. New York: Farrar Straus Giroux, 1989.

Isay R. The homosexual analyst: Clinical considerations. *The Psychoanalytic Study of the Child* 46:199-216, 1991.

Kleber H. *Harm Reduction or Production*. Presented at the 1997 annual meeting of the American Psychiatric Association. San Diego, CA: 1997.

Krafft-Ebing R. *Psychopathia Sexualis*. (1898). Reprinted by Brooklyn Physicians and Surgeons Book Company, 1922.

Kurtz E. *Not-God: A History of Alcoholics Anonymous*. Center City, MN: Hazelden, 1979.

McDowell D, Kleber H. MDMA, its history and pharmacology. *Psychiatric Annals* 24(3):127-130, 1994.

McDowell D, Spitz H. *Substance Abuse: From Principles to Practice*. New York: Brunner Mazel, 1999.

McKirnan D, Peterson P. Psychological and cultural factors in alcohol and drug abuse: An analysis of a homosexual community. *Addictive Behavior* 14:555-563, 1989.

Richardson J. The science and politics of gay teen suicide. *Harvard Review of Psychiatry* 3(2):107-110, 1995.

Spitz HI, Spitz ST. *A Pragmatic Approach to Group Psychotherapy.* Philadelphia, PA: Taylor & Francis Group, 1998.

Vannicelli M. *Group Psychotherapy with Adult Children of Alcoholics.* New York: Guilford Press, 1990.

Vickers MD. Gammahydroxybutyric acid. *International Anaesthesiology Clinics,* 75-89, 1969.

Wolfe A. The homosexual exception. *The New York Times Magazine,* February 8, 1998, p. 46.

Zweben J. Recovery-oriented psychotherapy. *Journal of Substance Abuse Treatment* 3:255-262, 1986.

Chapter 16

Multidimensional Family Therapy for Adolescent Drug Abuse: Making the Case for a Developmental-Contextual, Family-Based Intervention

Howard A. Liddle
Cynthia L. Rowe

INTRODUCTION

Much of family therapy's past has been estranged, intentionally so, from mainstream individual and group psychotherapy, from which it evolved. Family therapy's genuine and self-proclaimed differentness helped to sequester it from the influences of the mental health establishment. Although this position was functional and developmentally useful in its day, this separatist position is no longer viable (Coyne and Liddle 1992). There is a developing spirit of integration of methods in family therapy, and in group psychotherapy as well, to deal with pragmatic, clinical problems and population-specific treatment packages, using integrated treatment models.

Family therapy's roots in group therapy are clear, with similarities between the two approaches (Nichols and Schwartz 1998). In fact, early family therapists approached families as small groups with equality among their members (e.g., John Bell). First, family and group therapy are both very concerned with process at the level of etiology and intervention. Both assume that interactional and interpersonal processes and functioning are interconnected, with clinical implications. Modern family therapy approaches do not limit their boundaries to family process but extend diagnostic and intervention targets to include processes within the family, within individual family members, and among family members and extrafamilial sources of input and influence. Second, in both family and group therapy, the interactional process is the main target of change, using the interpersonal processes in group and in the family. Third, family and group therapy both utilize developmental aspects of group dynamics, understanding that groups and families in therapy go through natural, predictable developmental stages. Finally, both approaches focus on the roles members play in the family or group.

However, important differences exist among families and other groups, which explains why family therapists developed unique techniques and approaches (Nichols and Schwartz 1998). Families are not random groups of people, but instead family members share common histories and maintain long-term commitments to one another. Families are not democratic groups in which members can have equal power and status, nor is the family therapy environment always safe, supportive, and nonthreatening, as is often the case in group therapy. Family therapists must employ creative techniques to promote openness and honesty and generate new ways of relating that will break long-standing, ineffective interactional patterns. Family therapists regard the family as the core, and in certain developmental periods the most important, unit of socialization.

Family therapists may use aspects of group therapy; two major family therapy approaches maintained their group therapy roots: multiple family therapy (Laqueur 1972) and network therapy (Speck and Attneave 1972; Rueveni 1979). Multiple family therapy, as the name suggests, brings several families together as one supportive and often challenging group to deal with their problems jointly. The multiple family therapy approach was widely used by Murray Bowen (Nichols and Schwartz 1998) and has demonstrated efficacy with families of schizophrenics (Goldstein and Miklowitz 1995). Network therapy (Chapter 11) brings together everyone who is significantly involved with the family and/or individual who presents for treatment, including friends, extended family, neighbors, and members of external systems. The therapy network is directed by a team of two or three professionals whose primary goal is to "stimulate, reflect, and focus the potentials within the network to solve one another's problems" (Speck and Attneave 1972, p. 641). In both of these family therapy approaches, aspects of the therapeutic process parallel the dynamics of traditional group therapy.

This chapter presents an integrated intervention model that has broadened the scope of family therapy interventions, approaching adolescent substance abuse from a developmental-contextual, family-based perspective, using a working knowledge of the influence of group and family dynamics. This multidimensional approach places emphasis on the unique feelings, thoughts, and behaviors of the individuals within the system as well as the interactional patterns occurring within the system. Two questions organize this pursuit: (1) What is the role of the adolescent's family group in the development and maintenance of adolescent substance abuse? and (2) How are these developmental and contextual factors incorporated into and addressed within a multidimensional treatment for adolescent substance abuse?

Reviews of family therapy efficacy research articulate major advances in the field during the past two decades (Lebow and Gurman 1995; Liddle and Dakof 1995b). Manualized family-based approaches have been developed and tested in controlled trials with clinical populations of adolescent substance abusers by several research groups (e.g., Henggeler et al. 1991; Liddle and Dakof 1995b). Specific engagement strategies (Szapocznik et al. 1989) and therapist behaviors related to positive therapeutic alliance (Diamond and Liddle 1993, 1996) have been defined, clinically developed, and empirically tested to improve therapeutic alliances and cohesion and increase retention rates in family therapy with problem youth (Liddle et al. 1998). Family-based interventions have been tested against clinically viable treatment alternatives (e.g., Chamberlain and Reid 1991).

Family therapy has emerged as a promising but not exclusive approach to treating adolescent drug abuse and related problems (Liddle and Dakof 1995a). Family therapy approaches for problem adolescents have been shown to have effects in multiple domains in addition to reducing drug use, including improving school performance, externalizing problems, and reducing internalized distress. *Structural strategic family therapy* has been shown to effectively engage Hispanic adolescents and their parents, reduce drug use and behavior problems, and improve family relations up to one year following treatment (Szapocznik et al. 1989). Among delinquent adolescents followed up to four years, *multisystemic family therapy* (Henggeler et al. 1991) was associated with fewer drug-related arrests and less drug use compared with juvenile delinquents treated in individual therapy and those who refused treatment (Mann et al. 1990). *Multidimen-*

sional family therapy (Liddle, Dakof, and Diamond 1991) is more effective than a family group education intervention, peer group counseling, and individual treatment in reducing drug use and externalizing problems up to one year following treatment. Thus, positive results with clinically referred adolescent drug abusers have shown that family therapy holds great promise in treating this difficult population (Liddle and Dakof 1995a).

The onset and progression of adolescent substance abuse is multiply determined by the interaction of individual, family, peer, and community variables. Therefore, interventions must occur at several levels of the adolescent's functioning. The family-based model described in this chapter was developed specifically to attend to the multiple forces impacting upon the adolescent, intervening within the adolescent, as well as parental, parent-adolescent, and extrafamilal subsystems. Critical changes within each of these subsystems must occur in order to stop the cycle of chronic problem behaviors and heavy substance involvement.

THE FAMILY AND ADOLESCENT DRUG ABUSE

Family risk factors for adolescent drug use and antisocial behavior include parent and sibling modeling of substance abuse, parental attitudes that minimize the child's drug use, poor relationships with parents, and inadequate child-rearing practices (Brook et al. 1990). The close association between adolescent problems and family variables, which often predate the initiation of adolescent problem behaviors (Baumrind 1991; Farrington 1995), establishes the critical influence of families in mediating and/or moderating the development and maintenance of adolescent drug and other problem behaviors. However, changes in parenting practices can impact adolescents' drug initiation as well as their frequency of drug taking after initiation has begun (Steinberg, Fletcher, and Darling 1994), and interventions have been shown to change parenting practices of drug-involved and delinquent youths (Schmidt, Liddle, and Dakof 1996). The family's role in adolescent substance abuse includes (1) ineffective child-rearing practices, (2) family discord, and (3) poor parent-child bonding.

Ineffective Child-Rearing Practices

Baumrind (1991) reports that parents who are nondirective and permissive have children with the highest level of drug use. Lack of both clear limit setting and rules against drug use have been correlated with relatively high levels of drug use among adolescents (Brook et al. 1990). Negative communication patterns (criticism, blaming, lack of praise), unrealistic parental expectations of children, and inconsistent or harsh discipline are strongly correlated with delinquency (Farrington 1995). Parents who do not monitor and structure their children's behaviors and activities place them at high risk for substance abuse and delinquency (Chilcoat, Dishion, and Anthony 1995). Children raised by "authoritative" parents, who are consistent and firm in disciplining the child but also warm, responsive, and respectful of the children's needs and ideas, are less likely to use substances (Steinberg, Fletcher, and Darling 1994). Coombs and Landsverk (1988) described the nonuser's parent as more likely to provide praise and encouragement, set down guidelines and rules about the adolescent's activities, and play an active role in the teenager's life than the user's parents, who are seen as emotionally distant, less helpful, and less likely to establish limits.

Family Discord

A second familial factor associated with adolescent problem behavior is family discord. It is not the disruption of the family due to divorce that contributes to adolescent problems, but the level and management of parental conflict (McCord 1979). Stanton et al. (1982) were among the first researchers to link drug abuse to families in which parental conflict prohibited a strong primary parental coalition. Marital instability both affects child development and makes an independent contribution to adolescent problem behavior and illicit drug use.

Poor Parent-Adolescent Relations

Numerous studies have found that a lack of parental warmth and involvement are positively correlated with drug use (Jessor and Jessor 1977; Brook et al. 1990). Poor relationships among family members may be more important than parental drug use or parental control in determining adolescent drug use. Parental warmth, support, and interest in the children protects adolescents from drug abuse problems and delinquency (Brook et al. 1990).

The family-based model described in this chapter places primary emphasis on reestablishing the critical connection that is frequently damaged in families of drug-abusing youth. Family members must feel respected and trust that their side of the story will be heard. Individual work with both parents and adolescents addresses the unique issues and concerns of each family member, and prepares the adolescent and parents to come together for the work of repairing strained and often disconnected relationships. The next section presents some clinical interventions describing the role of the family during adolescence and the factors that place adolescents at risk for continued problems, using examples of interventions prescribed in each of the modules of this family therapy approach to correct disruptions in the development of the adolescent.

CLINICAL IMPLICATIONS

This final section offers guidelines for the practical translation of some of the previously outlined research findings within a family treatment approach (MDFT) for adolescent drug abuse (Liddle, Dakof, and Diamond 1991). The interventions described were developed and refined according to empirical findings within the domains of adolescent development, drug abuse risk and protection, as well as adolescent treatment research. Examples of interactions from actual therapy sessions with drug-abusing adolescents and their parents are provided in order to illuminate specific points.

Contemporary thinking endorses interventions that are comprehensive (targeting multiple levels or areas of problem behavior), coherent, and intensive, finding ways to enhance existing treatment models, sometimes by combining various components of existing, empirically based approaches. A multidimensional perspective suggests that change can occur via *multiple pathways or mechanisms* (e.g., cognitive restructuring, affective clarification and expression), *in different contexts* (individual, familial, and extrafamilial), and *through different mechanisms* (e.g., development of a new cognitive framework and acquisition of new skills). The format used an interconnected series of sessions/interactions between therapist-adolescent, therapist-parent(s), therapist-extrafamilial systems (e.g., probation officers, school personnel), which gives access to these multiple domains.

Specific Therapeutic Guidelines

Working with families as small groups does not mean abandoning individual therapeutic work. Individual sessions, in which the adolescent and parents are seen separately, comprise up to 40 percent of the total treatment protocol. The therapist organizes therapy by introducing several generic themes (Liddle, Dakof, and Diamond 1991). These are different for the parents (e.g., feeling abused and incapable of finding a way to influence their child) and the adolescent (e.g., feeling disconnected and angry with parents). The therapist uses the generic themes of parent-adolescent conflict as assessment tools and as a way of developing workable content in sessions. Sometimes, interactions with the teenagers or parents are intended to prepare them for a conversation that they will have with the other family member ("what do you need to talk with them about?" and "what can we do now to plan it out?"). Individual work with family members is conducted in accordance with assumptions about mechanisms of change: adolescents and parents will change if they have the motivation, opportunity, skills, and practice to interact in new ways.

Individual Work with the Adolescent

Engaging adolescents in the therapy process is extremely challenging, particularly with adolescent drug abusers, who frequently have been coerced into therapy, do not believe that they have a problem, and are not necessarily motivated to make any significant changes in their lives. It is important to attend to interventions designed to engage the adolescent during the critical first phase of therapy (Diamond and Liddle 1997). Specific therapist behaviors have been identified that relate to the quality of the adolescent-therapist alliance, or therapeutic relationship. Therapists who are able to establish a positive therapeutic alliance with the adolescent present themselves as an ally, help the adolescent to formulate personally meaningful goals, and attend to the adolescent experience (Diamond and Liddle 1997). These techniques may be helpful in improving therapeutic relationships with unengaged adolescents.

In the first several sessions, the therapist spends a significant amount of time with the adolescent alone in order to hear the adolescent's story, and to provide the adolescent with the opportunity to share things with the therapist privately. Alliance-building techniques are the main focus of early interactions with the adolescent. In the following example of a first session with a drug-abusing adolescent, the therapist notes that the parent has offered most of the information about why the adolescent and she are coming to therapy, and the adolescent has been withdrawn and seemingly frustrated with being forced to come for therapy. The therapist uses time alone with the adolescent to hear about the things that upset him most about his current situation, and the adolescent explains to the therapist that whenever he tries to talk to his mom about his problems, they end up arguing. The therapist offers the following statement to the adolescent in an attempt to show him that there is something in this therapy for him:

> One of the things that we do here, and that I'm going to try to help you to do, is to try to have these kinds of conversations without arguing, to find a way to sort of negotiate so that you feel that you get your story out. This isn't just about what your mom or your probation officer have to say—you have a story to tell. You have a perspective. You started to say some of that today, and that's going to be really important. I want to help you say some of those things in a way that your mom and your probation officer and the people at school can hear. I hear you saying some important things, like "I want to build Mom's trust back," and "I want to be able to talk to Mom about some of these things that are important to me and feel like I'm being heard." I hope that I can help you do that in here.

The adolescent responds to this intervention by sharing more about his frustration with being treated like a child, and the therapist is able to offer the suggestion that therapy can be about negotiating with his mother to gain back some of his privileges.

Drug abuse derails adolescent development (Kandel and Davies 1996). Adolescent drug abusers have profound feelings of meaninglessness, low self-efficacy, and tend to lack commitment to and involvement in normative, prosocial activities and bonds. The individual subsystem sessions focus on important tasks of development, such as decision making, developing effective communication skills, and problem-solving. Drug use is discussed from a perspective of the negative ways in which it impacts one's health and one's perceptions of the world. Drug use is seen as an ineffective solution for bad feelings about oneself and the world, and the therapist helps the adolescents to identify the ways in which their drug use fails in meeting their needs. The therapist takes advantages of opportunities throughout the therapy process to explore with the adolescent how drug use makes these short-term gains difficult or impossible, reminding the adolescent of the "big picture."

The overall themes of individual work with the adolescent pertain to identity formation issues, self-efficacy, and the development of the adolescent as an individual and as a participant in multiple other interpersonal contexts. Change for the adolescent and the parent is both intrapersonal and interpersonal, and neither is more important. Helping the adolescent prepare for a conversation with parents increases self-efficacy and feelings of competence. Exploration of new ways of communicating thoughts and feelings is also critical because it increases the likelihood of more positive responses from the parent. In many cases, parents have given up hope of being able to talk honestly with the adolescent, or feel that they have no way of reaching the adolescent in any meaningful way. When adolescents act in new ways, the parents' feelings and beliefs about them change, and their commitment and involvement can be resuscitated, which is critical to treatment success (Dishion, Patterson, and Reid 1988). Parents who can experience the new behaviors and attitudes of their adolescent are then more likely to develop the attitudinal set necessary to renegotiate the parent-adolescent transition (Schmidt, Liddle, and Dakof 1996).

Individual Work with Parents

Running parallel to these adolescent subsystem sessions are sessions or parts of sessions with the parental subsystem. Parenting styles are directly related to adolescent drug abuse (Baumrind 1991; Brook et al. 1990), and thus are a direct intervention target. Parental belief systems pertaining to adolescents are addressed in order to propose fresh perspective skills for parenting adolescents. Parents are helped to examine the consistency between their parental philosophy (policy) and the implementation of this policy (in the form of their parenting styles), examining parental influence that is appropriate for adolescence. Parents learn to decide more appropriately which "battles" to choose, and engage the adolescent in more effective interactions.

The alliance between the therapist and parents is critical in promoting change during therapy. Interventions designed to bring parents into collaboration with the therapist are called "Parental Reconnection Interventions" (PRI). The ultimate aim of PRI is to have the parent reconnect on an affective level with the adolescent, and hence recommit to trying to help him or her (i.e., reclaim their parenting role and functions). The following techniques comprise the PRI:

1. *Focusing on parents' stress and burden,* acknowledging the difficult circumstances that impede parenting, as well as acknowledging that the parent has individual issues and problems.
2. *Identifying and supporting previous or current parenting efforts,* confirming examples of successful parenting behaviors and abilities.
3. *Enhancing feelings of love and commitment,* including therapist behaviors that facilitate a parent's experience and feelings of love, caring, and commitment toward the adolescent.
4. *Addressing important events, core issues, or themes* in the parent-adolescent relationship to bring issues of conflict and hurt out into the open.
5. *Enhancing beliefs in parental influence,* including planned discussions about the degree to which parents believe they can influence their adolescent's life for the better.
6. *Generating hope: Therapist as an ally,* involving interventions instilling hope that the therapist is willing to work with, stand by, and support the parents in their attempts to influence the adolescent. These interventions are critical in changing parenting behaviors.

Parents of problem youth present with both strengths and weaknesses (Schmidt, Liddle, and Dakof 1996). Parental strengths, or positive parenting practices, are identified early in therapy, and the therapist utilizes these behaviors during sessions and makes suggestions for building these behaviors outside of sessions. These behaviors include positive discipline and communication, monitoring and limit setting, positive affect and commitment, and interparent consistency. Negative parenting behaviors fall into categories defined by power, assertive discipline, problems in monitoring and limit setting, inconsistency between parents, negative affect and disengagement, and cognitive inflexibility. It is easier to replace negative parenting practices by introducing new, positive parenting behaviors than it is to focus solely on getting rid of negative behaviors. Most parents show significant improvements over the course of MDFT, including an increase in positive parenting behaviors and a decrease in less effective parenting practices. These improvements have been linked to reductions in adolescents' drug use and externalizing problems (Schmidt, Liddle, and Dakof 1996).

This vignette shows how parenting behaviors are frequently closely tied to the emotional climate of the parent-adolescent relationship. Parenting style, or the emotional context in which parenting practices are delivered, largely determines the impact and effectiveness of parenting behaviors upon the adolescent (Darling and Steinberg 1993). The father's "preaching" is examined as the father's basic parenting tool as well as the main way that the father interacts with his son. The therapist suggests that a different, more fulfilling, and more effective way of communicating with his son might exist.

T: I'm really interested in two things you just said. You feel like you've been doing a lot of preaching. Let me ask you—what kind of response do you get when you preach?

D: I get the sense that most of the time it's going in one ear and out the other. But I resolved myself a long, long time ago that I don't care if it does or not—I'm going to do it anyway. You know? At least he's going to hear how I feel about this—my principles and what I expect. It's up to him if he wants to take it and go with it or not, but at least I'm going to let him know. Maybe it's preaching, but we interact.

T: When you're preaching about important things like his future plans, or how he's dealing with his life now, you say he doesn't really get a chance to talk.

D: Right. He doesn't say much. He doesn't give much input back.

T: Is that something you're interested in? Would you like to hear his thoughts?

D: Oh yeah! 'Cause I'd like to help him along in what he wants to do. But up until this point I always felt that he didn't know what he wants to do.

T: Preaching doesn't lead to the kinds of conversations you want to have with him. I think you're right—it goes in one ear and out the other. But there is a different way of having a conversation with Jim. It would be more satisfying for you, because you'd be heard. He's not going to do everything you say, but I think he's going to consider what you say in a different way.

D: Right—that's the important thing—I just want to know that I have tried to tell him what I think about the things he's doing. But I know when it comes out, it's not coming out in that way—that loving, caring way. I don't know how it comes out, but I know it doesn't come out the way I think it comes out. . . . I want to help him, but I must come off like I'm yelling at him. He gets afraid. . . . The next thing I know, he's got tears in his eyes. I start out trying to help him, and I'm hurting the kid.

T: It sounds to me like you're an involved, caring father. I think that's a great thing and I want to help you reach out in a way where you don't feel frustrated. We're going to have to think about that together—how to do that. I think there's a way for you to be there for Jim and help him grapple with these things, without doing it all for him.

Bringing Parents and Adolescents Together

Facilitating new methods of relating and opening lines of communication that have been shut down due to years of disappointment and conflict are important goals of work with parents and adolescents. Once the therapist has joined with each family member and has helped the parent and adolescent individually to "sign on" to the therapeutic process, significant work in the parent-adolescent relational domain can begin.

Specific interventions can break impasses that frequently occur during individual and group sessions with adolescents and their parents and block in-session progress (Diamond and Liddle 1996). Therapists use three basic techniques in successful resolutions of in-session impasses: (1) actively blocking or diverting, or working through negative affect, blame, and resistance; (2) implanting, evoking, and amplifying thoughts and feelings that promote constructive dialogue; and (3) crafting an emotional treaty using "shuttle diplomacy." These techniques have been found to be more difficult to utilize, and failure to resolve impasses has been shown to be more likely in families that were initially more conflicted and pessimistic. The process of resolving therapeutic impasses between the parent and adolescent involves several critical interventions. First, the therapist transforms parents' blaming and hopelessness by focusing on feelings of regret and loss, bringing the parents to a more vulnerable position in which they can be open to and listen to the adolescent. In order to engage the adolescent in this process, the therapist asks the adolescent if he or she believes that the parent is actually concerned. This provides the opportunity for the adolescent to share his or her experience. The therapist moves the conversation into the parent-adolescent relationship domain, asking the parent to listen and respond to the adolescent's belief and/or disbelief. Finally, the therapist amplifies the parent's empathy by offering support and admiration, which helps to facilitate further disclosure by the adolescent and an open dialogue between family members. The resolution of therapeutic impasses is one example of how therapists work in the relational domain.

The following segment offers an example of how the therapist works through an impasse, pulling for a different emotional tone and reaching a new level of openness between the parent and adolescent. In this session, the adolescent is angry and refuses to talk about a fight he and his mother had after she realized his girlfriend had spent the night in their home. The mother in this session insists that she is happy with how she handled the situation and feels that the issue is resolved. The adolescent, however, is clearly very angry about the argument. The therapist has the option of letting the issue die, but decides to push the mother to use this as an opportunity to find out more about her son's feelings and thoughts about intimacy and sexuality.

T: Let's go a little bit further and let's find out—I mean this is a big topic for a kid his age. He's starting to be sexually active and he's got to make decisions about this. Could you help him think through some of this? Does he want to be a father? Doesn't he? If he was a father, what would he do?

M: Do you want a child?

A: Not now.

M: If you keep having sex and someone comes to you and says they're pregnant, what would you do?

A: I would be there for her as the father . . . but I don't know . . .

T: Follow that up. Find out what he means.

M: What does it mean to be with someone?

A: To me to be with someone is to go places together, talk over the phone, do things together. Like that.

T: Have you ever had a relationship like that?

A: Just once—it was like five months.

T: [To mom] Did you know her? Did you like her?

M: Yeah—she was a sweet girl and she cared about him. He cried over her. Even this one now—I see that he really cares about her.

T: It sounds to me like you like being in a relationship. [Mom and adolescent both nod yes. Therapist turns to Mom.] You say yes. How do you know that? You think he enjoys being with someone?

M: He just likes having a girl he can talk with, laugh with, go places with. I see he gets real emotional about the girls he's with.

T: [To mom] You sound impressed about your son's sensitivity with women and relationships. It sounds like there's a lot more going on with him than just sleeping around and wanting his girlfriend to sleep over. I think he must have learned that sensitivity somewhere, and I'm thinking he has ideas and memories about what it was like for you to go through your relationships. Can you ask him what he remembers about you being in relationships?

The adolescent and his mother talk for the rest of the session about her relationship with his father, and how his father was not able to show him how to be in a stable, caring relationship. As they share their memories of this time in their lives, the adolescent talks more about what type of husband and father he would like to be. The adolescent and his mother have talked for the first time about the most important things in the adolescent's life, and they have opened lines of communication that were closed with hostility and resentment. The therapist moves the conversation into the realm of their relationship, and helps the adolescent and parent find a new way of talking about an issue that is and will continue to be central in each of their lives.

In summary, working in this way requires many conceptual and personal challenges for the therapist. A deep knowledge of the developmental issues of the adolescent period, family risk factors for adolescent substance abuse problems, and the transformations that typically occur in the parent-adolescent relationship, including changes in group cohesion in the family, provides a conceptual foundation for family-based interventions with adolescents. Comfort and knowledge in building and maintaining separate therapeutic alliances with the parent and the teenager is essential in this process. The ability to conceptualize family therapy and individual sessions in a stage-specific sense guides therapy in each domain.

REFERENCES

Baumrind D. The influence of parenting style on adolescent competence and substance use. *Journal of Early Adolescence* 11:56-95, 1991.

Brook JS, Brook DW, Gordon AS, Whiteman M, Cohen P. The psychosocial etiology of adolescent drug use: A family-interactional approach. *Genetic Social and General Psychology Monographs* 116(2):111-267, 1990.

Chamberlain P, Reid JB. Using a specialized foster care community treatment model for children and adolescents leaving the state mental hospital. *Journal of Community Psychology* 19:266-276, 1991.

Chilcoat HD, Dishion TJ, Anthony JC. Parent monitoring and the incidence of drug sampling in urban elementary school children. *American Journal of Epidemiology* 141:25-31, 1995.

Coombs RH, Landsverk J. Parenting styles and substance use during childhood and adolescence. *Journal of Marriage and the Family* 50:473-482, 1988.

Coyne J, Liddle HA. The future of systems therapy: Shedding myths and facing opportunities. *Psychotherapy: Theory, Research, and Practice* 29:44-50, 1992.

Darling N, Steinberg LD. Parenting style as context: An integrative model. *Psychological Bulletin* 113:487-496, 1993.

Diamond GM, Liddle HA. Improving a negative therapist-adolescent alliance in family therapy. In *101 Interventions in Family Therapy,* Second Edition, edited by Trepper T, Nelson T. Binghamton, NY: The Haworth Press, 1993, pp. 87-95.

Diamond G, Liddle HA. Resolving a therapeutic impasse between parents and adolescents in multidimensional family therapy. *Journal of Consulting and Clinical Psychology* 64(3):481-488, 1996.

Dishion TJ, Patterson GR, Reid JR. *Parent and Peer Factors Associated with Drug Sampling in Early Adolescence: Implications for Treatment* (NIDA Research Monograph No 77). Rockville, MD: National Institute on Drug Abuse, 1988, pp. 69-93.

Farrington D. The development of offending and antisocial behavior from childhood: Key findings from the Cambridge Study in Delinquent Youth. *Journal of Child Psychology and Psychiatry and Allied Disciplines* 36:1-35, 1995.

Goldstein MJ, Miklowitz DJ. The effectiveness of psychoeducational family therapy in the treatment of schizophrenic disorders. *Journal of Marital and Family Therapy* 21:361-376, 1995.

Henggeler SW, Borduin CM, Melton GB, Mann BJ, Smith LA, Hall JA, Cone L, Fucci BR. Effects of multisystemic therapy on drug use and abuse in serious juvenile offenders: A progress report from two outcome studies. *Family Dynamics of Addiction Quarterly* 1:40-51, 1991.

Jessor R, Jessor SL. *Problem Behavior and Psychosocial Development: A Longitudinal Study of Youth.* San Diego, CA: Academic Press, 1977.

Kandel DB, Davies M. High school students who use crack and other drugs. *Archives of General Psychiatry* 53:71-80, 1996.

Laqueur HP. Multiple family therapy. In *The Book of Family Therapy,* edited by Ferber AJ, Mendelsohn M, Napier A. New York: Science House, Inc., 1972, pp. 618-636.

Lebow JL, Gurman AS. Research assessing couple and family therapy. *Annual Review of Psychology* 46:27-57, 1995.

Liddle HA, Dakof GA. Efficacy of family therapy for drug abuse: Promising but not definitive. *Journal of Marital and Family Therapy* 21:511-544, 1995a.

Liddle HA, Dakof GA. Family-based treatments for adolescent drug use: State of the science. In *Adolescent Drug Abuse: Clinical Assessment and Therapeutic Interventions* (NIDA Research Monograph No 156, NIH Publ No 95-3908), edited by Rahdert E, Czechowicz D. Rockville, MD: National Institute on Drug Abuse, 1995b, pp. 218-254.

Liddle HA, Dakof G, Diamond G. Adolescent substance abuse: Multidimensional family therapy in action. In *Family Therapy Approaches with Drug and Alcohol Problems,* edited by Kaufman E, Kaufmann P. Boston: Allyn & Bacon, 1991.

Liddle HA, Rowe CL, Dakof GA, Lyke T. Translating parenting research into clinical interventions for families with adolescents. *Clinical Child Psychology and Psychiatry* 3:419-443, 1998.

Mann BJ, Borduin CM, Henggeler SW, Blake DM. An investigation of systemic conceptualizations of parent-child coalitions and symptom change. *Journal of Consulting and Clinical Psychology* 58:336-344, 1990.

McCord J. Some child-rearing antecedents of criminal behavior in adult men. *Journal of Personality and Social Psychology* 37:1477-1486, 1979.

Nichols MP, Schwartz RC. *Family Therapy: Concepts and Methods,* Fourth Edition. Boston, MA: Allyn & Bacon, 1998.

Rueveni U. *Networking Families in Crisis.* New York: Human Sciences Press, 1979.

Schmidt S, Liddle HA, Dakof GD. Changes in parenting practices in multidimensional family therapy. *Journal of Family Psychology* 10:1-16, 1996.

Speck R, Attneave C. Network therapy. In *The Book of Family Therapy,* edited by Ferber A, Mendelsohn M, Napier A. New York: Science House, Inc., 1972, pp. 637-665.

Stanton MD, Todd C. *The Family Therapy of Drug Abuse and Addiction.* New York: Guilford Press, 1982.

Steinberg LD, Fletcher A, Darling N. Parental monitoring and peer influences on adolescent substance abuse. *Pediatrics* 93:1-5, 1994.

Szapocznik J, Santisteban D, Rio A, Perez-Vidal A, Santisteban D, Kurtines WM. Family effectiveness training: An intervention to prevent drug abuse and problem behavior in Hispanic adolescents. *Hispanic Journal of Behavioral Sciences* 11:3-27, 1989.

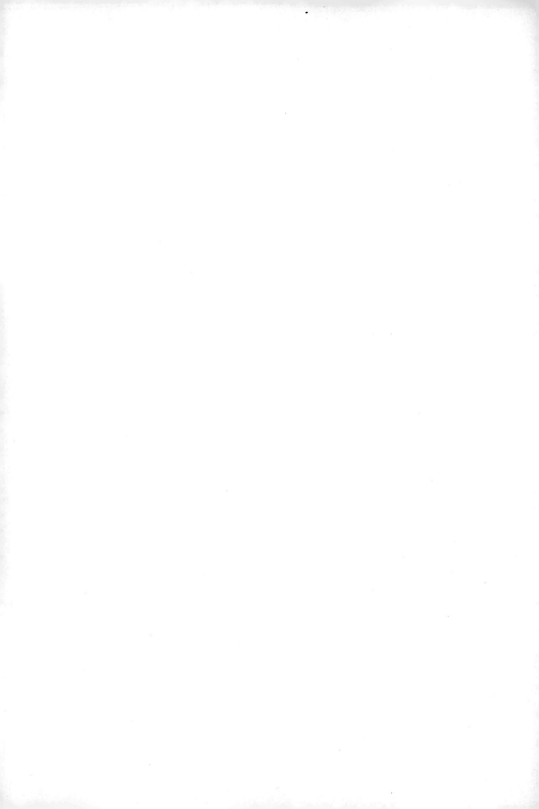

Chapter 17

Group Psychotherapy with Drug-Dependent, Dually Diagnosed Adolescents in a Residential Setting

Thomas Edward Bratter

DIAGNOSIS: ITS RELATIONSHIP WITH TREATMENT OUTCOME

Diagnosing the psychoeducational characteristics of gifted, deceitful, drug-dependent adolescents is never a benign therapeutic act. Using provocative rhetoric, Szasz (1974) rightfully contends that a diagnosis can reflect the bias of the therapist (and institution), which poses not only a stigmatization but also a justification to prescribe medication. To make an accurate assessment is difficult. Gediman and Lieberman (1996, p. 3-4) state that "deception is ubiquitous in everyday life ... psychoanalysts have not studied deceptive phenomena." Psychotherapists recognize denial, mistrust, and paranoia as defense mechanisms of drug-dependent adolescents, but they are not trained to discern or confront deceit.

The degree of dysfunctional behavior complicates the distinction between a *normal* and a *self-destructive* diagnosis. Kreisman and Straus (1989, p. 3) contend, "a normal adolescent may listen to gloomy music, write pessimistic poetry, glorify suicidal celebrities, dramatically scream, cry, and threaten[;] however, the normal adolescent does not cut ... wrists, binge and purge several times a day, become addicted to drugs, or attack [parents]; and it is these extremes that herald BPD" (Borderline Personality Disorder). Clinicians need to recognize acute or chronic drug abuse because drug dependence and addiction can impede personality development. An accurate DSM-IV diagnosis can be complicated by the mimicking of schizophrenic symptoms by some psychoactive substances. Amphetamines can cause a temporary psychotic state that can be confused with a schizophrenic psychosis. Cannabis and amphetamines, when combined with other hallucinogens, can produce paranoid symptoms. The primary problem of the drug-dependent adolescent is the antisocial attitudes, not the use of psychoactive substances. To assess adolescent responses, capricious and unpredictable behavior, conflict, testing of limits, anger, mistrust, and rejection of authority should be considered with age-appropriate measures contingent on degree. It is neither unusual nor unhealthy for adolescents to mistrust treatment personnel who can seem threatening because they possess the power to incarcerate.

Ponce and Jo (1990) discuss the clinical challenges for residential programs posed by those who are dually diagnosed. In an attempt to organize and clarify this problem, Ryglewicz and Pepper (1996, pp. 74-75) identify four groups of dually diagnosed persons:

> *Group 1:* A major mental illness and a major problem with alcohol and/or drug abuse.
> *Group 2:* A major mental illness and a special vulnerability to the effects of alcohol and other drugs.
> *Group 3:* Personality disordered and/or other mental/emotional problems that are complicated and aggravated by alcohol and/or street drug use, but no major mental illness, that would produce psychotic episodes or require hospitalization.
> *Group 4:* Diagnosed or identified alcohol/drug abuse, dependence, or addiction, plus personality disorder or other mental/emotional/cognitive problems that are masked by substance use and may increase during withdrawal.

After making a preliminary diagnosis, the final assessment should be delayed until after detoxification to ascertain whether symptoms will continue or abate. Care needs to be exercised to refrain from absolving the chemically dependent adolescent of responsibility for antisocial attitudes and acts attributed to psychopathology. Insisting that the adolescent accept accountability for such behavior rather than using psychiatric nomenclature, which abets the abdication of control of behavior, makes more treatment sense. Personal problems that precede self-medication need to be confronted and resolved prior to positive identity formation.

Drug-dependent, dysfunctional, deceitful, destructive adolescents need no justification for behavior that a DSM-IV diagnosis may inadvertently provide. Often adolescents perceive these diagnoses to be a tacit approval to insulate themselves from reality and to continue self-destructive, drug-related conduct, and they become passive (innocent) and vulnerable (impotent) to control thoughts, feelings, and behavior. This negates the viability of psychoanalytic diagnoses that obfuscate the problem by suggesting that in the analytic model, patients subtly are relieved of any responsibility for acts and behavior.

This chapter is a plea never to forget *patients* are *people* who *consciously choose* not only to abuse psychoactive and psychotropic substances but also to perform masochistic and sadistic acts—in other words, these adolescents are individuals capable of controlling their own behavior.

MEDICATION: NOT A PHARMACOLOGICAL PANACEA

Biological theories can be reductionistic. Neurotransmitter research remains a heuristic technique, not a psychopharmacological panacea. Dysfunctional behavior can be ameliorated by selective serotonin inhibitors such as fluoxetine, and by tricyclic antidepressants such as imipramine and amitriptyline, and by antidepressants such as maprotiline, amoxapine, and monoamine oxidase (MAO) inhibitors (Dipiro et al. 1993). Tanouyc (1997, p. B1) warns that "no medications have been approved by the Food and Drug Administration to treat depression in patients under 18 years old."

By definition, an alcoholic or addict lacks the capacity to regulate consumption of psychoactive and psychotropic substances after ingesting the first dose. The convoluted thinking of the drug-dependent adolescent results in the belief that abuse will produce euphoria. Mendel (1966, p. 95) believes that prior to entering into a treatment alliance, patients attempt to convince the therapist that they are "victimized by unconscious needs . . . which . . . lead to self-defeat . . . [; they are] not responsible and [do not] understand...[; they are] the victim." Karp (1996, p. 73), concurs: "acceptance of a victim's role, while diminishing a sense of personal responsibility, is . . . enfeebling. To be a victim of biochemical forces beyond one's control gives . . . definition of oneself as a helpless, passive, object of injury."

Clinicians may ignore that isolation, feelings of inadequacy, rejection and/or failure can cause depression. Beeder and Millman (1995, p. 85) warn that "in patients with major depression, dysthymia, bipolar disorder, and related disorders, it is difficult to determine whether mood states are the cause or the sequelae of protracted drug use. Affective symptoms can represent a distinct illness and/or a result of antagonistic effects of the drug." The gifted know they are abusing their talents.

Many who attend the John Dewey Academy had been diagnosed as defiant, exacerbated by ADD/ADHD. Many arrived medicated on fluoxetine, alprazolam, lithium, sodium valproate, methylphenidate, and bupropion. All become drug free. The John Dewey Academy contends that psychotropic medicine does not modify attitude problems.

THE JOHN DEWEY ACADEMY

Bratter et al. (1998) have noted that the John Dewey Academy traces its antecedents to the divergent therapeutic community (TC) movements that arose concurrently but operated independently. TC inpatient psychiatric hospitals utilize an educational process that stresses social learning in a group for (re)habilitation (Jones 1968). This process is unique compared to other treatment programs.

The John Dewey Academy mobilizes positive peer pressure. This structure, stressing role expectations and individual empowerment while minimizing the number of rules and regulations, differentiates the Academy community from other residential approaches. Regardless of time spent in the program and their position, students share in the daily management of the community (Collabolletta, Gordon, Kaufman 1999).

The John Dewey Academy determines rewards and consequences for its members. Encouraging adolescents to evaluate one another's behavior helps them internalize the guiding principles of the caring community. The John Dewey Academy is a residential, college preparatory, therapeutic, voluntary high school (Bratter 1993; Bratter et al. 1998). This residential therapeutic caring community provides "a safe, structured, supportive treatment environment" (Bratter et al. 1993, p. 299). It also provides an unrelenting, uncompromising, and stressful environment where escalating expectations demand that everyone improve by changing rather than continuing dysfunctional, deceitful, destructive patterns of behavior.

Prior to admission, 33 percent of the adolescents have been hospitalized for at least two months, 80 percent have been treated by a psychiatrist, and 40 percent are admitted with an addiction to potent psychotropic medication. Students are expected not only to take control of their lives but also to accept responsibility for their acts and attitudes. Consequently, the rigid atmosphere of institutions that stress the four "Cs" of care, custody, conformity, and control is condemned. Four different "Cs" of change, communication, cooperation, and care, are stressed. Moreover, change, of a constructive and creative nature, is demanded. Bratter, Bratter, and Bratter (1995, p. 59) write that "the most important goal of therapy is to help adolescents (re)gain their self-respect [by becoming responsible and productive]."

PSYCHOSOCIAL-EDUCATIONAL CHARACTERISTICS OF GIFTED, SELF-DESTRUCTIVE ADOLESCENTS

The majority of the John Dewey Academy adolescents are chemically dependent. Wexler (1991, p. 78) describes these adolescents as "troubled" for they have "abused drugs and alcohol, fought with family members . . . run away . . . truant . . . stolen . . . [yet,] they are [not] a serious danger to society . . . [nor] do they suffer from severe psychological or organic dysfunctions." They are at risk simply because they may return to abusing if the changes they have made to their lifestyle are not heeded.

Although gifted, alienated adolescents are usually diagnosed as being *unmotivated,* unwilling to change, and unable to perform, this appraisal is incorrect. Drug- and alcohol-dependent adolescents are *unconvinced.* Although psychotherapists and educators often view them as untreatable, uneducable, uncivilized, and untrustworthy, when placed in an environment with high expectations for improvement, and when convinced change will be salubrious, they will work diligently, emotionally, and academically.

These students have similar family histories. During formative years, some have suffered from parental acts of benign neglect or emotional/physical abuse. Gifted adolescents feel cheated and their self-esteem is impaired by parents who deprive them of emotional nourishment. Kohut (1987) explains that shame occurs when there are no ego-gratifying opportunities to experience self-esteem. Bright adolescents understand that their current behaviors place them in a lose-lose labyrinth that jeopardizes their future options. This reaction can produce resentment, jealousy, and anger camouflaged to conceal painful feelings of an enfeebled, inadequate, and/or negative sense of self. Often, sensitive and gifted adolescents compensate with a voracious sense of entitlement accompanied by rage. Frequently, the sense of powerlessness is expressed "I can't," when the real feeling is "I won't and you can't make me!" These tyrannical teens dehumanize others to satisfy their wants. They defend themselves by projecting an aura of hostility to insulate themselves from intimacy and being hurt. Whether they are victims or perpetrators is irrelevant because the pain of rejection is debilitating. They have been bruised, betrayed, battered, and bloodied by their choices. They conceal wounds from those whom they mistrust, because they fear that others have the power to inflict more intense suffering. In an effort to protect themselves against this kind of morbid rumination, these adolescents project facades of grandiosity to hide inadequacy, confusion, and fear.

Salinger's fictional character Holden Caulfield personifies the angry alienation and nihilistic attitudes typical of those who attend the John Dewey Academy. Holden's teacher, Mr. Antolini, accurately describes the plight of these lost souls, "this fall . . . is a special kind . . . a horrible kind. The man . . . just keeps falling and falling[; t]he whole arrangement is designed for men who . . . were looking for something their . . . environment couldn't supply them with[; s]o they gave up looking[; t]hey gave up before they ever really even got started" (Salinger 1951, p. 253).

IMPLICATIONS OF PSYCHOPATHOLOGY FOR TREATMENT

All pathological beliefs and behaviors can be modified with therapy. There are two phases in the psychotherapeutic process, unlearning and learning. Unlearning precedes learning more positive and healthy responses. Wolpe (1958, p. ix) emphasizes this two-phase model "since neurotic behavior . . . originates in learning, it is only expected that its elimination will be a matter of unlearning"; through a corrective emotional experience one can transcend past self-destructive acts and attitudes by achieving the greatness of which one once was thought capable.

For dually diagnosed, comorbid, deceitful, drug-dependent adolescents specifically, it makes sense to attribute the etiology of psychopathology and pathogenic attitudes to a distorted learning process that produced flawed reality testing. These adolescents engage in extreme behavior. The group experience makes it difficult to escape from the reality of responsibility yet still provides a therapeutic milieu, and demonstrates to the group members the irresponsible and self-defeating aspects of their behavior and the consequences of their acts. This fosters the growth of responsibility.

Adolescents can transcend their past experiences. Patterson (1966, p. 466) explains that the adolescent "cannot . . . control the conditions [by] which he is confronted, but can control his responses . . . choices, and his actions."

RENEGOTIATING THE PARAMETERS OF CONFIDENTIALITY

Writing about the American Socialist and utopian communities, Noyes (1870), the founder of the Oneida Community (1848), noted that public confession encouraged individuals to relate misdeeds and then take corrective action. Serendipitously, the community was transformed into a curative therapeutic force. According to Clark (1951), the progenitor of Alcoholics Anonymous, the Oxford Community may have been the first to recognize the cathartic value of public confession as a prerequisite for change. Alcoholics Anonymous discontinued public confessions that had a certain negative impact on the individual as well as the group. Bill W. (1957) believed that the tenets of the Oxford Group were excessive for AA. In 1957, AA excluded recovering addicts who were confrontational. Dederich started Synanon, which utilized ex-addicts as primary treatment agents, as described by Casriel (1964) and Yablonsky (1965). Unlike AA, members were confronted in front of the community not only to humiliate, but also to force compliance with a rigid set of behaviors.

Distinguishing self-help therapeutic communities from more traditional treatment programs, De Leon (1997, pp. 4-6) states, "the purposive use of the peer community is to facilitate social and psychological change in individuals . . . the public nature and shared experiences in the community is used for therapeutic purposes."

Spitz and Spitz (1995, p. 270) present the traditional view of confidentiality in outpatient group psychotherapy with adolescent substance abusers that any "breach of confidentiality . . . [would be] grounds for dismissal." Rather, drug-dependent adolescents, whose reckless behavior terrifies them, wish to be stopped, and their disclosures need to be viewed as desperate pleas for therapist and/or group intervention. Once a therapeutic alliance has been established and predicated on trust, drug-dependent adolescents are candid, and discuss voluntarily current and future acts, which confirms their wish to be stopped. If viewed within this perspective, the therapist, who maintains confidentiality in a residential setting, enters into the "conspiracy of silence" by becoming an "enabler" who unwittingly condones dangerous behavior. An evaluation and a revision of the parameters of confidentiality in residential settings is needed.

GROUP PSYCHOTHERAPY:
TREATMENT OF CHOICE FOR DUALLY DIAGNOSED,
DRUG-DEPENDENT ADOLESCENTS

Blaustein and Wolff (1972) were the first to suggest that group psychotherapy is the most effective modality for hospitalized adolescents. Alienated and angry adolescents need to be held accountable for predicaments caused by their immature, irresponsible, illicit, and impulsive choices, with a major goal of treatment defined as helping the patient to accept responsibility. Initial therapeutic interventions would therefore need to help annihilative adolescents take control of their lives. This can best be achieved within a group setting where no one either excuses mediocrity or commiserates how unlucky and unjust life is. Bratter (1989, p. 176) states, "until the group leader can convince adolescent addicts that there can be a more rewarding existence than using drugs, it is unlikely they will modify their attitudes." Relying on her work with dually diagnosed, drug-dependent persons, Director (1995, p. 386) adds "group psychotherapy . . . is not solely devoted to behavior change and education[; t]here is a . . . need to address the characterological problems and difficulty with feelings that form the root causes of their use of drugs."

Most students are antiauthority. The group leader is advised to empower the group to become a catalyst for constructive change. Positive peer pressure will motivate members to convert painful criticism into creative change. Group psychotherapy is the modality of choice for such dually diagnosed, destructive, drug-dependent adolescents. Stein and Kymissis (1989) emphasize that the institutionalized adolescent may more easily accept help from peers. The group helps members identify negative attitudes and avoid placing themselves in no-win situations. By confronting dysfunctional thinking, members become more aware of behavior, feelings, and attitudes. Brook (1996) provides justification for group therapy as the most potent psychotherapeutic modality for drug-dependent adolescents because it sets behavior limits, which help adolescents develop internal controls and accept responsibility for their actions.

TREATMENT STRATEGIES: THE ACT OF ADVOCACY

Drug-using adolescents are demoralized because they have compromised their futures. Until there is hope, students will not contemplate changing. The restoration of hope after they assume responsibility serves as an incentive. Bratter (1973) notes that such adolescents may be motivated to enter into a therapeutic alliance by the hope that the therapist may act as an advocate and may help the adolescent's continued growth into a more optimistic future. It is the burden of the leader to convince members who no longer dream about success to have hope that their futures can be optimistic—i.e., pleasurable, without pain and drugs.

Adolescents who have frustrated, alienated, and polarized the adults in their lives who could have helped them, make it necessary for a credible person to intercede as an advocate. The act of advocacy is salutary for adolescents who have failure identities. Before agreeing to become an advocate, the therapist shares decision-making power with the group by mobilizing its collective resources to appraise achievement. To ensure candor and cooperation, the therapist notifies the group that his or her reputation is their asset, but if this trust were lost, the chance to deliver vital service in the future would be decreased. If the group decides a member does not deserve special consideration, the therapist should inquire why. When realistic reasons are given, the leader can appoint peers to serve as consultants to prescribe specific strategies that coopt negative attitudes. Becoming partners with an adolescent helps the therapist and the group to encourage the adolescent to realize his or her full potential.

TRANSFERENCE AND COUNTERTRANSFERENCE

One of the most powerful, but least studied, phenomena for adolescent therapists is countertransference. Many authors do not discuss countertransference issues. Bloch (1995) discusses transference, but excludes countertransference. Gifted, acting-out adolescents evoke the most intense countertransference reactions of any treatment population because of the ubiquitous experience of adolescence. Therapists should be aware and guard against gaining gratification from the adventures and exploits of emancipated adolescents whose lives seem exciting. The group leaders must recognize that they can encourage amoral activity if the youth perceives any vicarious thrill in the therapist during their discussion of dangerous behavior. This is especially true for those therapists whose adolescence predates the drug and sexual revolutions. If therapists "envy" the adolescent, who engages in dangerous and exciting acts, they need to be aware that this behavior would signal a negative countertransference. The phenomenon of parents who unconsciously encourage their adolescent to act out for their own gratification is well known. The voracious, vicarious, unconscious needs of parents unwittingly can encourage erratic and dangerous behavior, which prompts adults to become either domineering or overly permissive and indulgent. The converse is also true when the therapist feels the need to punish. Imhof, Hirsch, and Terenzi (1983, pp. 501-502) explain the psychodynamics of creating a good-bad dichotomy, which threatens the ego formation of the adolescent who "provokes, cajoles, humiliates, and deceives the therapist."

Adolescents gain identities by interacting with others. Guntrip (1975, p. 155) states that psychoanalytic psychotherapy can be a nurturing, human relationship which enables the repressed traumatized child to become healthier in the "security of a new real relationship." This dynamic often is misunderstood or minimized by psychoanalysts. Those psychotherapists who believe the rescue fantasy is pathogenic need to disqualify themselves from working with this adolescent population who engage in life-threatening behavior. Palmer, Harper and Rivinus (1983, p. 122) incorrectly view an "adoptive process" in the residential treatment of adolescents as acting out the rescue fantasy of practitioners who have not resolved their conflicts or who seek to become parental surrogates due to unfulfilled needs. Shay (1987) also wrongly attributes the need to rescue as an unresolved countertransferential reaction.

The potential for abuse exists when the leader competes for the control and/or the affection of the adolescent, minimizes psychopathology, fantasizes about becoming the good parent, and deems the family incapable of changing and excludes them from treatment. Indeed, a goal of psychotherapy is to offer the adolescent a healthy replacement for a pathogenic family, giving the adolescent a safe base from which to explore the world. Grotjahn (1972, p. 197), suggests that the group psychotherapist "accept in himself a considerable amount of maternal identification . . . [for] maternal attitude facilitates the experience of weaning and individuation[;] the breaking of the mother-infant symbiosis may amount to an experience of rebirth in the group."

CLINICAL CHALLENGES: SELF-DISCLOSURE

While working in a residential environment, the psychotherapist at times will be tired, sick, angry, discouraged, depressed, and disgusted. Due to daily contact, it is impossible to camouflage, hide, retreat, and regenerate. The clinician needs the stamina to continue despite painful personal problems; adolescents are privy to all of the personal issues of the practitioner. The leader needs to encourage adolescents to relate honestly.

Gifted, chemically dependent adolescents can frustrate, infuriate, insult, and defy the psychotherapist who must not become punitive. Living together, adolescents will bond against the authority of the group leader, forming a countertherapeutic "we-they" dichotomy. The burden to prove trust resides with the therapist, not the adolescent. Whenever possible the leader is advised to elicit peer input in the group regarding consequences for irresponsible, deceitful, unproductive behavior, rather than retain the power to make unilateral decisions. Rather than interpret motives and feelings, the therapist can ask, "What can we do to help you to help yourself?"

Once a therapeutic alliance has been formed, dysfunctional, drug-dependent adolescents can overwhelm the therapist by escalating their demands. The leaders need to defend themselves from being drained by adolescent needs for dependence. The clinical challenge, therefore, is to maintain the balance between therapeutic giving and acquiescing to adolescent demands. More than any other treatment population, inpatient groups with dually diagnosed narcissistic adolescents need an explanation why it is impossible to fulfill their needs to avoid reinforcing their feelings of unworthiness.

The therapist can relate to a personal, painful past, including failure and rejection to convince adolescents that no one can win and succeed all the time. At times, the leader can extend the treatment alliance by permitting adolescents to relate to and identify with him or her. Self-disclosure can be a therapeutic benefit to adolescents, though it must not be for the self-aggrandizement of the practitioner. Exhibitionistic and grandiose tendencies need to be eliminated. Sharing past experiences involves risk, because these adolescents will confront the hypocrisies of the therapist. When adolescents gained leverage, then personal disclosures post hoc were deleterious. The therapist needs the strength to permit personal values to be criticized, but to relate so that adolescents can clarify issues and can begin to determine solutions while internalizing beliefs. When the leader seeks the support or advice of adolescents, self-disclosure is detrimental. Adolescents can gain insight and strength, however, when a group leader reveals painful and depressing events that can substantiate resilience and the determination to remain responsible even if overwhelmed by adversity and failure. Being transparent can convey a potent therapeutic message that life can be painful and unpleasant but that it is possible to remain both responsive and responsible.

CONCLUSION

Before working with adolescents who abuse dangerous, psychoactive substances, Amodeo and Drouilhet (1992, p. 305) suggest that therapists be aware of "visceral reactions to these patients . . . [for] some clinicians will struggle with feelings of moralism, anger, and anxiety." Practitioners, who dehumanize (and want to punish) dually diagnosed, drug-dependent youth, need to refer them elsewhere. Rather, a therapist should feel pride possessing the expertise, energy, optimism, toughness, tenderness, and resilience to work with this most difficult-to-engage population. With the group leader's assistance, they can transcend their pasts and, in so doing, justify their existences to themselves to use, rather than continue to abuse, their abilities. Bratter et al. (1993) assert that once these adolescents trust the therapist, they can change.

Creating conditions conducive for constructive change, which help these adolescents (re)claim their lives from chemical oblivion, rejection, and failure, is fascinating work. There are, however, occupational hazards in working with gifted, self-destructive, drug-dependent youth who refuse to play by anyone's rules but their own. Under the most optimal conditions, there are no guarantees of treatment success. Bratter (1997, p. 51) warns that "there are two unalterable realities working with gifted, drug-dependent, adolescents: Rule 1: Some will die of drug overdoses, commit suicide, or be murdered; Rule 2: There will be cases when the concerned clinician cannot change Rule 1." When treatment outcomes are painful, the therapist must possess the resilience to prevail.

The group therapist has a choice either to assume the analytical, benign observer stance or become active and directive. Those wishing to remain overly analytic probably will be ineffective, because dually diagnosed, drug-dependent, gifted adolescents know that self-medication can produce temporary relief and euphoria with little effort. Without clinical intervention, drug abuse will escalate to dangerous levels, rendering the group therapist impotent. When the therapist opts to be active and directive, the chances of creating the conditions necessary for change and improvement are maximized, and "burnout" and negative countertransference issues are minimized.

Like the surgeon whose expertise can improve and prolong the quality of life, it is an invigorating challenge to create the catalytic conditions that can help dually diagnosed adolescents to redirect nihilistic passions into positive directions by accepting responsibility for dysfunctional behavior. The group helps members not only to make decisions when they resist, but also to recognize that gaining self-respect is more important than is the pursuit of pleasure. It is gratifying to know that one has helped an adolescent transcend a painful, unproductive, and wasted past. There can be no finer reward than to help adolescents to help themselves survive and succeed.

REFERENCES

Amodeo M, Drouilhet A. Substance-abusing adolescents in countertransference. In *Psychotherapy with Children and Adolescents,* edited by Brandell JR. Northvale, NJ: Jason Aronson, 1992, pp. 285-314.

Beeder AB, Millman RB. Treatment strategies for comorbid disorders: Psychopathology and substance abuse. In *Psychotherapy and Substance Abuse: A Practitioner's Handbook,* edited by Washton AM. New York: Guilford, 1995, p. 85.

Bill W. *Alcoholics Anonymous Comes of Age: A Brief History of AA.* New York: Alcoholics Anonymous Press, 1957.

Blaustein F, Wolff HB. Adolescent group: A "must" on a psychiatric unit—problems and results. In *Adolescents Grow in Groups: Experiences in Adolescent Group Psychotherapy,* edited by Berkovitz IH. New York: Brunner/Mazel, 1972, pp. 181-190.

Bloch HS. *Adolescent Development, Psychopathology, and Treatment.* Madison, CT: International Universities Press, 1995.

Bratter BI, Bratter CJ, Bratter TE. Beyond reality: The need to (re)gain self-respect. *Psychotherapy: Theory, Research and Practice* 32:59-69, 1995.

Bratter BI, Bratter CJ, Bratter TE, Maxym C, Steiner KM. The John Dewey Academy: A moral caring community, an amalgamation of the professional model and self-help concept of the therapeutic community. In *Community As Method: Modified Therapeutic Communities for Special Populations and Special Settings,* edited by De Leon G. Westport, CT: Praeger, 1998, pp. 179-195, 272-274.

Bratter TE. Treating, alienated, unmotivated drug-abusing adolescents. *American Journal of Psychology* XXVII:585-598, 1973.

Bratter TE. Group Psychotherapy with alcohol and drug addicted adolescents: Special clinical concerns and challenges. In *Adolescent Group Psychotherapy,* edited by Azima FJC, Richmond L. Madison, CT: International Universities Press, 1989, pp. 163-189.

Bratter TE. The John Dewey Academy: A residential quality school for self-destructive adolescents who have superior intellectual and intuitive potential. *Journal of Reality Therapy* XII:42-53, 1993.

Bratter TE. Major challenges of working with gifted, suicidal adolescents. *Psychiatric Times* XIV:50-53, 1997.

Bratter TE, Bratter BI, Radda HT, Steiner KM. The residential therapeutic caring community. *Psychotherapy—Theory, Research and Practice* 30(2):299-304, 1993.

Brook DW. Adolescents who abuse substances. In *Group Therapy with Children and Adolescents,* edited by Kymissis P, Halperin DA.Washington, DC: American Psychiatric Press, 1996, pp. 243-264.

Casriel D. *So Fair a House: The Story of Synanon.* Englewood Cliffs, NJ: Prentice-Hall, 1964.

Clark WH. *The Oxford Group.* New York: Bookman Associates, 1951.

Collabolletta EA, Gordon D, Kaufman, SD. The John Dewey Academy: Motivating unconvinced, ADD/ADHD, oppositional students to use, rather than contrive to abuse, their superior assets. *International Journal of Reality Therapy* 19(2):38-45, 2000.

De Leon G. Therapeutic communities: Is there an essential model? In *Community as Method: Therapeutic Communities for Special Populations and Special Settings,* edited by De Leon G. Westport, CT: Praeger, 1997, pp. 3-18.

Dipiro JT, Talbert RL, Hayes PE, Matzke GR, Posey LM. *Pharmacotherapy: A Pathophysiologic Approach,* Second Edition. Norwalk, CT: Appleton & Lange, 1993.

Director L. Dual diagnosis: Outpatient treatment of substance abusers with coexisting psychiatric disorders. In *Psychotherapy and Substance Abuse: A Practitioner's Handbook,* edited by Washton AM. New York: The Guilford Press, 1995, pp. 375-393.

Gediman HK, Lieberman JS. *The Many Faces of Deceit: Omissions, Lies, and Disguise in Psychotherapy.* Northvale, NJ: Jason Aronson, 1996.

Grotjahn M. The qualities of the group therapist. In *New Models for Group Psychotherapy,* edited by Kaplan HI, Sadock BJ. New York: EP Dutton, 1972, pp. 191-207.

Guntrip H. My experience of analysis with Fairbain and Winnicott. *International Review of Psycho-Analysis* 2:145-156, 1975.

Imhof J, Hirsch R, Terenzi RE. Countertransferential and attitudinal considerations in the treatment of drug abuse and addiction. *International Journal of Addictions* 18:491-510, 1983.

Jones M. *Beyond the Therapeutic Community—Social Learning and Social Psychiatry.* New Haven, CT: Yale University Press, 1968.

Karp DA. *Depression, Disconnection, and the Meanings of Illness: Speaking of Sadness.* New York: Oxford University Press, 1996.

Kohut H. Narcissism as a resistance and as a driving force in psychoanalysis. In *Techniques of Working with Resistance,* edited by Milman DS, Goldman GD. Northvale, NJ: Jason Aronson, 1987.

Kreisman JJ, Strauss H. *I Hate You—Don't Leave Me.* Los Angeles: The Body Press, 1989.

Lennard HL. *The Psychiatric Hospital: Context, Values and Therapeutic Process.* New York: Human Sciences Press, 1986.

Mendel WM. Psychotherapy and responsibility. *American Journal of Psychoanalysis* 26:91-96, 1966.

Mowrer OH. Therapeutic groups and communities in retrospect and prospect. In *Proceedings of the First World Conference on Therapeutic Communities,* edited by Vamos P, Devlin JJ. Montreal: The Portage Press, 1977, pp. 2-62.

Noyes JH. *History of American Socialisms.* Philadelphia, PA: JB Lippincott, 1870.

Palmer G, Harper G, Rivinus T. The "adoptive process" in the inpatient treatment of children and adolescents. *Journal of the American Academy of Child and Adolescent Psychiatry* 22(3):286-293, 1983.

Patterson CH. *Theories of Counseling and Psychotherapy.* New York: Harper & Row, 1966.

Ponce DE, Jo HS. Substance abuse and psychiatric disorders: The dilemma of increasing incidence of dual diagnosis in residential treatment centers. *Residential Treatment for Children and Youth* 8:5-15, 1990.

Pruyser PW, Menninger K. Language pitfalls in diagnostic thought and work. In *Diagnosis and the Difference It Makes,* edited by Pruyser PW. New York: Jason Aronson, 1976, pp. 11-28.

Ryglewicz H, Pepper B. *Lives at Risk: Understanding and Treating Young People with Dual Disorders.* New York: The Free Press, a Division of Simon & Schuster, 1996.

Salinger JD. *The Catcher in the Rye.* Boston: Little, Brown, & Co., 1951.

Shay JJ. The wish to do psychotherapy with borderline adolescents—and other common errors. *Psychotherapy—Theory, Research and Practice* 24:712-719, 1987.

Spitz HI, Spitz ST. A five-phase model for adolescents who abuse substances. In *Group Therapy with Children and Adolescents,* edited by Kymissis P, Halperin DA. Washington, DC: American Psychiatric Press, 1995, pp. 265-279.

Stein MD, Kymissis P. Adolescent inpatient group psychotherapy. In *Adolescent Group Psychotherapy,* edited by Azima FJC, Richmond LH. Madison, CT: International Universities Press, 1989, pp. 69-84.

Szasz T. *Ceremonial Chemistry: The Ritual Persecution of Drugs, Addicts, and Pushers.* Garden City, NY: Doubleday, 1974.

Tanouye E. Antidepressant makers study kids' market. *The Wall Street Journal,* CCXXIX:62 B1, B6, 1997.

Wexler DB. *The Adolescent Self: Strategies for Self-Management, Self-Soothing, and Self-Esteem in Adolescents.* New York: WW Norton & Co., 1991.

Wolpe J. *Psychotherapy by Reciprocal Inhibition.* Stanford, CT: Stanford University Press, 1958, p. ix.

Yablonsky L. *The Tunnel Back: The Story of Synanon.* New York: Macmillan & Co., 1965.

Chapter 18

Group Psychotherapy for Elderly Substance Abusers

Eloise Rathbone-McCuan
Roy Nelson

INTRODUCTION

Over the past twenty years there has been an increased amount of clinical attention and research activity on substance misuse and abuse among older people (American Medical Association (AMA) Council on Scientific Affairs 1996). With the continuously expanding aging population, in a society impacted with the consequences of drug addiction throughout the life span (Dufour 1996), concern about later life alcohol abuse and dependence and other substance addictions should be a priority in the geriatric, mental health, and substance abuse fields (Brennan and Moos 1996).

The focus of this chapter is group treatment approaches applicable to older people who experience biological, psychosocial, and environmental factors that influence the development and continuation of a progressive disease known as alcohol abuse. Older people with this disease are similar to younger people in that they share symptoms of impaired control over drinking, preoccupation with alcohol, use of alcohol despite adverse consequences, and distortions in thinking, including denial of the disease (Wiseman, Souder, and O'Sullivan 1996).

Alcohol abuse and its treatment is the specific substance abuse to be considered in this discussion; however, many of the assessment, treatment, and recovery issues related to alcohol abuse apply to other forms of substance abuse. Any type of substance dependence (prescribed drugs, over-the-counter [OTC] medications, or illicit substances) can produce life-threatening dependence among older people (Barnea and Teichman 1994).

DEVELOPMENT OF INTEREST IN AGING
AND SUBSTANCE ABUSE

Interest in the field of alcohol abuse and dependence among older Americans has increased rapidly over the past twenty years as the interdisciplinary knowledge of mental health and aging has expanded (Fink, Hays, and Moore 1996). During the 1960s and 1970s the most commonly applied psychiatric diagnosis applicable to patients of advanced age with a history of chronic alcohol abuse was Wernicke-Korsakoff's syndrome. As more mental health specialists entered practice with older people, evidence showed that conditions such as substance abuse and violence victimization were more prevalent than ever anticipated.

Today issues of alcohol abuse and aging are more widely understood across many service systems. For example, home health care agencies and adult protective service workers know how self and caregiver neglect can be the result of the addiction of the caregiver or the care-receiver. More aware of the problem, greater numbers of care providers are searching for places in the community to where they can refer the addiction-impaired older persons they support daily. The intensified effort to direct older people to treatment delivered by experienced professionals is often a dead-end process because too few resources exist. Even now Alcoholics Anonymous (AA) remains the most utilized source of help available to older alcoholics (Washburn 1996).

Nearly two decades ago the AMA established guidelines for the treatment of alcohol abuse/dependence. At that time 11 percent of the U.S. population was older than sixty-five years of age. By the year 2002 it is estimated that the proportion may grow to over 20 percent of the population. As suggested in a recent AMA report on alcoholism and the elderly (1996), even if the rate of alcohol dependence remains constant, there will be 50 percent more elderly alcoholic patients at the turn of the century compared to the estimated rates thirty years ago.

Prevalence rates are unclear because current estimates of alcohol abuse among the older population vary according to definitions of the disease and its symptoms, measurements used to study the disease, and the sampling approaches applied in conjunction with numerous research methodologies. Elderly living in the community are reported in various studies to have a prevalence rate of less than 1 percent for women and up to 6 percent for men (Szwabo 1993).

The Epidemiologic Catchment Area (ECA) survey is the most frequently referenced data source for estimating prevalence rates for older women living outside institutional settings (Schonfeld et al. 1993). Even with the low estimate rate of chemical dependence, older women have special risk factors for substance abuse such as living alone, suffering from isolation and depression, disabling physical conditions, below poverty incomes, and misuse/dependence on prescription and nonprescription drugs (Szwabo 1993).

According to Goldstein, Pataki, and Webb (1996) the lifetime rate of alcohol dependence among males sixty-five years and older is 14 percent, in contrast to 27 percent for those aged eighteen to twenty-nine, 28 percent for those thirty to forty-four, and 21 percent for those forty-five to sixty-four years of age. In the Veterans Administration (VA) health care system, the largest single treatment source for men with substance abuse problems, about 25 percent of substance abusers are fifty-five years and older (Moos, Mertens, and Brennan 1993). Much of the addiction treatment of older alcohol-dependent men takes place in VA hospitals.

Among the elderly patient population living in nursing homes, the prevalence rate estimates are from 2.8 to 15 percent depending on the setting, method of case identification, and the inclusion of primary and/or secondary diagnoses of alcohol abuse. Rates dramatically increase when data is given for elderly in medical settings. Hospitalization of elderly people with alcohol and/or other drug-related problems increase the estimates to 7 to 22 percent of the older patient population in medical facilities. The estimate of elderly people with alcohol and other drug problems in psychiatric facilities is more than double the estimated rates of medical inpatients, with between 28 percent and 44 percent of older psychiatric patients carrying an alcohol abuse diagnosis (Adams et al. 1992; Joseph, Ganzini, and Atkinson 1995; Liberto, Oslin, and Ruskin 1992). Evidence shows that elderly alcohol abusers have a high rate of such psychiatric disorders as depression, dementia, and other long-standing psychiatric conditions as bipolar disorder and schizophrenia.

Disease Onset Studies

Another variable considered in estimating alcohol problem prevalence in later life is the onset of the alcohol problem. The distinction between early-onset and late-onset alcohol abuse is often defined according to the chronological age when problem usage is determined. It is estimated that two-thirds of the older population with alcohol problems evidenced their problem earlier in life, while the remaining third develop the abuse problem at a later life stage (Brennan and Moos 1996).

According to Fink, Hays, and Moore (1996), 80 percent of men sixty years and older consume alcohol. The average onset of alcohol dependence for men sixty years and older is reported to be thirty-one years of age. Kostyk et al. (1994) suggest that the shorter length of problem drinking found among late-onset abusers can be associated with more successful treatment outcomes. In the late-onset pattern the denial system may not be so deeply entrenched, and individual and group interventions may contribute more quickly to problem acceptance. The biomedical aspects of addiction to alcohol may be less severe, and related medical problems less serious, because higher amounts of alcohol have been consumed for shorter time periods compared to those with the disease onset earlier in adulthood.

Prescribed and Over-the-Counter Drugs

Medication misuse, including combining prescription and over-the-counter medication intentionally or unintentionally with alcohol, is a complex and dangerous aspect of the illness-related behavior. Ruppert (1996) notes that the noninstitutionalized elderly consume about 50 percent of all OTC drugs. It is estimated that at least one drug is prescribed during 60 percent of the physician visits made by persons sixty-five years and older, and that individuals in this age group use about 30 percent of all prescribed drugs (Solomon et al. 1993). Given the high availability of cardiovascular medications, sedative/hypnotics, tranquilizers, analgesics, and psychoactive drugs, it is ironic that dependence and addiction to these prescribed medications, possibly combined with alcohol misuse, continue to go undetected and unaddressed among the elderly under active and consistent medical care (Schonfeld et al. 1993).

Common problems resulting from prescribed and OTC drugs used inappropriately by elderly persons can produce problems that require interventions from the physician, family, in-home health workers, and mental health clinicians. During individual or group therapy sessions it is appropriate for the clinician to raise the topic of medications and explore the attitude held about medication usage, understanding of all the medications prescribed including benefits and risks, and general attitudes toward compliance with medication regimens and other health care prescriptions.

SCREENING TOOLS AND ASSESSMENT PROCEDURES

The identification of older persons at risk of substance abuse relies on a variety of information sources including the use of screening instruments, conducting an interdisciplinary clinical assessment involving the patient and other caregivers, and the use of an alcohol and drug abuse history process that may be applied in a variety of settings as part of the assessment and evaluation process given to older people by health and mental health providers.

Screening Instruments for Older People

A useful part of the assessment process may be to include the application of one of several screening instruments used to determine alcohol abuse risks in the elderly. The CAGE Screening Questionnaire (Ewing 1984) is a short, four-question assessment tool designed to determine alcohol abuse. It can be included in a multidimensional assessment of a structured psychosocial history completed during the interview process.

The thirteen-question Short Michigan Alcohol Screening Test (SMART) is another tool that is used frequently with older patients (AMA 1996). It examines both drinking and the consequences of drinking. A new tool has recently been adapted from the SMART, designated specifically for geriatric assessment, known as the MAST-G. The questions in the MAST-G are especially useful in helping to identify some of the specific conditions associated with abusive drinking such as bereavement periods and other interpersonal crises (Ruppert 1996).

Interdisciplinary Cognitive Focused Assessment

There is little discussion of assessment in the literature on aging and substance abuse. This is a clinical oversight and reflects the continuing lack of understanding that drug abuse is related to many of the problems that older people may encounter. Drug abuse has implications for medical treatment, cognitive functioning, and safety concerns in all aspects of daily life such as driving an automobile, caring for the needs of oneself or others, and judgment and decision making.

Medical history and physical examinations can provide vital information. Some common medical complications for older people with a long history of alcohol dependence include liver disease, hypertension, myocardial infarction, cardiac arrhythmia, strokes, peptic ulcer disease, immunosuppression, dehydration, electrolyte abnormalities, and falls. Many illnesses present different patterns in later life and obfuscate the association between alcohol dependence and age-prevalent disease. An evaluation of comorbid psychiatric illness is equally important as the presence of affective and anxiety disorders and other psychiatric illnesses that frequently accompany substance abuse in later life.

Cognitive dysfunction is a frequent, although not inevitable, consequence of aging and must be assessed. In addition, a plethora of cognitive deficits may result from alcohol abuse. Difficulties with visual-spatial processing, commonly seen in people who abuse alcohol, may be present following abstinence (Cohen-Mansfield 1995; Nixon 1995). Such difficulties, similar to those coexisting with acute alcohol abuse, may compromise the ability of the person to perform daily routines and self-care activities.

When the individual's ability to learn and retain new information is only minimally affected, the client should be considered for participation in group treatment modalities that are similar to those found in traditional inpatient treatment settings and outpatient programs (Rains and Ditzler 1993). Those individuals with greater cognitive deficits needing substance abuse treatment should be referred for evaluation and admission to a substance abuse program that is matched to their overall functional abilities, and does not demand more cognitive comprehension than is possible. There is no therapeutic value in group participation demands that leave the older patient frustrated because of cognitive abilities, and leave other group members distracted from learning and processing. Group therapists must assess whether a cognitively impaired member can fit into the treatment group. More severe disability often requires the assignment of clients to other groups where emphasis is on repetition and review in order to ensure that learning takes place. Although the patient may understand and demonstrate learning, impulsiveness may be so severe that the client cannot tolerate the behavioral conditions/expectations in traditional group therapy.

Motivational Issues in the Assessment Process

The motivational factors relevant to treatment participation must be assessed. One of the first dimensions to be explored is the source of motivation. Many older people are initially unable to motivate themselves to receive treatment out of self-interest. They agree to engage with an intervention plan because of the interest of others in them.

Motivation, derived from both self-interest and response to the vital concerns of other people, may be established for issues such as managing personal health, caregiving responsibilities, fear of dependence, fear of social abandonment, and other factors. These routine aspects of living may become the motivation for stopping substance abuse.

With time the sources of motivation for recovery may shift. Older people report this shift when they begin to be motivated by the individual benefits they receive from treatment, including participation in AA, because they want the better life they see as part of recovery. They have been able to attain self-esteem and retain it through sobriety and the day-to-day management of their chemical dependence. While the motivation reinforcement external to themselves is valuable, the internal sense of manageability can lead to regaining a better quality of life.

GROUP PSYCHOTHERAPY WITH OLDER MALE LONG-TERM ALCOHOLICS

Among the most challenging groups of older male alcohol addicts one can assist through psychotherapy are those with cognitive impairments. In addition to repeated failures to maintain sobriety, even though many treatment cycles have been completed, additional substance abuse or addiction, medical problems, and pervasive social network disconnections all combine to make therapy strategies often ineffective.

Several years ago the authors were asked to establish a psychotherapy group for older male alcohol addicts. There was a need for a special group because some of these men had cognitive and physical impairments so that their ability to identify and interrelate within a group dominated by much younger men seemed very difficult. These men were without families, and they had been revolving in and out of inpatient settings for many years and looked to the hospital as a place where they could feel accepted.

Realizing that these older men had very little incentive to remain sober when they were discharged from the hospital, the clinicians attempted to organize a psychosocial support group directed toward helping them find some purpose for their lives that gave an additional incentive for sobriety. Using the hospital as an environment where new social connections could be made for these men through the therapy group and other volunteer roles, the therapists organized a self-esteem–building therapy group that attempted to:

1. *Emphasize that each human being, irrespective of age, addiction history, and other physical and/or cognitive limitation, could make a contribution to other persons.* To give these older alcohol addicts a focus on useful productive roles, they were given an opportunity to participate in specially designed volunteer activities that incorporated opportunities to assist elderly men in the nursing home section of the facility.
2. *Build relationship skills that focused on their strengths.* This was accomplished by helping the men to build socially appropriate group interaction skills learned and demonstrated within the group sessions. Issues of anger management, appropriate listening, and respectful/supportive dialogue during sessions were established as goals to be demonstrated within the group sessions and extended to other social interactions outside the group.

The experience of designing this group, which remains one of the geriatric mental health programs offered at the hospital, demonstrated that a purpose for sobriety had to be found for men who were without purpose. In order to tolerate the group context, the participants had to feel a level of social comfort in a group of very similar members. The common histories, physical and mental capacities, and long history with the hospital gave them confidence to interact around sobriety-reinforcing issues.

The organization of a therapeutic group for the type of population served in this particular treatment group can be delivered on an inpatient or outpatient basis. The group can help men to receive supports in making the transition from living in the hospital environment to community residency. The model can also be fostered in specialized day treatment programs or partial hospital settings, and therefore may be more available in view of managed care requirements for lowered costs for chronic disability treatment.

When patients are in need of continuing group therapy after discharge, part of the treatment plan is to provide continuity of treatment. When men from this group are scheduled to return home to families, considerable time is spent helping caregivers learn about managing their needs for care, and what might best reinforce the sobriety and improved self-esteem found through meaningful social engagement with others.

DESIGNING A TREATMENT GROUP FOR OLDER WOMEN

Group therapists need to be creative in their design of interventions for older substance abusers. This is especially applicable for older women for whom the stigma of alcohol abuse may be greater than for older men. Once a substance abuse problem is identified, preferably through a comprehensive needs assessment of the older woman, denial continues, even if the chemical abuse is life threatening. Societal perceptions of older women, strongly reinforced in family systems and service delivery networks, actually play into denial. Older women with substance abuse issues may possibly get involved in more general mental health directed groups (Fredriksen 1992; Glantz and Backenheimer 1988; Rathbone-McCuan 1988; Ruyle 1988).

The Twilight Ladies Group

Older women with substance abuse issues become identified through many formal and informal channels. For instance, an alcohol abuse problem can be identified by the primary care physician in the process of doing a medical evaluation; a wife with alcohol or other drug dependencies can self-identify in a caregiver support group; alcohol abuse as an issue for an elderly woman can surface during intergenerational family therapy; or managers and staff in senior retirement settings can identify older female residents with alcohol problems. These and other case identification routes lead to sources of referral to the Twilight Program established within a women's comprehensive health center.

Programs for women that have a tradition of serving younger women, such as mental health services, domestic violence programs, and community educational institutions, are now beginning outreach to older women. Health, mental health, and social/educational programs are being created and adapted to better fit the experiences of aging women. The Twilight Program, a community-based psychotherapy-oriented group for older women, is an illustration of a comprehensive medical/behavioral health care response to the substance abuse treatment needs of older women.

The program is designed to offer both short-term and long-term group therapy opportunities for women fifty years and older struggling with substance abuse and the mental health issues that challenge sobriety. The group leaders, two women mental health clinicians with shared experience within gerontology and substance abuse, established the program because of an unrecognized and unmet need in women's health care. The group members were often connected to AA and Al-Anon groups that reinforced the work of the group therapy.

Illustration of the Group Process

A major therapeutic theme among group members was how issues of social emotional isolation interfaced with chemical abuse/dependence and recovery. Over time group members identified and shared their experiences of isolation, loneliness, fears, and persistent sense of abandonment. These were the sorts of feelings they identified as having been part of the "bottom" of their drug abuse, and they were challenged to meet these ongoing social and emotional challenges while sober.

As the women in the Twilight group discussed the circumstances they faced, for example, being a cancer survivor, an Alzheimer's disease spouse caregiver, an impaired professional, and a mother of a son with AIDS, they were seeking support for living in recovery. The psychotherapy group was a source of ongoing reflection about coping with their sources of isolation without the numbing impact of drugs.

Presented next is a brief summary of a session where group members (four members' input summarized) shared emotional conflicts. The members were socioeconomically diverse, had very different lifestyles, and distinct substance abuse histories:

Anna, a fifty-year-old industrial designer, had survived breast cancer and then faced a bitter divorce that continued to keep her sobriety maintenance very precarious. Blanche, a seventy-three-year-old French-Canadian immigrant with years of sobriety and AA participation, had recently placed her husband in a specialized dementia care nursing home. Eleanor, a sixty-year-old Protestant minister, was adjusting to a pressured early retirement resulting from her impaired functioning in a clergy position. Carmelita, a fifty-five-year-old Latina, was in severe crisis because her only son was living with advanced AIDS.

During the session these four women focused on their spiritual conflicts and their feelings of isolation. The therapists were experienced and comfortable with religious themes, spiritual questions, and their place in the recovery journey of many older women.

Carmelita raised the topic with her peers: "The truth is, Eddie, my son, has been living with me since he was diagnosed with AIDS, and we live in my house like ghosts, haunting each other during the day. Before he knew that he could get access to the new medications for AIDS, he was killing himself with his drugs. I knew that he would shoot his drugs every morning and then I would start drinking my wines. We didn't connect at any level and now that a healthy life may be extended to him, he says that he wants to stop using. I prayed to have such a blessing and in gratitude I am in recovery, but I will pray all the time again that he is going to come into a program of healing his body and soul." A suggestion was offered by a group member that she consider going to Al-Anon to help her find ways of handling her expectations of her son.

Anna then shared with the group: "Did you ever bargain with God that you would stop drinking if Eddie received a miracle cure for his disease? I have found myself bargaining with God to have both of my breasts saved from cancer and then I would stop drinking . . . breasts went, then the husband went, and I kept drinking and felt overwhelming anger toward God. Now I know that bargaining with people is as misplaced as bargaining with God."

In a tearful voice Eleanor almost whispered, "God was my business seven days a week, twenty-four hours a day. I prayed, led prayers, wrote hymns, and delivered eulogies—always as near to God as I was to a drink. I stood at the pulpit for so many years in fear that I would be discovered as the depressed alcoholic I was at that time. When people in the congregation and the denomination reached out to me I could only deny my conditions."

Blanche reached out for Eleanor and said, "My own loneliness is lifted when I come into this group with all of you, and we can exchange our fears in safety and with compassion because we have all been there. I would probably relapse if it weren't for the supports I get from being with older women who are my friends and there for me . . . it has been years since my husband was there for me with any real mind left. I think my finding this group was an action of my higher power."

The general supportive psychotherapy approach maintained in the group offered the "least threatening" form of mental health care that these women had found and complemented the other aspects of their recovery. The above dialogue indicates how isolation was ongoing, and not merely the consequences of addiction. Most women in the group did have a commitment to the principles of AA; the reference to spiritual issues is a good example of how the strengths of self-help group participation can blend with the ongoing psychotherapy group process. The group committed its work to identification of, and support for, each older woman according to personal circumstances, values, and life goals. In addition, the supportive psychotherapy approach incorporated the goal of personal empowerment applicable to broad problem-solving skills. The group identified the unmanageability in members' lives, using the feedback of the group process.

OTHER TREATMENT CONSIDERATIONS

The age of the onset should not be used as a rigid criterion for helping to connect an older person with therapeutic resources. Although the recovery potential for chronic substance-abusing older people may seem minimal, especially if they have a long history of abuse and treatment, a crisis created by breakdown of health and self-care associated with illness can give new motivation for recovery.

Perspectives on Recovery

Moving from a phase of abusive self-endangering alcohol consumption to the point of abstaining from alcohol should be considered only the beginning of a recovery process, the first step most frequently specified in treatment groups. The maintenance of and evolution in the spiritual, social, and emotional realms of life indicate that the person is in an active recovery process. The process is never linear, never easy, and frightening at any age. It is chosen by those who want to arrest their disease because of the quality of life they experience.

Group interventions for developing controlled drinking may be possible in clinical treatment for some older people, especially those without a history of chronic abuse. The efficacy of controlled drinking is likely to be challenged even if it is demonstrated to have benefits for late-onset alcohol abusers, given the continued central effective influence of the AA philosophy of first-drink/one-drink, which established a pathway for relapse.

Older People and AA Participation

Older peoples' participation in AA is at least as beneficial as it is for younger alcohol abusers (Rathbone-McCuan 1988). The participatory value in the self-help group process available through AA meetings, sponsorship, and community forums can offer older people the following benefits:

1. connection to an accepting nonageist social network;
2. accessibility to members willing to help with individual transportation and in-home visitation during relapse risk periods;
3. no costs associated with participation;
4. support for stigma reduction in later life; and
5. exposure to other older peers who have effectively maintained sobriety in the midst of their unpredictable crises in later life.

RESEARCH DIRECTIONS

Numerous areas of clinical research need to be undertaken to better understand the treatment approaches that have value for older substance-abusing adults. Clinical research should be established as initial and ongoing components of the treatment options developed for this at-risk group. The need for knowledge about treatment innovations and effectiveness is becoming greater as the demands for effectiveness and outcome measures are being required through managed care reimbursement monitoring.

Retirement and Substance Abuse Risks

Research is needed to provide more information about the interrelationship of retirement as an aging stressor and substance abuse as a dysfunctional coping mechanism. The retirement process may be a period of crisis when heavy drinkers progress into alcohol addiction because of retirement-related events. For example, the individual can experience decreased retirement income, loss of self-esteem and established social supports, and other aspects of social dislocation. There are numerous possibilities for preretirement group interventions that give attention to substance abuse risks.

Dual Diagnosis Issues

Stewart and Hale (1992) suggest that a high frequency of affective disorders exists among older alcohol abusers. Those older people with dually diagnosed conditions already consume an unknown proportion of medical care and mental health services. The normal physical processes of aging, the common diseases of the elderly and their treatments, the social and psychological losses of aging, and stigmatizing responses to older people with mental illness and addiction problems need to be examined through research.

CONCLUSION

In this chapter, data on prevalence has been presented even though the current data available may underestimate the scope of the problem and does not offer a confident estimate of need among the older alcohol-abusing population. Too little is known about how drug addiction profiles of the baby boomer cohort will emerge when they carry their drug usage patterns into later life. It is reasonable to anticipate, however, that there will be greater demand for substance abuse treatment as this cohort ages.

The authors have emphasized that age and some of the medical and psychiatric conditions in later life are not sufficient reasons for assuming older alcohol abusers will not benefit from traditional group intervention. Assessment, specifically neuropsychological assessment to determine cognitive impairment, followed by treatment planning, should be employed. Caregivers should always be involved in order to understand how substance abuse increases physical and mental age-related decline.

Gender is another important factor upon which to design group interventions. Older women benefit from processing and problem solving in all-women's groups. Whenever possible they should have access to other older women devoted to helping better the quality of life in old age. Specialized groups for older men needing supports for substance abuse recovery should also be available, thereby creating an opportunity for men to discuss the fears and limitations of aging among a male-only group.

The gaps in research are many, and the advancement of knowledge for effective intervention has been limited by the slow pace of creative clinical programming. The value of clinical descriptive studies, combined with empirical studies, can advance the work of treatment and prevention as applied to the spectrum of issues related to addiction and recovery in later life.

REFERENCES

Adams WL, Magruder-Habib K, Trued S, Broome HL. Alcohol abuse in elderly emergency department patients. *Journal of the American Geriatrics Society* 40:1236-1240, 1992.

American Medical Association Council on Scientific Affairs. Alcoholism in the elderly. *JAMA* 275:797-801, 1996.

Barnea A, Teichman M. Substance misuse and abuse among the elderly: Implications for social work intervention. *Journal of Gerontological Social Work* 21:133-148, 1994.

Brennan PL, Moos RH. Late-life drinking behavior: The influence of personal characteristics, life contact, and treatment. *Alcohol Health and Research World* 20:197-204, 1996.

Cohen-Mansfield J. Assessment of disruptive behavior/agitation in the elderly: Function, methods, and difficulties. *Journal of Geriatric Psychiatry and Neurology* 8:52-60, 1995.

Dufour M. Risk and benefits of alcohol use over the life span. *Alcohol Health and Research World* 20:145-151, 1996.

Ewing JA. Detecting alcoholism using the CAGE questionnaire. *JAMA* 252:1905-1907, 1984.

Fink A, Hays RD, Moore AA, Beck JC. Alcohol-related problems in older persons. *Archives of Internal Medicine* 156:1150-1156, 1996.

Fredriksen KI. North of market: Older women's alcohol outreach program. *Gerontologist* 32:270-272, 1992.

Glantz MD, Backenheimer MS. Substance abuse among elderly women. *Clinical Gerontologist* 8:3-26, 1988.

Goldstein MA, Pataki A, Webb MT. Alcoholism among elderly persons. *Psychiatric Services* 47:941-943, 1996.

Joseph CL, Ganzini L, Atkinson RM. Screening for alcoholic use disorders in the nursing home. *Journal of the American Geriatrics Society* 43:368-373, 1995.

Kostyk D, Lindblom L, Fuchs D, Tabisz E, Jacyk WR. Chemical dependency in the elderly: Treatment phase. *Journal of Gerontological Social Work* 22:175-191, 1994.

Liberto JG, Oslin DM, Ruskin PE. Alcoholism in older persons: A review of the literature. *Hospital and Community Psychiatry* 43:975-984, 1992.

Moos RH, Mertens JR, Brennan PL. Patterns of diagnosis and treatment among middle-aged and older substance abuse patients. *Journal of Studies on Alcohol* 54:479-487, 1993.

Nixon SJ. Assessing cognitive impairment. *Alcohol Health and Research World* 19:97-103, 1995.

Rains VD, Ditzler TF. Alcohol use disorders in cognitively impaired patients referred for geriatric assessment. *Journal of Addictive Diseases* 12:55-64, 1993.

Rathbone-McCuan E. Group intervention for alcohol-related problems among the elderly and their families. In *Group Psychotherapy for the Elderly,* edited by MacLennan BW, Saul S, Bakus MB. New York: International Universities Press, 1988, pp. 139-148.

Ruppert SD. Alcohol abuse in older persons: Implication for critical care. *Critical Care Nursing Quarterly* 19:62-70, 1996.

Ruyle J. Group therapy with older alcoholics: How it can happen and work. *Alcoholism Treatment Quarterly* 4:81-85, 1988.

Schonfeld L, Rohrer GE, Zima M, Spiegel T. Alcohol abuse and medication misuse in older adults as estimated by service providers. *Journal of Gerontological Social Work* 21:113-125, 1993.

Solomon K, Manepalli J, Ireland GA, Mahon GM. Alcoholism and prescription drug abuse in the elderly: St. Louis University Grand Rounds. *Journal of the American Geriatrics Society* 41:57-69, 1993.

Stewart RB, Hale WE. Acute confusional states in older adults and the role of polopharmacy. *Annual Review of Health* 13:415-430, 1992.

Szwabo PA. Substance abuse in older women. *Clinics in Geriatric Medicine* 9:197-208, 1993.

Washburn N. AA through the eyes of its older members. *Journal of Geriatric Psychiatry* 29:185-204, 1996.

Wiseman EJ, Souder E, O'Sullivan P. Age and denial of alcoholism severity. *Clinical Gerontologist* 17:55-58, 1996.

SECTION IV:
SPECIFIC DIAGNOSTIC POPULATIONS

Chapter 19

Group Treatment for Patients with Substance Abuse and Schizophrenia

Richard N. Rosenthal

INTRODUCTION
AND BRIEF HISTORICAL PERSPECTIVE

Since and before the advent of neuroleptic treatment, much has been written on group treatment of schizophrenia (Kanas 1993). There is also a wealth of literature on group treatment for substance use disorders (Flores 1993). By comparison, there is a small amount of clinical and research literature regarding group treatment of comorbid substance abuse and mentally ill patients, and even less concerning substance abusers with schizophrenia-continuum disorders. The lack of such work is due, in no small measure, to the historical bifurcation in the treatment of traditional mental disorders and addictions. Clinicians generally have been trained to treat either mental disorders or addictions. Despite the conservative estimate of 47.0 percent for lifetime prevalence of substance use disorders among persons with schizophrenia (Regier et al. 1990), comorbidity is most certainly underrecognized and undertreated.* For patients with both comorbid substance use disorders and schizophrenia, integrating substance abuse and mental health treatment components into one seamless approach will have efficacy and efficiency (Hellerstein, Rosenthal, and Miner 1995). Without this integration, patients typically do not fare well.

---

*Comorbid is the research term; dually diagnosed is used more frequently in clinical settings.

TREATMENT PLANNING

Evaluation, DSM-IV Issues

In an initial evaluation of a substance abuser, it is important to rule out substance abuse as a cause of psychotic symptoms (APA, 1994), for the treatment and course of schizophrenia is different from that of substance-induced psychotic symptoms (Szuster et al. 1990; Brady et al. 1991). In patients with schizophrenia, substance abuse may precede, coemerge with, or follow the onset of symptoms of the illness during the first psychotic episode (Hambrecht and Hafner 1996). It may be difficult, therefore, to establish a reliable diagnosis of schizophrenia upon cross-sectional analysis (Rosenthal and Miner 1997).

Clinicians should not be content with making only the two diagnoses of substance use disorder and schizophrenia (SUD/S).* The presence of comorbid antisocial personality disorder (ASPD) can have a negative impact upon the treatment of SUD/S patients, similar to the reaction between this disorder and other addicted groups (Mueser et al. 1997; Drake et al. 1996).

Assessment of Abuse Severity

Although substance abuse severity must be assessed as part of a proper approach to the treatment of SUD/S patients, the presence of a primary psychotic disorder will have an overarching impact upon the course and outcome of treatment. In fact, the degree of psychiatric impairment has a greater impact on the outcome of addiction treatment than does the severity of the substance abuse. For the patient with schizophrenia, it is useful to determine if the use of substances, including alcohol, is at the level of occasional use, abuse, or dependence. Drake, McHugo, and Noordsy (1993) have demonstrated that even alcohol use at a level subthreshold for an abuse diagnosis has a negative impact upon the course of schizophrenia. As substance use has such a negative effect upon the trajectory of illness (Kovasznay et al. 1997), clinicians should have a low threshold for treating patients with a diagnosis of abuse or dependence in a group that integrates substance abuse and mental health services.

---

*For the sake of brevity, the diagnosis of comorbid substance use disorder and schizophrenia will be denoted hereafter as SUD/S.

The specific assessment of severity measured by standardized means, such as the Addiction Severity Index (ASI) (McLellan, Luborsky, and Cacciola 1985), provides a higher likelihood of uncovering abuse of multiple substances than routine clinical interviews (Rosenthal, Hellerstein, and Miner 1992).

Stages of Recovery

Traditional models for addiction recovery establish sobriety as the first major step and subsequently differentiate early, middle, late and/or maintenance recovery stages, which typically span many years. Most attention has thus been focused on the components of treatment that come into play after abstinence has been established. This outlook fits well with and is reinforced by the programmatic approach that addiction treatment starts only with the attainment of sobriety. Because the SUD/S population is well known for its extreme difficulties with maintaining early treatment compliance and for frequently exacerbating illness, more attention has been recently given to the early stages of treatment.

Osher and Kofoed (1989) used Prochaska, DiClemente, and Norcross' (1992) stages to model a similar configuration of recovery phases with an interpersonal and behavioral frame for the treatment of mentally ill substance abusers: *engagement, persuasion, active treatment (maintenance),* and *relapse prevention.* In the engagement phase, much like the precontemplation stage, the patient does not see an intrinsic problem and must be motivated toward contact with a therapist. The persuasion phase is like contemplation, but it frames the motivational issue interpersonally. Active treatment is the stage of moving toward sobriety; it essentially covers the preparation and action stages of the Prochaska, DiClemente, and Norcross model. Relapse prevention is a version of the maintenance of abstinence phase.

Although debatable, it is probably more important for the SUD/S population to maintain frequent contact with treatment specialists than it is to establish absolute sobriety, especially over the short-term. Some patients may have great difficulty achieving full abstinence from drugs or alcohol, but will stay in early active treatment. As such, a harm reduction model is the appropriate therapeutic stance, rather than insisting on abstinence before group treatment.

Retention is often half the battle with SUD/S patients in treatment. Treatment that meets the interventions appropriate for an individual patient's motivational state is likely to allow for a higher rate of retention and thus, through more exposure to treatment, a better outcome.

As group members develop and implement methods for maintaining stable sobriety and compliance with medical treatment, they will begin to reassess their assumptions about their lives. Typically, lives will change with respect to the aspects of daily living (with whom, where, and how they spend their time), a vocational or educational opportunity, or an intimate relationship. Each change, however, should be discussed with respect to the amount of stress it might cause if acted upon, so that an anticipatory examination of specific triggers for relapse can be made and the potential benefits versus risks of making the change can be assessed. When SUD/S patients are in a phase of advanced recovery, they must still attend to issues concerning relapse prevention, avoidance of high-risk situations, and maintenance of therapeutic gains.

Indications for Specific Treatment

Choice of Techniques

In group therapy with SUD/S patients, several useful categories of techniques are derived from the dynamic, behavioral, cognitive, interpersonal, and self-help traditions.

Role of Group Treatment

SUD/S patients are often lacking in social skills, a supportive interpersonal environment, and a culture of recovery. Group therapy offers a chance to relate to and form supportive bonds with others who have similar problems, with more flexibility than in individual therapy.

A group also offers the opportunity to understand one's own attitudes toward and denial of addiction by allowing discussion of common attitudes and defenses in substance-abusing patients (Flores 1993; see Chapter 2). Although SUD/S patients in early group therapy are typically not adept at self-observation of interpersonal style, with continued participation in group, recovery from psychosis, the establishment of early sobriety, and the development of more adaptive behavioral skills, these patients begin to better observe their own and others' interpersonal behavior.

Concomitant Use of Adjunctive Treatment

Medications

Presently, it is difficult to justify the participation of patients who are not being prescribed adequate doses of antipsychotic medications in SUD/S therapy groups. There may be instances in which the need for therapy outweighs immediate compliance with antipsychotic medications. However, treatment that reduces the intrusion of psychotic symptoms (positive symptoms) and increases hedonic capacity and energy (negative symptoms) will prove beneficial for the individual member and will help to put the group process into focus. SUD/S patients should usually be treated with second generation antipsychotic medications if feasible (Albanese et al. 1994; Buckley et al. 1994).

Use of Other Assessment Methods

Urine Screens

For clinicians, weekly urine screens are objective checks on drug abstinence claimed by patients. With a group member's informed consent, this information can be used in the clinical setting as feedback, to enlist group support for sobriety. Alcohol use is usually more difficult to ascertain. Missed urine samples are counted as positive. Furthermore, a patient's self-report of drug abuse should supersede a negative result on a urine screen.

Psychological Testing

The results of psychological testing are not normally considered treatment adjuncts but, rather, are used by clinicians to understand cognitive or other psychological deficits and to assist in determining a proper course of treatment. Miller and Rollnick (1991) in describing the methodology of motivational interviewing, on the other hand, support the verbal and graphical feedback of medical examinations and laboratory results for precontemplation-stage patients. For example, teaching patients in a group about the toxic effects of alcohol and the possibility of resulting short-term cognitive impairment can bolster an individual patient's resolve to engage in treatment.

Curative Factors

From his therapeutic experience, Yalom (1995) derived elemental factors that could contribute to therapeutic change. Several of these, as well as other factors, are discussed below with respect to group therapeutic treatment of SUD/S patients.

Instillation of Hope

Patients suffering from the ravages of substance use disorders are frequently demoralized. In such patients, concurrent schizophrenia typically creates further damage to life expectations by distorting those expectations in unrealistic ways, or by creating a sense of profound disability and ennui when patients in treatment gain a modicum of self-awareness.

Group treatment for SUD/S patients is a powerful medium for increasing self-efficacy. Group members gain real-life exposure to others struggling for recovery from both illnesses. Therapists who champion recovery-oriented treatment increase the motivation of group members to begin and continue the arduous process of change.

Universality

Undoubtedly, SUD/S patients may feel utterly alone and misunderstood by virtue of their having such profound problems. Group therapy, therefore, can provide support in combating feelings of isolation, despair, and hopelessness, and increases the possibility for change. Patients become aware that others in the group have had similar thoughts, feelings, and life events.

Imparting Information

Variously labeled and appropriate recovery-oriented psychotherapy for SUD/S patients, such as psychoeducation, cognitive restructuring, or substance abuse counseling, contain elements that teach about the symptoms and course of disorders, the disorders' effects, and the early symptoms of relapse, to increase cognitive mastery and self-esteem. Supportive psychotherapy, a foundation for the construction of appropriate therapies for SUD/S patients, typically includes both information and direct advice as suitable (Pinsker, Rosenthal, and McCullough 1991).

Altruism

Beneficence should be modeled for group members to adopt with respect to one another. The development of gratitude in addiction recovery often engages patients to use what they have learned to support others in recovery in more intimate and less isolated ways, communicating concern, care, and support, which can lead to increased self-efficacy and a sense of meaning (Yalom 1995).

Development of Socializing Techniques

In a SUD/S therapy group, individuals with deficits in social skills have the opportunity to receive honest feedback about inappropriate or ineffective behavior in a safe and modulated fashion, which cuts through distortions and supports the generation of adaptive skills. In addition, specific attention to skills training and practice within the group provides a means for behavioral adaptation.

Imitative Behavior and Interpersonal Learning

Group therapy for SUD/S patients offers at least two modalities in which members can learn normalizing behaviors. First, the concerned, empathic, mature, and informative responsiveness of the therapist sets a standard with which patients identify and emulate to encourage an interactive mode. Participants alternately express their thoughts or experiences while the others listen. This cooperation models appropriate and adaptive social skills. However, not all groups require that every member speaks in turn.

Second, by observing others in similar situations, group members can discover novel adaptive behaviors and values and real-world strategies, as opposed to maladaptive drug- or psychosis-related actions.

Group Cohesiveness

Like other addiction recovery groups, identification with other group members in SUD/S groups increases support for recovery and compliance with treatment. Attention in group concerning the shared experience of the illness of schizophrenia, its symptoms, its common impact, and coping strategies supports the development of common values, real camaraderie, and cohesion.

Existential Factors

Although the early stages of the group process often center around individual, here-and-now concerns, later stages begin more and more to offer members the opportunity to address expectations they have about the course of their lives in the context of chronic illness. The process of the group then begins to resemble those of somewhat higher functioning groups.

PRETREATMENT ISSUES

Motivation for Treatment

Clinicians frequently have the belief that patients who do not muster the requisite control over substance intake are not yet "ready" for treatment. Instead, these people are sent back to their environment to experience more negative consequences ("hit bottom"), which will hopefully drive them into active treatment. Unfortunately, this method drives many addicted persons away from the sphere of treatment and sustains the high risk of morbidity and mortality in the SUD/S population.

Current views on motivation enhancement (Rollnick and Miller 1995) frame the patient's lack of enthusiasm for change (resistance) as feedback regarding therapist behavior (i.e., as the therapist's problem). Thus, the use of active clinical interventions to engage SUD/S patients into treatment is appropriate. The use of positive reinforcement and privileges, such as unescorted passes, should be made contingent upon attendance at group treatment or maintenance of drug-free urine samples. Motivation for treatment should be built up by educating potential group members about the course of the addictive illness, the effects of drugs on mood, thinking, and behavior, and the real-life damage to psychosocial functioning.

Rationale for Choice of Treatment

Although individual therapy can provide support and assistance with problem solving, group therapy more readily provides SUD/S patients with a climate for sharing and exploring mutual concerns, accepting addictive and mental problems, and acknowledging and celebrating the achievement of goals.

Group therapy for SUD/S patients must integrate psychiatric and substance abuse treatment. When addiction and mental health services are provided separately to schizophrenic patients, misinterpretation, confusion, and mixed messages occur too often. Therefore, the most appropriate treatments are conducted by a therapist who is cross-trained in the treatment of both substance abuse and mental illness. Another reasonable model uses cotherapists, each of whom focuses either on addiction or mental illness but has some training and a level of comfort with the other domain.

Selection and Preparation of Patients

In group therapy for schizophrenia and addiction, patients at any stage should be able to abide by certain ground rules, such as no physical aggression, no verbal abuse, and no intoxication while in the group. Due to the special nature of the positive symptoms of schizophrenia which can distract, confuse, and distort the reception of information, it is useful to select patients who have some anxiety tolerance and who are unlikely to become either physically or verbally disruptive, or leave without returning during a therapy session. Nonetheless, patients with active delusions and hallucinations can still make use of therapy and the reality-orienting responses of other members, as can patients with strong negative symptoms (Miner, Rosenthal, and Hellerstein 1997).

Groups will often take place within inpatient service and partial hospitalization programs, but outpatient groups may also have patients in the precontemplation and contemplation stages. SUD/S patients often cycle through various motivational phases, and at different times may demonstrate behavior in the group commensurate with an earlier stage of change.

At the outset, the therapist should meet with the prospective group member several times alone in order to ascertain the patient's motivational stage, increase motivation for engagement in group treatment, explain the ground rules and goals of treatment, answer questions about the conduct of treatment, clarify the role of the therapist (e.g., who is the responsible party for medication management), and map out the expected course of therapy. Moreover, in cases where the payer system and logistics will allow, an initial visit to the group prior to discharge may help SUD/S patients connect with outpatient group treatment by enhancing familiarity and decreasing anticipatory anxiety (Rosenthal, Hellerstein, and Meyer 1992).

Suitability

Some patients may be unable to benefit from the group's support network, or at least may not be able to use it in the initial approach to treatment. Some characteristics of these patients might include severe paranoid persecutory delusions that reference those with whom the patient has contact, inability to control physical aggression, inability to remain seated due to anxiety or agitation, and phobic avoidance of groups. After an interval of individual treatment, in which the focus is the reduction of the symptom or characteristic that impedes group entry, however, some of these patients may be able to make use of group therapy.

Therapist Characteristics

The group leader must be a trained, skilled professional who is able to be supportive, charismatic, and evocative in early sessions, instructive in middle sessions, and supportive and attentive in later sessions.

STAGES OF GROUP DEVELOPMENT

Group Dynamics

Supportive group psychotherapy is an active, reality-based treatment that applies direct methods to promote abstinence, ameliorate symptoms, and maintain, restore, or improve self-esteem, coping, adaptive skills, and psychological function. Examination of interpersonal issues and relationships and both past and current patterns of emotional response/behavior is utilized as necessary to accomplish treatment objectives. These tenets of supportive psychotherapy should be used in the group therapy of SUD/S patients unless clinical requirements warrant a departure from that model.

The therapist is an important role model for patients who typically have severe deficits in social interaction. In order to summarize, paraphrase, and organize the patients' statements, the therapist clarifies extensively without elaboration or inference. This feedback is essential for the development of the therapeutic alliance because it makes patients feel understood by the therapist. Through careful listening, accurate clarification, and active empathic responses on the part of the therapist, patients build an alliance and increase their willingness to consider change.

Because the therapeutic alliance is so critical for the maintenance of the group, positive transference is typically not interpreted within supportive group psychotherapy unless it is grossly pathological (e.g., erotomania). Similarly, negative transferences, unless they are grossly pathological (e.g., persecutory delusion) or threaten the integrity of the group, are not interpreted. In supportive group psychotherapy, transferences that are recognized by dynamically aware therapists can be used to guide therapist interventions, but they are not generally discussed within the group.

In the beginning of treatment, more emphasis is placed on simple messages and the development of adaptive, concrete skills, which help patients to engage in and comply with treatment. Defenses are generally supported to maintain or improve patients' functioning. Defenses are not challenged in any patient without an appraisal of the potential impact upon the ego organization of that patient or upon others in the group.

Resistance in SUD/S patients is frequently demonstrated by means of withdrawal and noninteraction. Thus, conversational responsiveness on the part of the therapist is a characteristic tactic of supportive group therapy. As such, the therapist should not wait for discussions to unfold if the group is sitting quietly, for this may support resistance and increase anxiety.

Countertransference issues are always imminent for therapists who work with addicted patients who can be impulsive, seductive, or sociopathic. Due in part to the especially high frequency of episodes of noncompliance and relapse in SUD/S patients, therapists are frequently frustrated and/or disappointed, making access to peer support or professional supervision indispensable. Therapists may become bored with the provision of care, or overly confrontational. Keeping one's distance from empathic connection is a common therapist response to patients' projective identifications.

Initial Entry into Group

The initial phase is essentially one of engagement and evaluation. First, the therapist observes the patient's speech content and behavior. After a few sessions, the therapist formulates the case in the context of a functional assessment of the patient's problems with drug use, motivation, high-risk situations, patterns of dealing with urges, denial, and problems of daily living. Therapists should coach the group about helping new members.

SUD/S patients frequently have cycles of relapse and early recovery before they are able to implement a stable approach to sober, medication-compliant functioning. When a previously sober group member returns to group after a relapse, new patients and returning patients alike may benefit from the cohesion, structure, and interpersonal support of a group that understands the symptoms of addiction and schizophrenia, and consistently values sobriety and recovery. Nonetheless, a patient in precontemplation will likely be a poor match with a more advanced recovery group (e.g., maintenance).

Conduct of Initial Sessions

Support is given by the group to discuss substance abuse, including both positive and negative experiences and consequences. SUD/S groups emphasize that therapy is a rational, collaborative process. During a didactic segment, an agenda is usually set by the therapist (see Table 19.1). However, if appropriate, the therapist may use content from the current group session and add educational material to the issue at hand. The therapist must be flexible because patients may reject the proposed agenda, yet, typically, patients will adapt to a therapist's style of teaching.

Since the first priority of group therapy with SUD/S patients is engagement in treatment, patients are not rejected if they continue substance use, provided that they accept some responsibility for addressing problems related to substance use. If patients come to group intoxicated, they are asked to leave but, at the same time, they are in-

TABLE 19.1. Basic Concepts and Skills for Managing Substance Abuse

Basic Concepts	Specific Behavioral Skills

Damage control/harm reduction
  Abstinence violation effect
  Escaping high-risk situations
	Report a slip to a support person.
	Stop before a slip becomes a relapse.
	Refuse drugs from an aggressive dealer.

Avoiding high-risk situations
  U-turns at warning signs
  Removing triggers
  Money management
	Refuse drugs from a friend or relative.
	Get an appointment with a busy person.

Seek healthy pleasures
  Healthy habits
  Healthy pleasures
  Schedule activities
	Find and enlist a support person.
	Discuss symptoms/side effects with a psychiatrist.

Support persons	Get someone to join in a healthy pleasure.

Drug abuse is learned
  Triggers, craving
  Reinforcement, extinction of habit
	Negotiate with a representative payee.

Decisional balance
  Advantages/disadvantages
    of drug use
  Advantages/disadvantages
    of abstinence	

Source: Adapted from Roberts, Shaner, and Eckman 1997.

vited to the next session with the request that a substance not be taken beforehand.

Concurrent with the focus on continuous engagement in treatment, attention is directed at fostering acceptance of the reality of drug problems and mental illness, addressing maladaptive and impaired behaviors, denial, improving functioning, and preventing early relapse. Significant impairment must be the initial focus of treatment along with the substance abuse problem.

Middle Phases of Group

Attention must be paid to engagement on an ongoing basis because during the course of treatment some patients will relapse, stop attending group, and then show up again after an interval. Rerecruitment with the reestablishment of the therapeutic alliance, therefore, becomes the primary focus of treatment for those patients. Once this is accomplished, they often will move more rapidly through the motivational stages than they initially did at the start of group.

In the middle phases of group therapy, both group cohesion and the therapeutic alliance are present, with the therapeutic alliance having primacy early in treatment and group cohesion developing and assuming prominence in the middle phase of therapy. To facilitate the development of group cohesion, the therapist purposely shifts the process away from a patient-therapist interaction toward a patient-patient interaction.

Although attention in supportive group therapy must be directed at self-esteem issues, adaptive skills, or psychological function, frequently patterns of behavior and feelings that lead to addictive behavior are explored. Patients with acute relapse or chronic difficulty in maintaining sobriety find themselves under increasing peer pressure to take the appropriate steps to address their substance use. The therapist and the group help each patient to develop a concrete plan of action if relapse should occur. With the therapeutic alliance, group cohesion, and the positive effects of peer support, these patients can often find their way to higher functioning.

Termination

Termination proves variable in time-limited and goal-focused therapy groups for SUD/S patients. Since schizophrenia is a chronic illness, the traditional approach to group treatment is to prescribe an indefinite length of stay in the group. As the group matures, it becomes a mainstay for patients who suffer from chronic isolation and poor psychosocial function and need enduring professional support for sobriety over the long term. However, many patients are able to advance their recovery and social functioning. In fact, many need to leave the group in order to fulfill work obligations or pursue educational goals. In such cases, the mature SUD/S group may choose to meet less frequently (i.e., an alumni group) or change its focus to more maintenance-oriented goals. Given the relative dearth of constant, positively held objects in most of these patients' lives, it is futile to get patients to end their relationship with the therapist or other members of the group.

Although recovery is an expectation actively promoted, cure is not. Schizophrenia is a chronic illness and substance use disorders are also framed as chronic as well as relapsing. SUD/S patients need to be reassured that if they should need more of the treatment provided in group, it will always be available. As such, the door is forever open and the welcome mat is always in its place.

TECHNIQUES

Choice and Timing of Interventions

In the integrated approach to group therapy with SUD/S patients, there is a reliance on techniques derived from various traditions: supportive psychotherapy, motivational enhancement techniques, psychoeducation, behavioral, and cognitive-behavioral strategies. Certain techniques of supportive psychotherapy are used frequently throughout the course of treatment. Enhancement of self-esteem and self-praise is appropriate at each step of recovery, often dealt with by the group itself as it develops cohesion and a capacity for active peer support. Thus, supportive techniques, originally developed in the context of individual treatment, prove useful in SUD/S groups where the patient-therapist process predominates over the group-oriented process for a longer period than it does in higher functioning groups.

General and Stage-Specific Interventions

Techniques of Supportive Group Therapy for SUD/S

The supportive techniques described next are given an in-depth explication in *A Primer of Supportive Psychotherapy* (Pinsker 1998; Rosenthal, Pinsker, and Winston 1993).

Contain or reduce anxiety. Interaction between therapists and patients is modeled on conversation rather than on interrogation or passive listening. Awkward, anxiety-provoking silences are avoided. Interjections, or comments, are made proactively by the therapist in order to normalize the verbal interchange. The therapist asks the group questions to demonstrate active listening and, if a patient answers, the therapist acknowledges what has been said in some way.

Indirect suggestion is used to advance ideas that might otherwise be rejected by the group members.

Enhance self-esteem. The therapist's stance should be accepting, nonjudgmental, and aimed at maintaining a collaborative relationship with the explicit objective of improving self-esteem. SUD/S patients tend to be very sensitive to rejection, enmity, and insincerity; they often feel mistrustful or judged, especially those with schizoid styles or paranoid persecutory ideas.

High expressed emotion (EE) is a major predictor of relapse in schizophrenics, and substance abuse is a major predictor of relapse in SUD/S patients with high-EE families (Linszen et al. 1997). As such, questions that will have a challenging and attacking impact are avoided or softened in the group treatment of SUD/S patients.

Maintain/improve psychological functions. Faulty impulse control is a serious deficit found in SUD/S patients. Therapeutic efforts are directed toward establishing cause and effect relationships, without making critical comments, to illuminate what happens to patients and their relationships. An emphasis should be made on strengthening psychological functioning (e.g., reality testing, logical appreciation of cause and effect, adaptive defensive functioning) to aid cessation of drug use. Later, in the action and maintenance stages, the patient learns to look for "using signals"—the emotions, interoceptive cues (e.g., craving), and thoughts that precede drug use. The goal is to get the group to recognize substance use as a predictable behavior, and then to develop strategies to be employed when previously unrecognized predictors recur. Psychoeducation (discussed later) increases the patients' knowledge base and range of choices with respect to assessing events, and it falls within the construct of improving psychological functioning through cognitive restructuring.

Defenses can be adaptive or maladaptive. For example, projection, frequently used by SUD/S patients and often reinforced by the patient's peers, is a typically maladaptive defense. The focus of an intervention should be placed on what the patient must do, but should not include an assessment of the correctness of his or her impressions. Maladaptive defenses must be gently confronted, at times by challenging the group as a whole.

Improve adaptive skills. Many SUD/S patients are basically competent in their lives and interpersonal relations, but they usually have

---

Case Example: Cognitive Disorganization

Verbal Content	Process Evaluation
PT: They said they smell it on me the other day. You know maybe he's got a problem! I don't want to be there, and now he's leaving. I didn't use anything.	Therapist clarifies that the patient is stating he was falsely accused of using marijuana. Then he states that the patient may assume a connection between the accusation, his anger, and a staff member's resignation.
T: So you're upset that staff said you were using when you weren't. It makes you angry enough to leave. Now you hear that the staff member is leaving. Do you think there is some connection?	

---

not mastered some of the adaptive and social skills taken for granted by most people. The teachings of Alcoholics Anonymous are consistent with goals for improving adaptive skills.

Clarification. This technique is used extensively in supportive group psychotherapy with SUD/S patients to confirm that the therapist is listening and understands. This summarizing, paraphrasing, and organizing of a patient's statements, without elaboration or inference, is often useful both for the specific patient and the other group members, and can specifically facilitate the therapeutic alliance, group cohesion, and increased self-reliance.

Confrontation. This technique, which brings attention to a behavior or communication that the patient is avoiding or not attending, can be useful when constructed and delivered in a nonpunitive manner appropriate to the individual patient or the whole group. Confrontation can be used to make patients aware of a situation that is high risk for substance use, as well as the patients' use of maladaptive defenses.

Rationalization. Although this is a defensive maneuver, in supportive therapies it is a legitimate technique if done knowingly, and for a reason. The therapist should make patients aware of rationalizations in the service of drug use and involvement in high-risk situations, using the group for reality testing.

Case Example: Confrontation

Verbal Content	Process Evaluation
PT1: He's going next week, so I'm fine with it! I don't know why they get in my face. I wasn't using! Now I hear they were talking about me leaving! It's bullshit, why even try to be sober?	Therapist clarifies that the patient is stating he was falsely accused of using marijuana. Then he states that the patient may assume a connection between the accusation, his anger, and a staff member's resignation.
T: Let's assume you didn't use marijuana. Is there something about how you acted with the staff that made them consider having you move out?	Patient angrily assumes a victim's position. Therapist points out that the patient may have communicated in an angry way, implying it may have had a negative effect. The confrontation is framed supportively by normalizing the
PT1: They're just on my case! [Shakes clenched fists, rocks in seat]	patient's emotional reaction.
T: Maybe you were angrier than you realized when you responded that night, just as you look angry right now. I know I'd sure be angry if I was accused by staff of using when I didn't!	Patient 2 joins with both the therapist's and patient 1's position. Patient angrily rejects therapist's position. Patient 3 feeds back his experience of patient 1 in a supportive way.
PT2: Me too! They didn't treat him fair.	
PT1: [Loudly] I'm *not* angry!	
PT3: Man, you look angry. It's okay with me [assured smile], but maybe you scared 'em.	

Encouragement. This supportive technique includes reassurance, praise, or the empathic comments and subtle encouragements that are bestowed in daily life by people who have positive regard for one another. The therapist should actively seek opportunities to add empathic words that help the patients to feel good about themselves. With encouragement, the therapist not only offers support to a particular patient, but also models how to be supportive to the rest of the group. However, praise and reassurance must be data based (i.e., directed to something the patient considers worthy of praise), within the context of the discussion. Misapplied, praise may belittle the patient and may have a damaging effect upon the therapeutic alliance because the therapist may be perceived as insincere.

Advice. In work with SUD/S patients, due to the patients' deficits in self-care, cognition, and interpersonal skills, giving data-based advice can be appropriate, related to the therapist's expert knowledge and the topics of treatment, including daily life.

Anticipatory guidance. This technique of planning and rehearsal allows patients to move through new situations hypothetically, with the help of other group members, while considering possible events and ways to respond to them. This allows the patient to become acquainted with the context of a future event, and helps to reduce some of the anticipatory anxiety associated with such an event.

Ventilation. Unburdening may be a useful tool for the patient who feels guilty or anxious about something important or has undergone a traumatic event. If the group members and the therapist have heard the patient's story and have not rejected him or her, this reception may be the essence of support.

Psychoeducation

Basic topics concerning mental illness and substance abuse that should be included in psychoeducational content for SUD/S patients are prepared in advance, and brief written or graphic materials support the learning experience and act as jumping-off points for discussion. Topics can be addressed during formal didactic intervals (ten to fifteen minutes), and can be woven into the fabric of the group process. In framing a psychoeducational module, it is important to allow adequate time for repetition of important concepts, discussion, feedback, and questions. Topics can include aspects of craving, withdrawal, drug cues, risky situations, and stopping use.

Skills Training/Relapse Prevention

Roberts, Shaner, and colleagues (1997), among others (see Ziedonis and Trudeau 1997), have developed a structured group skills training approach by adapting standard cognitive-behavioral relapse prevention strategies that are most acceptable and readily understood by SUD/S patients. A less structured approach delivered as a component of a group psychotherapy session should still prove beneficial to patients.

RELEVANT RESEARCH

Despite the fact that the group therapy model is a mainstay of outpatient treatment in the public sector and that a high comorbidity of schizophrenia and substance abuse exists, notably little empirical research has been conducted specifically addressing the efficacy of group therapies for SUD/S patients. Recent reviews of research on group psychotherapies for schizophrenia suggest that reality-based supportive treatments may have benefits over expressive therapies regarding the likelihood of relapse and reducing the severity of psychopathology (Kanas 1993; Scott and Dixon 1995), but overall the reviews demonstrate that no clear and convincing empirical evidence exists for improvement in rehospitalization rates, psychopathology, psychosocial functioning, or work functioning. Clear evidence for the efficacy of group therapy of schizophrenia may be lacking because of methodologic flaws in many prior studies (American Psychiatric Association 1997).

A few pilot studies in the mid 1980s suggested that group treatment with an integrated focus on recovery from mental illness and substance abuse is beneficial for certain diagnostic groups including schizophrenia (Kofoed et al. 1986; Hellerstein and Meehan 1987).

More recently, group therapy interventions have been studied specifically in SUD/S patients. Using a sufficient services model that would allow for the elucidation of specific factors that contribute to outcome (Rosenthal, Hellerstein, and Miner 1992), sixty-three inpatients diagnosed with schizophrenia and psychoactive substance use disorder, using DSM-III-R criteria, were randomly sent either to outpatient group therapy in an addiction setting, with medications monitored at an off-site mental health clinic, or to the Combined Psychiatric and Addictive Disorders program (COPAD), an outpatient group therapy program that integrated substance abuse and psychiatric services and met twice weekly at the same outpatient mental health clinic. The COPAD integrated model successfully retained 69.7 percent of patients in treatment at four months and 60.6 percent at eight months, significantly more than those retained in the standard, nonintegrated treatment program. Patients who remained in group treatment had significant reductions in the severity of psychiatric and substance use disorder symptoms (Hellerstein, Rosenthal, and Miner 1995).

Further research addressing the effectiveness of a variety of group treatment approaches for these difficult-to-treat patients should prove useful in formulating methods of treatment that provide good, cost-effective treatment outcomes.

REFERENCES

Albanese MJ, Khantzian EJ, Murphy SL, Green AI. Decreased substance use in chronically psychotic patients treated with clozapine. *American Journal of Psychiatry* 151:780-781, 1994.

American Psychiatric Association. *Diagnostic and Statistical Manual of Mental Disorders,* Fourth Edition. Washington, DC: American Psychiatric Association, 1994.

American Psychiatric Association. *Practice Guidelines for the Treatment of Patients with Schizophrenia.* Washington, DC: American Psychiatric Press, 1997.

Brady KT, Lydiard RB, Malcolm R, Ballenger JC. Cocaine-induced psychosis. *Journal of Clinical Psychiatry* 52:509-512, 1991.

Buckley P, Thompson P, Way L, Meltzer HY. Substance abuse among patients with treatment resistant schizophrenia: Characteristics and implications for clozapine therapy. *American Journal of Psychiatry* 151:385-389, 1994.

Drake RE, McHugo GJ, Noordsy DL. Treatment of alcoholism among schizophrenic outpatients: 4-year outcomes. *American Journal of Psychiatry* 150:328-329, 1993.

Drake RE, Mueser KT, Clark RE, Wallach MA. The course, treatment, and outcome of substance disorder in persons with severe mental illness. *American Journal of Orthopsychiatry* 66:42-51, 1996.

Flores PJ. Group psychotherapy with alcoholics, substance abusers, and adult children of alcoholics, area D.5. In *Comprehensive Group Psychotherapy,* Third Edition, edited by Kaplan HI, Sadock BJ. Baltimore, MD: Williams and Wilkins, 1993.

Hambrecht M, Hafner H. Substance abuse and the onset of schizophrenia. *Biological Psychiatry* 40:1155-1163, 1996.

Hellerstein DJ, Meehan B. Outpatient group therapy for schizophrenic substance abusers. *American Journal of Psychiatry* 144:1337-1339, 1987.

Hellerstein DJ, Rosenthal RN, Miner CR. A prospective study of integrated outpatient treatment for substance-abusing schizophrenic patients. *American Journal on Addictions* 4:33-42, 1995.

Kanas N. Group psychotherapy with schizophrenia. In *Comprehensive Group Psychotherapy,* Third Edition, edited by Kaplan HI, Sadock BJ. Baltimore, MD: Williams and Wilkins, 1993, pp. 407-417.

Kofoed L, Kania J, Walsh T, Atkinson RM. Outpatient treatment of patients with substance abuse and coexisting psychiatric disorders. *American Journal of Psychiatry* 143:867-872, 1986.

Kovasznay B, Fleischer J, Tananberg-Karant M, Jandorf L, Miller AD, Bromet E. Substance use disorder and the early course of illness in schizophrenia and affective psychosis. *Schizophrenia Bulletin* 23:195-201, 1997.

Linszen DH, Dingemans PM, Nugter MA, Van der Does AJ, Scholte WF, Lenior MA. Patient attributes and expressed emotion as risk factors for psychotic relapse. *Schizophrenia Bulletin* 23:119-130, 1997.

McLellan AT, Luborsky L, Cacciola J. New data from the addiction severity index: Reliability and validity in three centers. *Journal of Nervous and Mental Disorders* 173:412-423, 1985.

Miller WR, Rollnick S. *Motivational Interviewing.* New York, Guilford Press, 1991.

Miner CR, Rosenthal RN, Hellerstein DJ. Prediction of non-compliance with outpatient treatment referral in substance-abusing schizophrenics. *Archives of General Psychiatry* 706-712, 1997.

Mueser KT, Drake RE, Ackerson TH, Alterman AI, Miles KM, Noordsy DL. Antisocial personality disorder, conduct disorder, and substance abuse in schizophrenia. *Journal of Abnormal Psychology* 106(3):473-477, 1997.

Osher FC, Kofoed LL. Treatment of patients with psychiatric and psychoactive substance abuse disorders. *Hospital and Community Psychiatry* 40(10): 1025-1030, 1989.

Pinsker H. *A Primer of Supportive Psychotherapy.* Hillsdale, NJ: Analytic Press, 1998.

Pinsker H, Rosenthal RN, McCullough L. Supportive dynamic psychotherapy. In *Handbook of Short-Term Dynamic Therapy,* edited by Crits-Christoph P and Barber J. New York: Basic Books, 1991, pp. 220-247.

Prochaska JO, DiClemente CC, Norcross JC. In search of how people change: Applications to addictive behaviors. *American Psychologist* 47:1102-1114, 1992.

Regier DA, Farmer ME, Rae DS, Locke BZ, Keith SJ, Judd LL, Goodwin FK. Comorbidity of mental disorder with alcohol and other drug abuse: Results from the Epidemiologic Catchment Area (ECA) Study. *JAMA* 264:2511-2518, 1990.

Roberts LJ, Shaner A, Eckman T. Substance abuse management module (SAMM): Skills training for people with schizophrenia who are also addicted to drugs and alcohol. In *Substance Abuse Management Module* (West LA VA Medical Center and Department of Psychiatry and Biobehavioral Sciences), edited by Roberts LJ, Shaner A, Eckman T. Los Angeles: UCLA, 1997.

Rollnick S, Miller WR. What is motivational interviewing? *Behavioural and Cognitive Psychotherapy* 23(4):325-334, 1995.

Rosenthal RN, Hellerstein DJ, Miner CR. A model of integrated services for outpatient treatment of patients with comorbid schizophrenia and addictive disorders. *American Journal on Addictions* 1(4):339-348, 1992.

Rosenthal RN, Miner CR. Differential diagnosis of substance-induced psychosis and schizophrenia in patients with substance use disorders. *Schizophrenia Bulletin* 23:187-193, 1997.

Rosenthal RN, Pinsker H, Winston A. *Supportive Group Psychotherapy and Counseling Manual for Patients with Substance Abuse and Schizophrenia: COPAD Program.* Unpublished Manual. New York, Beth Israel Medical Center Department of Psychiatry, Psychotherapy Research Program, 1993.

Scott JE, Dixon LB. Psychological interventions for schizophrenia. *Schizophrenia Bulletin* 21:621-630, 1995.

Szuster RR, Schanbacher BL, McCann SC, McConnell A. Underdiagnosis of psychoactive-substance-induced organic mental disorders in emergency psychiatry. *American Journal of Drug and Alcohol Abuse* 16:319-327, 1990.

Yalom ID. *The Theory and Practice of Group Psychotherapy,* Fourth Edition. New York: Basic Books, 1995.

Ziedonis DM, Trudeau K. Motivation to quit using substances among individuals with schizophrenia: Implications for a motivation-based treatment model. *Schizophrenia Bulletin* 23:229-238, 1997.

Chapter 20

Smoking Cessation Treatment Groups

Timothy P. Carmody

INTRODUCTION

Cigarette smoking is the major cause of preventable deaths in the United States, accounting for more than 400,000 deaths per year or about 1,000 deaths per day (DHHS, 1988, 1990). Cigarette smoking causes lung and other cancers, chronic obstructive pulmonary disease, cardiovascular disease, peptic ulcers, gastrointestinal disorders, and maternal/fetal complications. It is estimated that almost one-half of the 50 million Americans who are currently regular smokers will eventually die of a tobacco-induced disorder (DHHS, 1988). Furthermore, secondhand smoke causes the deaths of many nonsmokers, including the children and other relatives of smokers, with estimates of mortality ranging up to 53,000 nonsmokers per year.

The prevalence of cigarette smoking in the United States, which had been decreasing about 1 percent per year, has now plateaued. Approximately two-thirds of current smokers have made three or more attempts to quit (Schelling, 1992). Most smokers who quit smoking do so on their own. However, only one-third of these self-quitters remain abstinent for more than two days and fewer than 5 percent are ultimately successful on any given quit attempt (Cohen et al., 1989). Moreover, two-thirds of smokers who quit with the help of some intervention relapse within the first three months after quitting. Just as with other forms of substance abuse, the lifetime of a long-term regular smoker is characterized by cyclical episodes of quitting and relapsing (Carmody, 1990).

Approximately 80 to 90 percent of regular smokers meet the DSM-IV (APA, 1994) criteria for nicotine dependence (e.g., occurrence of withdrawal symptoms during quitting attempts). Among smokers who try to quit, about one-half experience many of the symptoms of nicotine withdrawal, including anxiety, depression, insomnia, irritability, restlessness, weight gain, difficulty concentrating, and decreased heart rate (APA, 1994). Nicotine withdrawal symptoms usually begin within one to two days after cessation.

To summarize, cigarette smoking is a highly prevalent and often lethal addiction. Because of the large disease burden associated with cigarette smoking, reducing the percentage of Americans who smoke is an important public health goal (DHHS, 1990).

In this chapter, smoking cessation groups will be described within the context of the overall treatment of nicotine dependence. This discussion will focus on the stages of group development and specific intervention techniques used within and in conjunction with smoking cessation groups. Research on the role and efficacy of smoking cessation groups and other issues in the treatment of nicotine dependence will also be reviewed.

OVERVIEW OF SMOKING CESSATION TREATMENT

Smoking cessation treatment methods vary from the use of self-help educational materials to intensive multicomponent intervention programs. Many smoking cessation programs use a stepped-care approach in helping a smoker to quit (AHCPR, 1996), starting with less costly and low-intensity treatment procedures and moving to more costly and high-intensity treatment programs. Less intensive smoking cessation treatments may involve only a few minutes of advice and distribution of educational materials. More intensive smoking cessation programs typically include multiple intervention techniques utilized over several sessions (either individual or group), cognitive-behavioral therapy, and use of one or more medications such as nicotine patches. Smokers who fail initial low-intensity treatments for smoking cessation are subsequently provided with more intensive treatments.

Smoking cessation interventions are conducted by a variety of health care providers, including primary care physicians, nurses, public health educators, psychiatrists, psychologists, and other mental health professionals. The National Cancer Institute has sponsored training programs for health care professionals in smoking cessation treatment and has funded large-scale research studies testing the effectiveness of major community-based public health interventions aimed at reducing the prevalence of cigarette smoking.

In viewing smoking cessation treatment from a public health perspective, both "reach" and "efficacy" are considered in determining the impact of specific interventions. Public health "reach" refers to the number of smokers that can be reached by a specific treatment. Public health education campaigns utilizing mass media directed at entire communities have enormous "reach" but little impact on heavily addicted smokers. Only a small percentage of smokers who attempt to quit smoking participate in smoking cessation treatment programs or groups. For this reason, major trends in the field of smoking cessation include the use of public health campaigns with a large "reach" (i.e., community-based and population-based interventions) and training health care professionals (i.e., primary care physicians) to counsel their patients to quit (Lichtenstein and Glasgow, 1992). A third area in the antitobacco field remains the use of formal smoking cessation treatment programs in which intervention groups are conducted. These treatment programs are particularly helpful in facilitating smoking cessation in heavily addicted smokers.

Smoking Cessation Treatment Groups

Group interventions represent a core component of most formal smoking cessation treatment programs. Smoking cessation groups typically provide support, education, and behavioral skills training for smokers trying to quit smoking. In groups that focus on education, smokers may simply be provided with information about the dangers of smoking. In other groups, the emphasis is on support for cessation. Smoking cessation groups that provide both support and education are offered by a number of public and private health-related agencies and organizations. For example, Nicotine Anonymous, which is based on the twelve-step approach, offers group meetings to anyone interested in quitting smoking. Other nationwide health organizations include the American Cancer Society's Fresh Start, American Lung Association's Freedom from Smoking, and the Seventh-Day Adventists' Smoking Cessation Program. In addition, various commercial smoking cessation programs such as Smokenders include group meetings as an important part of their interventions. The kinds of groups offered by these organizations and agencies utilize both group support and education on the dangers of smoking and quitting skills.

Many smokers join smoking cessation groups after they have tried other methods or have tried to quit on their own without success. Some smokers participate in smoking cessation groups as part of formal smoking cessation treatment programs. Others join smoking cessation groups because they have found groups to be helpful in overcoming other addictions or other mental health problems. Although some smokers seek out groups to help them to quit, others agree to join such groups only after this option has been recommended by a health care professional.

TREATMENT PLANNING ISSUES

Smoking cessation programs vary in terms of the range of pharmacological and psychosocial interventions they offer and the degree of flexibility in tailoring treatment to individual smokers. Most smoking cessation programs emphasize the importance of thorough evaluation, screening, and negotiation of a treatment contract with the patient.

Assessment and Selection of Patients

An important area of assessment in evaluating patients for smoking cessation treatment and screening them for smoking cessation groups is their motivation for quitting. During the intake assessment for smoking cessation, smokers are typically asked to estimate the strength of their desire to quit and to describe their reasons for wanting to quit. Smokers who indicate that they realize the need to quit but are not ready to quit may not be appropriate to participate in smoking cessation groups.

Most smokers are readily able to identify their reasons for wanting to quit. They are also able to describe their reasons for continuing to smoke. Most smokers want to quit smoking for health reasons. However, some smokers decide to quit for other reasons (e.g., cost of cigarettes, increasing social stigma of smoking). The answers to these questions provide important clues for tailoring treatment for each patient.

Smoking history also provides information that is useful in planning treatment. Smoking history includes factors associated with the onset and progressive course of regular cigarette smoking, methods used in previous attempts to quit, previous experience of nicotine withdrawal symptoms during quit attempts, factors triggering relapse, relationships between smoking and use/abuse of other substances, and previous participation in smoking cessation treatment. Preference for specific treatment modalities (e.g., group versus individual format) and past benefit or lack of benefit from groups or other treatments provide additional information for treatment planning.

Degree or severity of nicotine dependence is another important area of assessment, and is used primarily in the planning of nicotine replacement component of treatment. One commonly used method for assessing nicotine dependence is the Fagerstrom Tolerance Scale (FTS) (Fagerstrom, Heatherton, and Kozlowski, 1992), a brief self-report instrument. The current number of cigarettes smoked per day and past occurrence of nicotine withdrawal symptoms during previous quitting attempts are important indicators of nicotine dependence that are included on the FTS. Another FTS question that is useful in evaluating nicotine dependence is: How soon after you wake up do you smoke your first cigarette? The smokers who indicate that they smoke the first cigarette within thirty minutes after waking are more likely to be highly nicotine dependent.

Stages of Behavior Change

The Transtheoretical or Stages of Change model (Prochaska and DiClemente, 1992) has provided a conceptual framework for understanding the processes of behavior change across several forms of substance abuse. This model has been used extensively in developing and implementing smoking cessation treatment methods, whether low-intensity advice and self-help educational materials or high-intensity intervention programs involving pharmacological agents, behavioral skills training, and groups (Perz, DiClemente, and Carbonari, 1996). Five stages of change are included in this model: precontemplation, contemplation, preparation, action, and maintenance (Perz, DiClemente, and Carbonari, 1996; Prochaska and DiClemente, 1992). Precontemplation is characterized by a lack of desire to quit smoking. Contemplation involves an awareness of the dangers of smoking and the decision-making process of weighing the benefits and drawbacks of quitting. Smokers in the preparation stage have begun to make some behavioral adjustments to prepare for quitting. This stage serves as a bridge between the considerations of the contemplation stage and the behavioral work of the action stage in which the smoker attempts to quit. Maintenance involves the long-term adjustment to the more acute changes made during the contemplation, preparation, and action stages.

Comorbid Depression and Substance Abuse

Another important area of assessment in evaluating patients for smoking cessation pertains to the presence and/or history of depression and substance abuse disorders. A high proportion of smokers have comorbid psychiatric conditions, particularly depression (Carmody, 1989). A history of major depression is quite common among smokers seeking help to quit (Carmody, 1989). Glassman (1993) reported that 25 to 40 percent of patients seeking treatment for nicotine dependence had a history of major depression or dysthymic symptoms. These smokers are two to three times less likely to be successful in quitting smoking and generally require more intensive treatment. Considerable evidence shows dysphoric mood at the time of the quit attempt is predictive of continued smoking (Hall, Munoz, Reus, et al., 1996). In addition, individuals with persistent nicotine withdrawal symptoms following cessation of tobacco use have also been found to be at increased risk for depressive episodes (Covey, Glassman, and Stetner, 1997).

The relationship between depression and nicotine dependence has several possible explanations (Carmody, 1989). Some smokers may smoke to elevate their mood. For other smokers, depression may be an obstacle to quitting or maintaining abstinence. Alternatively, neuroendocrine function may be dysregulated during nicotine withdrawal. The quit attempt is more likely to be successful when the psychiatric condition is stable. For these reasons, mood and blood levels of psychotropic medications are closely monitored during early cessation (APA, 1996).

Another important subgroup of smokers are those with other concurrent substance abuse disorders (Abrams et al., 1992; Hughes, 1993). Between 15 and 20 percent of heavy smokers have current alcohol dependence or abuse and 40 percent have a history of past alcohol abuse (Hughes, 1996). Approximately 80 percent of alcohol/drug abusers who are in chemical dependence treatment are smokers (Hughes, 1996). A critical issue for these smokers is the optimal timing of smoking cessation treatment in conjunction with treatment for their other substance abuse problems (Bobo, Slade, and Hoffman, 1995; Hughes, 1993). A common concern is that smoking cessation will cause relapse in the use of alcohol/drugs. However, studies support the treatment of smoking during or shortly after treatment of alcohol dependence (Hughes, 1995). Smoking cessation is now incorporated into some alcohol/drug treatment programs (Hughes, 1993, 1995).

Specific Forms of Group Treatment

Most smoking cessation groups are psychoeducational and use a uniform order of programmed content rather than open-ended process. Some smoking cessation groups utilize a rotating theme format. Smoking cessation groups vary in terms of the amount of support, education, process, and quitting skills training. Some of these groups simply provide support while others offer more intensive and systematic training in behavioral self-management skills. Most smoking cessation groups include didactic presentations and skills training aimed at helping smokers through the process of quitting and relapse prevention. In these groups, information is provided regarding the health consequences of smoking, importance of quitting, and recommendations regarding quitting strategies.

Most of the smoking cessation groups that have been studied in the research literature utilize behavioral self-management skills training (Carmody, 1993; Lichtenstein and Glasgow, 1992). These groups are designed to teach participants how to use basic principles of learning theory to facilitate smoking cessation. The specific treatment techniques used in these group interventions range from providing didactic information on the dangers of smoking to enhance motivation for quitting, to the use of hypnosis or behavioral self-management strategies such as contingency contracting. Just as with process-oriented groups, management of group process is an important component of these nonprocess psychoeducational groups.

The frequency, duration, and number of group sessions vary across smoking cessation programs. Most smoking cessation groups are conducted on a weekly basis. In some smoking cessation treatments, groups are conducted three or four times during the week of the quit attempt. Smoking cessation groups in inpatient settings may also be conducted several times a week. The importance of maintaining adequate support and close contact with the smoker during the week just before and after the quit date is emphasized in most smoking cessation treatment programs. Most behavioral smoking cessation groups meet on a weekly basis for eight to twelve weeks. Follow-up individual or group treatment sessions are also provided. In some programs, drop-in or ongoing maintenance groups are conducted to support ex-smokers in preventing relapse.

STAGES OF GROUP DEVELOPMENT

Group Format and Dynamics

In smoking cessation groups, participants are reminded that they are not alone or unique in terms of their nicotine dependence. This is the well-known "universality effect" of group therapy. Group participants have an opportunity to observe other smokers proceeding through the same quitting process, struggling with cigarette cravings, using similar strategies to quit, reminding themselves of the same reasons for quitting. They experience a relatedness and support, which is particularly helpful for those who lack support for quitting outside the group. Group members model various forms of skill-building for one another.

The degree of homogeneity versus heterogeneity of participants is an important issue in smoking cessation groups. One source of homogeneity derives from the common goal of participants to quit smoking, and shared experiences involved in the quit attempt and nicotine withdrawal. Some groups attempt to utilize this homogeneity of purpose by encouraging a common quit date for the entire group, and other groups allow participants to choose individual quit dates. Sources of heterogeneity derive from different reasons for wanting to quit, levels of nicotine dependence, smoking triggers, and strategies for quitting. Different perspectives about smoking and quitting can lead to disagreements and confusion as to which methods work best to facilitate quitting. Group participants are reminded that no single best method for quitting applies to all smokers.

Three Phases of Quitting

The process of quitting smoking is generally divided into three phases: preparation for the quit date, the quit date itself, and maintenance (relapse prevention), which starts at the moment of quitting. Groups are generally structured according to these three phases. During the preparation phase, the focus of group treatment is on motivational issues, facilitation of commitment for quitting, and setting a quit day. The focus of the group at the time of the quit date is for participants to implement a quitting ritual and cope with the first full day of cessation without smoking or even taking a puff. The maintenance phase addresses relapse prevention issues.

Conduct of Initial Sessions

Many smoking cessation programs begin with an orientation meeting in which potential participants learn about the program and decide whether to enroll. In other programs, the first group session serves this orientation function. Group members are introduced to one another and asked to discuss their reasons for participating in the group, reasons for wanting to quit, and specifics of their smoking history (e.g., previous attempts to quit, previous participation in smoking cessation treatment, etc.). Differences in level of commitment to quitting smoking among group members quickly become evident. Often, more committed participants, observing the ambivalence of other group members, try to encourage them to strengthen their commitment to quitting.

In general, during the initial sessions, an effort is made to develop group cohesiveness and to facilitate commitment to cessation. The goals, guidelines for participation, and expectations for treatment are discussed at length. For instance, in cognitive-behavioral groups, the expectation that participants will be assigned homework to practice quitting skills is emphasized during the initial session. At the same time, group members ask themselves whether the group intervention will be helpful for them and decide whether to commit themselves to becoming a part of the group and the treatment process.

Middle Phases of Group

The focus of discussion during the middle phases of smoking cessation groups is on setting and implementing a plan for the quit date, as well as on methods for coping with cravings for cigarettes and other nicotine withdrawal symptoms. There are two basic approaches to the task of setting a quit date. In one approach, group members decide on a singular and common quit date. In the other approach, group members select their own individual quit date. Whichever approach is used, differences quickly become apparent in the rate and success with which group members proceed through the steps of quitting.

As participants set quit dates and proceed through the quitting process, support and encouragement are provided at the time of the quit date and during the first week following the quit date. To this end, face-to-face contact in the group at the time of the quit attempt is often supplemented with phone contacts. Considering the intensity of nicotine withdrawal symptoms and high rate of relapse during the first week of cessation, it is generally recommended that some type of phone or face-to-face contact be scheduled within one to three days after the quit date.

During the middle phases of smoking cessation groups, the discussion, education, and skills training is focused on methods for resisting the urge to smoke and on coping with nicotine withdrawal symptoms. Participants share both common and unique aspects of their experiences with quitting, nicotine withdrawal, and coping efforts.

Differences also begin to emerge as some participants succeed in quitting while others continue to smoke or fail to make it through a complete day without smoking. An important task or challenge for the group leader is to utilize these differences to promote successful outcomes in as many participants as possible. Group members who are further along in the quitting process offer support, encouragement, and modeling of effective coping strategies to those participants who are experiencing more difficulty in quitting. Those group members who continue to struggle with quitting view more successful participants in a variety of ways. Some focus on the hope of their own success while others focus on their beliefs that they are more heavily addicted, lack the willpower to quit, and/or are doomed to continue to smoke. In most smoking cessation groups, most participants are able to quit, but less than half remain abstinent.

Termination, Follow-up, and Relapse Prevention

For those group members who are able to quit, postcessation follow-up and relapse prevention actually begin during the latter phases of the smoking cessation group. During this time, most group participants have quit smoking and are coping with nicotine withdrawal. When the group treatment is completed, the maintenance or follow-up phase of treatment is begun. The follow-up plan depends on the preferences, past history of cessation, psychiatric history, and need to monitor blood levels of medications that might increase with cessation. Follow-up treatment can be provided in group booster sessions or drop-in maintenance groups.

The steps involved in relapse prevention for smoking cessation are similar to those used in the treatment of any of the substance abuse disorders. High-risk situations are identified, ways of coping with those situations without smoking are discussed, and specific coping responses are rehearsed by role-playing these situations (i.e., behavioral rehearsal). During the first few days of cessation, relapse is usually triggered by nicotine withdrawal symptoms. Subsequently, relapse occurs most frequently in situations involving stress, negative affect, and/or use of alcohol/drugs (e.g., Carmody, 1989, 1990). Smokers who relapse and resume smoking on a regular basis may benefit most from returning to another smoking cessation group in which they can review what factors were involved in their relapse, make a commitment to quit again, and start the quitting process again.

Social support has been recognized as an important component of relapse prevention (Carmody, 1990; Lando, 1993). Smokers who receive more support from significant others tend to have more success in preventing relapse (Carmody, 1990). An additional source of social support for continued abstinence from smoking is provided in various kinds of intervention groups (e.g., self-help, support, educational, psychotherapeutic).

TECHNIQUES USED IN SMOKING CESSATION GROUPS

In most smoking cessation groups, a number of psychoeducational intervention techniques are used to facilitate motivation for cessation and to train on quitting skills to promote successful cessation and re-lapse prevention.

Motivation Enhancement

During the initial stages of smoking cessation groups, participants are asked to discuss their reasons for wanting to quit smoking, and to make a public commitment or contract with the group regarding their intention to quit. In some smoking cessation programs and groups, participants are instructed to list their reasons for wanting to quit on "quit cards," identify the quit date and coping responses to use in re-sisting the urge to smoke. Another method used to enhance motiva-tion is the use of a quitting ceremony in which group members plan and implement a quitting ritual. For instance, they might all bring empty packs of cigarettes and each in turn crumple the pack, toss it onto a pile of empty packs in the middle of the group, and proclaim "I am quitting for good!" Such ceremonies or rituals are thought to reinforce the importance of quitting and commitment to smoking cessation and to the group.

Behavioral Self-Management Skills

A number of behavioral interventions have been used in smoking cessation groups (APA, 1996; Carmody, 1990, 1993; Lichtenstein and Glasgow, 1992). These include stimulus control, aversive condi-tioning methods, contingency contracting, self-management skills training, and role-playing or behavioral rehearsal. Stimulus control refers to the identification of smoking cues or triggers, and efforts to avoid or minimize exposure to these cues during the quitting process. Aversive conditioning procedures such as rapid smoking are more commonly used on an individual basis, but can also be incorporated into treatment groups. In self-management skills training, partici-pants learn various cognitive and behavioral methods for resisting the urge to smoke. Smoking cues or triggers are identified. The group en-gages in problem solving to develop plans for avoiding or minimizing contact with smoking triggers and initiation of lifestyle changes. Substitute behaviors for smoking are identified. In contingency con-tracting, participants learn how to select and implement meaningful consequences for successful cessation and relapse. For example, in some programs, a refundable deposit system is used in which participants earn refunds for attending sessions, implementing quitting strategies, successfully quitting, and/or remaining abstinent. Self-management approaches include cognitive as well as behavioral techniques. For example, participants are taught how to identify and challenge specific "addictive" thoughts such as "I'll gain too much weight unless I smoke" or "I don't have the willpower to resist the temptation to smoke."

Hypnosis

Hypnosis is a technique that is typically used within individual treatment, but has also been incorporated into group interventions (Green, 1996). Lynn et al (1994) developed a cognitive-behavioral group treatment that utilizes hypnotic suggestion, education, motivation enhancement, self-monitoring, self-management, nicotine fading (i.e., gradual reduction of smoking or nicotine intake), and relapse prevention. The suggestions used during hypnosis focus on the themes of motivation enhancement, self-efficacy in resisting the urge to smoke, and improved self-esteem in becoming a nonsmoker. This particular group treatment is conducted in only two sessions.

Treating Depression Associated with Smoking Cessation

Depression represents one of the major obstacles to quitting smoking (Carmody, 1989). Smoking cessation treatment programs have been tailored for individuals who suffer from depression (e.g., Hall, Munoz, and Reus, 1994). These intervention groups utilize cognitive-behavioral procedures to identify and challenge cognitive distortions associated with depressed mood and behavioral methods for increasing pleasant activities. Without group support, it is particularly difficult for depressed smokers to quit or remain abstinent due to the relationship between nicotine use and their fragile mood states.

Case Example

The patient was a forty-two-year-old Hispanic male smoker with a history of alcohol dependence and dysthymia. He was divorced, had two grown children, and lived alone. He had smoked two packs of cigarettes per day since the age of fifteen and was heavily addicted. His score on the Fagerstrom Tolerance Scale was 9/10, indicating high nicotine dependence. He wanted to quit for health reasons. He was particularly concerned about the risk of lung cancer. He also wanted to quit smoking to improve his capacity to engage in physical activities. At intake, he rated his desire to quit as 9/10 and self-efficacy for quitting as 8/10. He was invited to participate in a cognitive-behavioral smoking cessation group that met weekly for eight sessions. In the group, he was provided with information and training in quitting skills and methods for resisting the urge to smoke. The group helped him to identify and challenge distorted beliefs or addictive thinking that was maintaining his nicotine dependence. He set a quit date together with the other group members. He was also provided with nicotine patches, following AHCPR guidelines, and reported that this medication was helpful in alleviating withdrawal symptoms and cigarette cravings. He was able to quit and remain abstinent for four weeks. Then, he was diagnosed with stomach cancer and underwent a total gastrectomy. During this stressful time, he relapsed. During a follow-up session with his primary therapist, he was encouraged to join another smoking cessation group. He enrolled in another smoking cessation group in which he explored the factors that triggered relapse, the difficulties he had experienced in coping with the diagnosis and treatment of his stomach cancer. He quit smoking again and has remained abstinent to the present time.

RELEVANT RESEARCH

Treatment Efficacy

Hundreds of studies have examined the effectiveness of a variety of smoking cessation treatments, varying in level of intensity, use of medication, and specific psychosocial approaches (e.g., AHCPR, 1996; Lichtenstein and Glasgow, 1992). In this research literature, the gold standard for determining the efficacy of treatment for smoking cessation is the biochemically verified abstinence rate at twelve months (AHCPR, 1996; APA, 1996). Self-reported abstinence is verified using cotinine levels in blood, urine, or saliva.

According to the AHCPR (1996), most evidence supports the use of nicotine replacement in combination with behavioral coping skills training. Interestingly, based on the meta-analysis conducted by the AHCPR, individual and group smoking cessation interventions appear to be equally effective. Interventions achieve more success when they involve at least four to seven sessions (AHCPR, 1996).

Effects of Group Support

One of the advantages of conducting smoking cessation treatment in a group format is the role of group support in facilitating behavior change (Lando, 1993). Interestingly, attempts to increase social support by setting up buddy systems, teaching spouses how to be more supportive, or increasing cohesiveness in treatment groups have not been found to increase quit rates (Carmody, 1993). At the same time, there are data to suggest that smokers who are high in negative affect benefit most from interpersonal support in smoking cessation treatment, which may serve to prepare them for future episodes of negative affect (Zelman et al., 1992). Thus, smoking cessation groups may be particularly beneficial for smokers who are depressed or suffering from other comorbid psychiatric conditions.

Comparisons of Different Types of Smoking Cessation Groups

Given the variety of approaches used in smoking cessation groups, there appears to be a consensus that cognitive-behavioral self-management approaches are the most efficacious (Lichtenstein and Glasgow, 1992). This consensus may be due to the fact that most of the research has focused on this type of treatment group. No series of research studies clearly and consistently indicate that one type of group is any more effective than other kinds of groups for smoking cessation. Several treatment outcome studies have compared various multicomponent behavioral treatments with waiting-list or no-treatment controls as well as placebo control conditions in which group support is sometimes provided (Lichtenstein and Glasgow, 1992). Discussion and/or support groups are often used as placebo control interventions in the treatment outcome literature and are found to be less effective than behavioral self-management groups. Most smoking cessation treatment groups use both didactic and process factors. In general, groups that utilize multiple behavioral self-management efforts have been found to yield the best long-term outcomes (AHCPR, 1996; APA, 1996).

SUMMARY AND CONCLUSIONS

Smoking cessation groups represent the core component of most formal intervention programs in the treatment of nicotine dependence. These groups typically use a behavioral self-management approach in which participants receive education and training in strategies for enhancing motivation, proceeding through the steps of the quitting process, coping with cigarette cravings, and preventing relapse. Smoking cessation groups are usually structured with an ordered sequence of agendas for providing information and skills training. Although these groups are typically not process focused, process factors or group dynamics are always present and represent an important part of the impact of this treatment modality. In general, groups provide the context for education, support, problem solving, and skills training that facilitate smoking cessation.

Many of the intervention techniques used in smoking cessation groups are also used in individual treatment. However, groups offer the advantage of utilizing social support to enhance commitment to quitting and learning methods for coping with nicotine withdrawal without giving in to the urge to smoke. Group members learn much from one another about the quitting process and coping strategies. Groups appear to be particularly helpful for heavily addicted smokers with a history of depression or substance abuse. Smoking cessation groups typically include intervention methods aimed at preventing relapse. However, relapse continues to be a major problem in the treatment of nicotine dependence, just as it is with other substance abuse disorders. A promising approach to smoking cessation treatment appears to be to combine group interventions with pharmacological approaches, particularly nicotine replacement.

REFERENCES

Abrams DB, Rohsenow DJ, Niarua RS, Pedraza M, Longabaugh R, Beattie MC, Binkoff JA, Noel NE, Monti PM. Smoking and treatment outcome for alcoholics: Effects on coping skills, urge to drink, and drinking rates. *Behavior Therapy* 23:283-297, 1992.

Agency for Health Care Policy and Research. Smoking cessation, clinical practice guideline number 18. DHHS Publ No AHCPR 96-0692. Washington, DC: U.S. Government Printing Office, 1996.

American Psychiatric Association. *Diagnostic and Statistical Manual of Mental Disorders,* Fourth Edition. Washington, DC: APA, 1994.

American Psychiatric Association. Practice guideline for the treatment of patients with nicotine dependence. *American Journal of Psychiatry* 153:1-31, 1996.

Bobo JK, Slade J, Hoffman AL. Nicotine addiction counseling for chemically dependent patients. *Psychiatric Services* 46:945-947, 1995.

Carmody TP. Affect regulation, nicotine addiction, and smoking cessation. *Journal of Psychoactive Drugs* 21:331-342, 1989.

Carmody TP. Preventing relapse in the treatment of nicotine addiction: Current issues and future directions. *Journal of Psychoactive Drugs* 22:211-238, 1990.

Carmody TP. Nicotine dependence: Psychosocial approaches to the prevention of smoking relapse. *Psychology of Addictive Behaviors* 7:96-102, 1993.

Cohen S, Lichtenstein E, Prochaska JO, Rossi JS, Gritz ER, Carr CR, Orleans CT, Curry S, Marlatt GA, Cumming KM, Emont SL, Giovino G, Ossip-Klein D. Debunking myths about self-quitting. *American Psychologist* 44:1355-1365, 1989.

Covey LS, Glassman AH, Stetner F. Major depression following smoking cessation. *American Journal of Psychiatry* 154:263-265, 1997.

Department of Health and Human Services. The Health Consequences of Smoking—Nicotine Addiction: A report of the Surgeon General. DHHS Publication No CDC 88-8406. Washington, DC: U.S. Government Printing Office, 1988.

Department of Health and Human Services. The Health Benefits of Smoking Cessation. DHHS Publication No CDC 90-8416. Washington, DC: U.S. Government Printing Office, 1990.

Fagerstrom KO, Heatherton TF, Kozlowski KT. Nicotine addiction and its assessment. *Ear, Nose, and Throat* 69:763-768, 1992.

Glassman AH. Cigarette smoking: Implications for psychiatric illness. *American Journal of Psychiatry* 150:546-553, 1993.

Green JP. Cognitive-behavioral hypnotherapy for smoking cessation: A case study in a group setting. In *Casebook of Clinical Hypnosis,* edited by Lynn SJ, Kirsch I, Rhue JW. Washington, DC: American Psychological Association, 1996, pp. 223-250.

Hall SM, Munoz RF, Reus VI. Cognitive-behavioral intervention increases abstinence rates for depressive-history smokers. *Journal of Consulting and Clinical Psychology* 62:141-146, 1994.

Hall SM, Munoz RF, Reus VI, Sees KL, Duncan C, Humfleet GL, Hartz DT. Mood management and nicotine gum in smoking treatment: A therapeutic contact and placebo-controlled study. *Journal of Consulting and Clinical Psychology* 64:1003-1009, 1996.

Hughes JR. Treatment of smoking cessation in smokers with past alcohol/drug problems. Special issue: Towards a broader view of recovery: Integrating nicotine addiction and chemical dependency treatments. *Journal of Substance Abuse Treatment* 10:181-187, 1993.

Hughes JR. Clinical implications of the association between smoking and alcoholism. In *Alcohol and Tobacco: From Basic Science to Policy* (NIAAA Research Monograph 30), edited by Fertig J, Fuller R. Washington, DC: U.S. Government Printing Office, 1995, pp. 171-181.

Hughes JR. Treating smokers with current or past alcohol dependence. *American Journal of Health Behavior* 20:286-290, 1996.

Lando HA. Formal quit smoking treatments. In *Nicotine Addiction: Principles and Management,* edited by Orleans CT, Slade J. New York: Oxford University Press, 1993, pp. 221-244.

Lichtenstein E, Glasgow RE. Smoking cessation: What have we learned over the past decade? *Journal of Consulting and Clinical Psychology* 60:518-527, 1992.

Lynn SJ, Neufeld V, Rhue JW, Matorin A. Hypnosis and smoking cessation: A cognitive-behavioral treatment. In *Handbook of Clinical Hypnosis,* edited by Lynn SJ, Rhue JW, Kirsch I. Washington, DC: American Psychological Association, 1994, pp. 555-585.*

Perz CA, DiClemente CC, Carbonari JP. Doing the right thing at the right time? The interaction of stages and processes of change in successful smoking cessation. *Health Psychology* 15:462-468, 1996.

Prochaska JO, DiClemente CC. Stages of change in the modification of problem behaviors. In *Progress in Behavior Modification,* edited by Hersen M, Eisler RM, Miller PM. Sycamore, IL: Sycamore Press, 1992, pp. 184-214.

Schelling TC. Addictive drugs: The cigarette experience. *Science* 255:430-433, 1992.

Zelman DC, Brandon TH, Jorenby DE, Baker TB. Measures of affect and nicotine dependence predict differential response to smoking cessation. *Journal of Consulting and Clinical Psychology* 60:943-952, 1992.

Chapter 21

Medically Ill Substance Abusers in Group Therapy

David J. Hellerstein
Lee Shomstein

INTRODUCTION

There is a surprising lack of literature on the group therapy of the medically ill substance abuser, primarily clinical descriptions, and almost no quantitative research. In general, substance abuse problems are barely mentioned in the literature on the group therapy of individuals with medical illnesses. Writings on group therapy of substance abusers generally mention medical issues only in passing, among the many other life problems that alcoholics or drug abusers may face.

Medical illnesses have often played a major role in the lives of substance abusers, and indeed it has been noted (Flores 1997) that medical crises commonly precipitate the individual substance abuser's entry into treatment. Historically, the development of medical illnesses such as cirrhosis of the liver, delirium tremens, cardiomyopathy, esophageal varices, and other life-threatening conditions have played a major role in providing motivation to stop drinking, to maintain abstinence, to set realistic treatment goals, and to determine prognosis. In the context of psychotherapy illnesses have also formed the matrix for psychological and interpersonal growth and for spiritual conversion experiences.

As such, medical illness has been a central but often unacknowledged focus in the group therapy of substance abusers. As new substances of abuse have entered common use, new medical problems or comorbid conditions become common (e.g., crack abuse, and consequent compulsive sexuality and increased risk of HIV infection), and group therapists have adapted their goals and treatment approaches to adjust to these realities—though often in an ad hoc and unsystematized fashion.

Obviously, group therapists must address medical illnesses among substance abusers (and address substance abuse among the medically ill). Substance abusers tend to have severe, multiple, and often chronic medical illnesses (Novick 1992). Habitual patterns of denial and self-neglect may lead to substandard medical care and thus unnecessary morbidity or mortality. The stress of unacknowledged or poorly treated medical illnesses may cause substance abuse relapse, even in the context of prolonged abstinence. Also, the medical illness of an individual group member is a stress upon the group itself: it may disrupt the group therapy process, leading to dropout or substance abuse relapse among other members.

The following chapter will summarize the existing literature in this area, and describe commonly used group treatment approaches when treating individuals with comorbid substance abuse and medical illnesses. In addition, an attempt will be made to clarify and systematize what are often ad hoc responses, and to provide a rationale for setting goals and making informed treatment decisions.

GENERAL ISSUES

Setting and Context of Treatment

In recent years, psychiatric and substance abuse clinicians have become increasingly aware of the frequent dual morbidities of co-occurring psychiatric and substance abuse disorders (Kaplan, Sadock, and Grebb 1994). This chapter describes populations who frequently have triple morbidities: substance abuse and medical comorbidity, and often psychiatric disorders as well. Given the complexity and heterogeneity of such clinical populations, it is essential to consider the specific contexts in which treatment occurs. Group therapy of the medically ill substance abuser may occur in clinics, hospitals, methadone programs, prisons, HIV programs, and other settings. The specific disease or diseases (whether acute, chronic, or recurrent; and the degree of mortality), and the specific substances abused (alcohol, cocaine, heroin, stimulants, etc.), similarly have a major impact on treatment. Fiscal and clinical realities may determine the scope of treatment, providing limits upon or incentives for certain treatment approaches. Thus, in order to set treatment goals, it is important to know the settings and constraints of treatment.

For group treatment of the medically ill substance abuser, key questions include: Is the group homogeneous or heterogeneous? Is the group a stand-alone entity or is it integrated into a treatment program? Is the duration of treatment brief or ongoing? What is the overall philosophy or approach to treatment? Furthermore, if the group is heterogeneous, in what way is it heterogeneous—by medical diagnosis or by the substance abused? For instance, one might provide group therapy for eight women with breast cancer in a cancer center, of whom two have a substance abuse disorder. In contrast, an ongoing group of ten alcoholics in an outpatient substance abuse rehabilitation program might include three members with hepatic failure. In the first instance, the primary treatment approach is that of group therapy for individuals with medical illness; in the second, the primary treatment approach is group therapy for individuals with substance use disorders.

Goals

Depending on the population treated, the clinical setting, and other factors, such as the severity of medical illnesses, a variety of different goals may be appropriate. They may include social goals (improving social support networks); medical goals (improving compliance with medical treatment regimens, decreasing dangerous behaviors such as impulsive sexuality, needle sharing, etc.); substance use goals (decreased substance use may be appropriate for one setting, complete abstinence for another); psychiatric goals (decreased symptomatology, dealing with grief or loss, improved life satisfaction or quality); or economic goals (decreasing unnecessary rehospitalizations, improved work functioning).

Clinicians may utilize appropriate measures (whether quantitative, subjective, or both) to help determine whether the group is achieving its goals. These measures should include specific measures (such as urine toxicologies or symptom inventories), global measures (life satisfaction), and measurements of the treatment process (patient satisfaction questionnaires, treatment alliance measures).

Time-Limited versus Ongoing Groups

Ulman (1993) points out pros and cons of time-limited versus long-term groups for the medically ill. The emphasis is on the here and now, with minimal exploration of historical issues and minimal interpretation of transferential material. In the instance of patients with comorbid substance abuse and medical illness, a few brief treatment models have been specifically described in the literature (Lenya 1994), but others could be developed. For instance, primary focus could be on adjustment to a new medical illness in a population of individuals with substance abuse, such as among cocaine abusers with newly diagnosed HIV infection, treated on an inpatient medical or rehabilitation unit.

The existing treatment literature for individuals with comorbid substance abuse and medical illness focuses primarily on ongoing or open-ended groups. While these could have a more traditional psychodynamic orientation such as that used with long-term group therapy of the medically ill (Rutan and Stone 1993), it is more likely that they would have the sort of recovery/relapse prevention approach (Flores 1997) commonly used in the group treatment of alcoholics and substance abusers. The latter treatment models can be utilized to meet the specific needs of addicted patients (Flores 1997), which in this case consists of significant physical illness, while not ignoring the individual and group psychodynamics commonly encountered among substance abusers (Khantzian, Halliday, Golden 1992; Yalom 1995).

Primary Focus

Beyond the time duration of the group treatment, an important issue is whether medical illness is the primary focus of the group or a secondary focus. In this chapter, the primary focus will be the heterogeneous group setting, in which substance abuse treatment is primary. This is probably the most common setting in which group treatment for these comorbidities occur. Homogeneous groups should also generally follow the model of substance abuse treatment as primary, in order to optimize the possibility of positive outcome, and to minimize the risk of substance abuse relapse.

PRETREATMENT ISSUES

Virtually any organ system may show significant disease as a result of chronic substance abuse (Novick 1992). Chronic medical disorders may present serious life difficulties to patients in group therapy (see Table 21.1). Since many, if not the majority, of substance

TABLE 21.1. Example of Chronic Medical Problems Commonly Found Among Substance Abusers and Addicts

Category	Condition
Cardiovascular	Myocardial infarction Hypertension Thrombophlebitis Cardiomyopathy
Endocrinological	Diabetes mellitus Pancreatitis
Gastrointestinal	Gastric ulcers and esophageal varices
Hepatic	Acute and chronic hepatitis Cirrhosis
Infectious	HIV/AIDS Tuberculosis, pneumonia Endocarditis Nephritis Abscesses, cellulitis Sexually transmitted diseases
Neoplastic	Lung cancer Oropharyngeal cancers Breast/ovarian cancer
Neurological	Seizure disorders Head trauma Cerebrovascular accidents Dementia Peripheral neuropathy
Neuropsychiatric	Insomnia Sexual dysfunction Hallucinosis
Renal	Nephrotic syndrome, renal failure, and glomerulonephritis
Respiratory	Emphysema Pulmonary hypertension

Note: For a more detailed account, see Novick 1992.

abusers have significant medical sequelae of substance abuse at some point during their lives, it makes more sense to think of a threshold of severity rather than presence or absence of illness when considering whether to include a physically ill substance abuser in group treatment, or whether to address physical illness as a major focus of group treatment. Many substance abusers are already in treatment when their medical illnesses begin to exacerbate in severity. Ideally, medical issues should be addressed throughout treatment (with psycho-education about health-maintaining behaviors and confrontation about self-neglect of health issues, and coordination of care with medical clinicians, both primary care and specialists). Health issues may develop clinical urgency, however, only when there is significant worsening. Often the seriousness of such a medical problem will first be evident to others (friends, relatives, health care providers, therapists) rather than to the substance-abusing individuals themselves.

Beyond the presence of such a medical illness, evidence should support that the individual might benefit from the social support, decreased isolation, and destigmatization that group psychotherapy can offer, and that some degree of motivation exists for participating in a group. For instance, the previously abstinent alcoholic who begins drinking heavily upon learning that he has lung cancer, and who becomes depressed and unable to stop drinking (despite attending twelve-step meetings), may benefit from group psychotherapy with other substance abusers with a focus on coping with medical illness.

Some medically ill substance-abusing patients are not suitable for group therapy. Severely or terminally ill patients may lack interest, motivation, or on a practical level be unable to attend group meetings on a regular basis. (However, many HIV patients and many patients with terminal illnesses may derive significant benefit from group treatment.) Patients suffering from significant dementia or other cognitive impairment may not be able to benefit from the group setting. Individuals with severe acting-out or exploitative behavior, or acutely suicidal impulses, may be too disruptive for some group settings. At times, patients present with compelling individual, personal, or family issues that they are unwilling to discuss in a group setting—or in a particular group setting. A former polysubstance abusing woman who had found benefit in talking about her esophageal cancer in a group setting, was unable to discuss issues raised by her later development of breast cancer, because the group included men. In her case, referral to CancerCare, a group program for cancer patients, was made, and she was able to discuss these issues in a group of women with breast cancer. Depending on clinical presentation, some patients with a history of substance abuse may benefit most from group therapy with medically ill (but non-substance abusing) individuals.

CONDUCT OF GROUP THERAPY

Individual Issues, Psychodynamic and Behavioral

Substance abusers often show characteristic, and maladaptive, responses to the development of medical illnesses (see Table 21.2). The most prominent of these is denial. New, evolving, or chronic medical symptoms may be ignored, just as the impact of drinking on work functioning or marriage has been ignored. IV drug abusers may prefer "not to know" their HIV status, refusing to take HIV tests, or may show little overt reaction to the diagnosis of AIDS or other life-threatening illnesses. Once illnesses are diagnosed, individuals may avoid doctors, or procrastinate in seeking treatment. These patterns, common during periods of active substance use, may also persist during periods of abstinence. Overwhelming feelings of victimization, shame, guilt, and fear can obscure and obfuscate life issues that need to be addressed. Commonly, medical illness may precipitate a relapse, whether into substance abuse or other compulsive behavior, such as sexual acting out, gambling, eating, etc. In other instances, medical illness may cause a combination of the above reactions, with increased cycling from abstinence to relapse to abstinence.

Conversely, medical illness may induce substance abusers to accept that they have a substance abuse problem, and may propel them into treatment, including AA, NA, or psychotherapy. For substance abusers already in treatment, a serious medical illness may augment the motivation to remain abstinent. Serious medical illness at times may precipitate conversion experiences, enabling addicted individuals finally to gain control over their substance abuse or other compulsive behavior. Stating "I don't want to die drunk," one HIV-infected man stopped his substance abuse and compulsive sexual behavior, and maintained through his final months that he was "grateful" to the illness that "allowed me to get sober and stay sober."

TABLE 21.2. Common Maladaptive Response to Illness Among Substance-Abusing Individuals and Possible Adaptive Alternatives

Maladaptive Responses	Adaptive Responses
Self-monitoring, self-appraisal	
Denial ("Nothing is the matter.")	Acceptance
Fantasy/false hope ("It will go away.")	Realistic appraisal
Rationalization ("I might as well drink.")	Honesty with self
Emotional reactions	
Victimization/anger ("Why me?")	Acceptance—illness is a part of life
Guilt ("Mea culpa." "I brought it on myself.")	Acceptance—addiction is also a disease
Punishment/penance ("God is punishing me.")	
Shame/avoidance ("I don't want anyone to know"—common with HIV.)	Selective disclosure—with appropriate people
Fear/panic ("What am I going to do?")	Management of feelings
Behavioral patterns	
Passivity/dependence ("Take care of me.")	Assuming responsibility
Procrastination ("I can't deal with this now.")	Setting and maintaining priorities and goals
Manipulation ("Give me a break; I'm sick.")	Honesty and mutuality
Acting out ("I can do whatever I want.")	Verbalizing, not acting on, negative impulses
Social withdrawal ("I don't need anybody.")	Developing better social supports
Relapse ("I might as well get high.")	Maintenance of sobriety

Group Responses to the Sick Member(s)

The group process is especially effective in dealing with the aforementioned psychodynamic issues (denial, anger/victimization, guilt/penance, shame/pariah, avoidance, fear/helplessness) as well as for forestalling substance relapse. The peer interactions of group therapy may be preferable to the therapist/client interactions of individual therapy, in that the group can provide a context of normalization ("we can all end up like this") and peer support ("we are here for you") as opposed to sharper role dichotomies ("you are sick and need to be taken care of ") inherent in individual therapy. These effects in turn can serve to reduce anxiety about neediness and dependency, and can increase a person's openness to social support. If several members have had the same or similar medical illnesses, the following additional benefits may accrue:

1. the sharing of information about disease treatment/recovery process;
2. the promotion of acceptance/hope;
3. the reduction of feelings of victimization; and
4. confrontation of nonproductive behavior.

The development of a medical crisis in one member may unify a group and provide a focus for supportive feelings. It can lead to increased cohesion and common effort. However, a concomitant risk is that the group will avoid dealing with other members' issues, that there will be overidentification with the sick member's dependent and needy feelings, and that members or the group leader may become overprotective of the sick member. The therapist may need to monitor this issue and make corrective interventions. By focusing on needs and problems of all its members, the group can help reduce the individual's tendency to amplify and magnify medical problems to the point where they are overwhelming, and help put medical problems in perspective.

Interventions and Clinical Examples

Phases of Group Treatment

When starting any new group, attention should be given to preparation of individual members.

For the development of a new group, especially one that is homogeneous, all members are "new" and thus the potential exists for immediate solidarity among them. For an ongoing group, or a heterogeneous group, leaders must be sensitive about introducing new members who may feel particularly vulnerable because of their illness. Often pairs of new members are introduced at one time in order to minimize this effect.

Depending on the context of the group, different issues may initially be prominent as treatment begins. For instance, in a women's

HIV group in a methadone program (Hardesty and Greif 1994), patients were secretive about revealing their HIV status to other members, and described an inability to trust other women with such information. In a heterogeneous group of medically ill patients, only some of whom may have substance abuse problems, leaders should be prepared for mistrust and stigmatization of the substance-abusing members. Medically ill substance-abusing individuals may be fearful of the confrontative approach often employed in substance abuse treatment (O'Dowd et al. 1991). All groups need clear ground rules about attendance, confidentiality, and rules about the prescription of abusable drugs (O'Dowd et al. 1991), i.e., benzodiazepines. O'Dowd describes the value of an open-house coffee hour in helping to break down negative ideas of potential group members, in that experienced group members may be able to assuage the fears of new potential members.

The general format will most likely follow this overall outline:

1. *Introduction of ill member/new illness of old member:* Extensive work may be required in order address the initial presentation and elicit reactions from other members in the group. Topics include the new member's goals, illness, attitudes, feelings, and behavior related to the illness and substance use;
2. *Development of group cohesion/solidarity:* Identifying:
   a. positive and negative adaptations to illness,
   b. unaddressed needs, including medical, psychological, and social/economic,
   c. feelings and attitudes impeding more positive adaptations,
   d. transference and countertransference issues, and
   e. techniques for developing and maintaining sobriety;
3. *Working through:* Identifying:
   a. more positive feelings, attitudes, behaviors,
   b. support for positive adaptations,
   c. positive responses to illness as examples of handling life problems, and
   d. positive responses to urges for relapse, and interventions to minimize the impact of slips;
4. *Termination/closure:* Identifying and dealing with issues including death, recovery, progression, or remission, members' and leader's reactions, and repeated/multiple losses.

The work of the group and its leaders. The phases of treatment just described, while roughly sequential, are often overlapping and may require repetition, return, and reinforcement. Crises and losses may require return to the introduction or group cohesion phases, and sudden death or loss of a member may require dealing with termination or closure before members are adequately prepared for such losses. The "working through" phase is ongoing, occurring throughout most of the course of therapy.

Developing a supportive environment. In addition to the therapeutic approaches discussed previously (recovery/relapse prevention and psychodynamic), model of supportive psychotherapy (Hellerstein, Rosenthal, and Pinsker 1994) may be valuable in underlying the approach of the group leaders. This model defines supportive therapy as a treatment that focuses upon:

1. strengthening the therapeutic alliance;
2. using direct measures (such as praise, psychoeducation, etc.) to relieve symptoms and to minimize development of anxiety within the therapy;
3. enhancing self-esteem, adaptive skills, and psychological (or ego) functions (measures may include reassurance, encouragement, praise, advice, reframing, clarification, confrontation, education);
4. attending to negative aspects of patient-therapist relationship when present, but in general not to positive transference; and
5. providing minimal interpretation of unconscious conflicts, except when necessary to maintain the frame of treatment.

Identifying changes in medical status. The group leaders must address medical issues with substance abusers in group *on an ongoing basis,* because patients are often not aware of their medical status, and/or new or worsening illnesses. For instance, one patient in ongoing group treatment was unaware of changes in his medical status despite a fifty-pound weight loss and development of focal weakness in one arm; subsequently, he admitted to recent head trauma and required neurological evaluation to rule out a cerebrovascular accident or subdural hematoma.

Monitoring and reinforcing compliance with medical treatment and coordination of care with other health providers. Compliance issues and problems are ubiquitous among medically ill substance abusers. A patient with chronic liver failure may take medication irregularly, thus becoming delirious. An HIV-infected alcoholic patient may miss medical appointments. The group leader may need to play a role of monitoring the status of members' medical problems, and reinforcing the importance of ongoing attention to medical problems. At times, the leader may choose to play a case management role, coordinating substance abuse, psychiatric, and medical treatment.

Identifying and handling medical illnesses as life challenges. Since substance abusers often initially experience medical illnesses as overwhelming and unendurable, one goal of group treatment is to help affected group members to put their medical illnesses in the perspective of other life difficulties and challenges—to help turn catastrophes into challenges (see Table 21.3). Within this context, the

TABLE 21.3. Stages of Illness and Response Among Substance Abusers with Medical Illnesses

Preaddictive Individual	Individual Substance Abuser	Development of Serious Illness	Group Treatment Goals
Varying premorbid levels of intrapsychic and interpersonal functioning	1. Compromised self-observation	Distortions in evaluation of condition	Correct perceptual distortions and evaluation of condition
	2. Low self-esteem; disturbed concept of self; difficulty in modulating and handling feelings	Narcissistic wound is amplified; despair, anger, guilt, shame	Reduce dimension of narcissistic wound; universalize condition
	3. Maladaptive defense mechanisms and behaviors	Denial, avoidance, procrastination, relapses, acting out	Reduce use of maladaptive defense mechanisms and improve coping with illness
	4. Development of destructive interpersonal modes of relating and loss of interpersonal ties	Isolation, overdependence, and manipulative use of illness	Reduce maladaptive interpersonal behaviors; develop constructive social support

group can help ill members to explore how they can deal with these challenges in adaptive, rather than self-destructive, ways. Helping physically ill members to adapt to the psychological impact of illness is an ongoing process, as they adapt to the requirements of medical treatment or physical impairment, as they search for productive responses to this life stress, and, in particular, as they struggle to maintain sobriety.

Keeping a focus on sobriety. Should substance abuse recur during a medical crisis, the group can play an important role in supporting the member's return to sobriety, encouraging attendance at twelve-step programs, etc., as needed. Members often rise to the challenge of assisting one another in maintaining sobriety, and addressing slips early, before they become full-blown relapses. In addition, leaders should be aware that in a patient dealing with a medical problem, relapse may occur *after* the crisis is over. As one patient put it, "I've been through so much, now I'll give myself a break." It may be helpful to return the focus to the "other disease" the patient has—drug or alcohol abuse.

Identifying and exploring the group's response to its sick members: confrontation versus support versus caretaking. Especially early in treatment, the medically ill substance abuser may present with a victim stance, and attempt to exploit other group members' sympathies, perhaps as a rationale for continued alcohol or substance abuse, or directly by attempting to get other members to provide money or procure drugs or alcohol. Perez and Pilsecker (1994) describe how expert some spinal cord-injured substance-abusing individuals are in manipulating family, friends, and caretakers by using a victim stance. The group may use such issues to integrate the patient into treatment; other members may reveal how they too have faced or currently face medical illnesses, and that they too have attempted to use a victim stance to enable further drug abuse. Although the group may rightly confront such behaviors, it may risk being trapped into taking care of a particularly ill member. If one patient is in a medical crisis, all attention may turn to addressing his or her issues, and the current problems of other members may be ignored.

Addressing transference and countertransference issues. The medically ill substance abuser may become extremely needy and dependent upon the group and its leaders. He or she may express rage or envy toward leaders who are healthy, and may describe fantasies of revenge (Perez and Pilsecker 1994). In the context of dealing with such difficult emotional issues and constantly changing clinical realities, group leaders will commonly experience a range of emotions, including anger, shame, guilt, the desire to provide caretaking, and, at times, emotional withdrawal from particularly ill or demanding members. In the case of acutely ill members, leaders may appropriately choose to change their therapeutic stance, for instance, being strict and limit-setting toward the acting-out and relapsing cocaine abuser, and at another time encouraging the group to become increasingly involved in the concrete needs of the member who is hospitalized with AIDS. With the dying patient, the therapeutic boundary is particularly fluid, and visits in the hospital, accompaniment to medical appointments, and attention to concrete needs may at times be indicated.

Adjusting therapeutic boundaries. As mentioned, particularly in dealing with progressive illness, it may be appropriate for the group leader to adjust therapeutic boundaries. This includes assessing the need for concrete services and caretaking, and encouraging contacts out of the group setting (Sageman 1989; Schwartz and Karasu 1977). A patient may be encouraged to visit a sick co-member at his apartment, to see if food is in the refrigerator, or to accompany another member to a medical appointment.

Facilitating positive adaptations. Getzel (1991) describes four possible "solutions" for patients with AIDS that may help them deal with its life-threatening aspects while simultaneously helping them live constructively in the present. These include the "beneficent solution" in which individuals focus on caring for others; the "heroic solution" in which the focus is on a contest or struggle against death; the "artistic-spiritual solution," which centers on faith in enduring beyond death; and the "rational-instrumental solution," which is characterized by a practical approach to living one day at a time. This conceptualization may be helpful for other terminal or progressive illnesses as well as AIDS—particularly among medically ill substance abusers, whose instinctive tendency may be to find less adaptive, more self-destructive "solutions."

Handling closure: termination, graduation, loss, death, and dying. Group leaders must pay particular attention to issues of closure and loss. The most difficult setting is generally the discussion of the death of a member or members, which may evoke a wide range of responses, including, of course, substance abuse relapse in other members. Losses of group members in general require working through feelings over an extended period of time. In addition there may be other aspects of closure, including termination (because of acting out or noncompliance) or "graduation" to other forms of treatment. There may also be gradual closure of the medical issue, in the months following the time that a serious illness has stabilized or gone into remission. Although the medical illness may still be present, it may no longer be a central and active issue for the patient, who is now ready to move on to other subjects. For example, now that more effective treatments are available for AIDS, many HIV-infected individuals may find themselves in a situation where their medical status is stabilized, and other life issues are more pressing.

CLINICAL EXAMPLES

Case 1

Mr. A. was a black homosexual man in his late forties, who had been treated successfully in group therapy for mixed addictions (alcohol, opiates, sedatives) but who continued to have problems in self-esteem, intimacy, and sexual acting out (promiscuity). He was a well-established member of the group, and had no difficulty in discussing his sexual behavior and compulsiveness. Issues of HIV-related problems were thoroughly explored in group, and Mr. A.'s usual response was one of *preferred ignorance* ("I'm probably positive but I don't want to know"). This reinforced his *continued promiscuity.* He engaged partners who were, like him, frequent participants in casual promiscuous sex, and rationalized his behavior with the idea that all of them were likely to be HIV positive already. He made a few attempts at sexual abstinence, most lasting less than a month. His use of "safe" sexual techniques was only partial.

Mr. A. was hospitalized at one point for pneumonia, but refused his physician's request that he take an HIV test. After a brief period of acting out (with promiscuous sex and gambling) his condition worsened, and he was diagnosed with carcinoma of the lung. This crisis led to his *decision to undergo HIV testing,* and notification of his positive status.

Once this was acknowledged, he received *considerable support in the group.* This helped him to cease all sexual behavior and to participate fully in medical treatment. Practical support was provided by a few members in dealing with concrete problems. Mr. A. was able to verbalize feelings about his *approaching death,* including his disappointment about unmet goals. Most important to him, he was able to maintain his goal of living each day to his best ability and maintaining sobriety. He remained sober and was "grateful" to the end. The entire group was deeply moved by the experience, and this helped some members to address issues of sobriety and procrastination more effectively. They attended an AA memorial service for him, which helped to provide closure. His positive example was cited in sessions long after his demise.

Case 2

Mr. B. was a forty-three-year-old white male with advanced and worsening cirrhosis. He had begun to abuse alcohol and drugs as a teenager, and used alcohol, cocaine, and marijuana heavily during his time in the military. His substance abuse continued during his years of working as an insurance adjuster, enabled by the loose schedule of his job. Following the development of cirrhosis, he quit alcohol and cocaine for the most part, but resumed heroin IV addiction and subsequently went on methadone maintenance.

Mr. B. became severely depressed following medical hospitalizations for esophageal varices and liver complications (encephalopathy) with increased ammonia levels. He also developed frequent panic attacks, with fears about esophageal varices rupturing and causing death. He had frequent suicidal ideation but no attempts; he related this restraint to his relationship with a grandson, to whom he felt a strong attachment and allegiance. Mr. B. took very quickly to a group composed of other methadone-treated patients, who shared varying problems, including intermittent/continual substance abuse, psychiatric symptomatology, medical problems, and interpersonal problems.

Mr. B. initially talked about his anger regarding his situation, often complaining about poor medical care. Obversely, he also blamed himself. These two dynamics served as the rationale for continued substance abuse. Other group members accepted him, identifying their own bouts with illness, past or present. They confronted his self-destructive behaviors, helping him to modulate his anger and raise his self-esteem. The group's support helped him to weather medical and family crises (including the death of his son), reducing emotional swings and crises, which in turn had played into continued substance abuse.

Group dynamics followed a characteristic pattern: Mr. B. would express angry or suicidal feelings or reveal recent substance abuse; the group would respond with support and acceptance of him as a person, normalizing his anger and other difficult feelings, and confronting his continued substance abuse. In addition, the group confronted his noncompliance with medical treatment, which had led to episodes of hepatic encephalopathy. The group leader also made outreach contacts with Mr. B.'s primary care physician and emergency room doctors, who routinely misinterpreted signs of encephalopathy as intoxication. The process reinforced the group's development of positive coping skills and increased members' self-esteem. It also reinforced other members' motivation for continued sobriety. The continued progression of Mr. B.'s hepatic failure, however, has been difficult for the group to handle, with frequent hospitalizations, fluctuating mental state, and increasing debility.

RESEARCH

Well-defined outcome studies for the group treatment of medically ill substance abusers are not found. Some authors have published clinical descriptions of treatment programs with a variety of medically ill substance abusers in several settings. Other writers have described the use of group therapy for HIV-positive substance abusers (Upadhya and Rosen 1989). Studies that represent the type of research being conducted in the field include the work of Hardesty and Greif (1994); O'Dowd and colleagues (1991); and Perez and Pilsecker (1994).

CONCLUSIONS

Medical illnesses are underrecognized as a topic in the group therapy of substance abusers, and few guides exist in the literature for approaching these topics. Whether homogeneous or heterogeneous, whether brief or long-term, group therapy has much to offer the medically ill with substance abuse problems. Group therapists must address and attempt to overcome common problems of denial, avoidance, and acting out, as well as the recurrence of active drug or alcohol use.

Thus, dealing with medical illness may be conceptualized as an extension of the substance abuse "recovery process," even in cases of terminal illnesses—at times with a spiritual as well as psychological aspect. A group's experience with illness can improve other members' self-esteem and problem-solving capacities, and as such can be experienced as a potential growth experience for physically ill and well members.

There is a need for more attention to medical issues among *all* substance abusers in group therapy whether they are overtly ill. The group therapy of the HIV-infected substance abuser may provide a model for other illnesses. Issues that are generally important to all substance abusers include the importance of health-maintaining behaviors (avoiding other substances of abuse such as tobacco, addressing the importance of a balanced diet, etc.), the importance of regular health screening and disease prophylaxis, and initiating and maintaining a connection with primary care physicians through regular medical checkups. Group therapy can provide a focus on health management in substance abusers and address the importance of early detection of medical problems, prompt interventions as illnesses emerge, and compliance with prescribed treatments. Such treatment approaches might be cost-effective ways of averting some long-term and chronic impairments for these populations.

With substance-abusing individuals who are acutely or chronically medically ill, group treatment programs could be developed in a large variety of settings. Therapists in these settings would face the clinical issue of how to best modify existing models for substance abuse group treatment (or the group therapy of medical illnesses) in order to optimally affect the course of both substance abuse and medical illnesses. This need is particularly compelling in the area of comorbid HIV infection and substance abuse, but would be relevant with many other illnesses as well.

Finally, research data must be developed on such group interventions. It would be important to develop manualized group therapy models for medically ill substance abusers, using standardized measures of alliance, treatment process, and outcome. Such studies should include measures for assessing medical illness, psychiatric impairment, substance abuse severity, quality of life, and mortality, as well as the possible impact of such interventions on health care costs and utilization.

REFERENCES

Flores PJ. *Group Psychotherapy with Addicted Populations,* Second Edition. Binghamton, NY: The Haworth Press, 1997.

Getzel GS. Survival modes for people with AIDS in groups. *Social Work* 36:7-12, 1991.

Hardesty L, Greif GL. Common themes in a group for female IV drug users who are HIV positive. *Journal of Psychoactive Drugs* 26:289-293, 1994.

Hellerstein DJ, Rosenthal RN, Pinsker H. Supportive therapy as the treatment model of choice. *Journal of Psychotherapy Practice and Research* 3:300-306, 1994.

Kaplan HI, Sadock BJ, Grebb JA. *Kaplan and Sadock's Synopsis of Psychiatry: Behavioral Sciences, Clinical Psychiatry,* Seventh Edition. Baltimore, MD: Williams and Wilkins, 1994.

Khantzian EJ, Halliday KS, Golden S, McAuliffe WE. Modified group therapy for substance abusers: A psychodynamic approach to relapse prevention. *American Journal of Addiction* 1:67-76, 1992.

Lenya RG. Quality of life: Outcome of TAPWAK group therapy counseling for PWAS and PWHIVS. *International Conference on AIDS* 10:410, 1994.

Novick D. The medically ill substance abuser. In *Substance Abuse: A Comprehensive Textbook,* edited by Lowinson JH, Ruiz P, Millman RB. Baltimore, MD: Williams and Wilkins, 1992, pp. 657-674.

O'Dowd MA, Natali C, Orr D, McKegney FP. Characteristics of patients attending an HIV-related psychiatric clinic. *Hospital and Community Psychiatry* 42:615-619, 1991.

Perez M, Pilsecker C. Group psychotherapy with spinal cord injured substance abusers. *Paraplegia* 32:188-192, 1994.

Rutan JS, Stone WN. *Psychodynamic Group Psychotherapy,* Second Edition. New York: Guilford Press, 1993.

Sageman S. Group therapy for people with AIDS. In *Group Psychodynamics: New Paradigms and New Perspectives,* edited by Halperin, DA. Chicago: Year Book Medical Publishers, 1989, pp. 125-138.

Schwartz AM, Karasu TB. Psychotherapy with the dying patient. *American Journal of Psychotherapy* 21:19-35, 1977.

Ulman KH. Group psychotherapy with the medically ill. In *Comprehensive Group Psychotherapy,* Third Edition, edited by Kaplan HI, Sadock BJ. Baltimore, MD: Williams and Wilkins, 1993, pp. 459-470.

Upadhya G, Rosen FM. Group psychotherapy with HIV+ drug users. *International Conference on AIDS* 5:787, 1989.

Yalom ID. *The Theory and Practice of Group Psychotherapy,* Fourth Edition. New York: Basic Books, 1995.

SECTION V:
INTEGRATION AND IMPLICATIONS

Chapter 22

Research in Group Psychotherapy for Substance Abuse: Fiction, Fact, and Future

Les R. Greene

THE FICTION, OR PREVAILING BELIEFS

Group psychotherapy is the treatment of choice—or at least the primary treatment in multimodal treatment programs—for drug-abusing and drug-dependent disorders. Such is the prevailing wisdom in the clinical-theoretical literature (Flores and Mahon, 1993; Margolis and Zweben, 1998). This long-standing opinion derives from and remains an integral part of the traditions of therapeutic communities and peer-based organizations such as Alcoholics Anonymous and accounts for its widespread, indeed ubiquitous, appearance in drug treatment programs throughout the country (Price et al., 1991). Interestingly, these views of the effectiveness of group therapy for treating substance abuse have been empirically and quantitatively documented in two recent large scale surveys. Burlingame, Fuhriman, and Taylor (1997) and Burlingame and Taylor (1998) solicited opinions from directors of training in the mental health disciplines of psychiatry, psychology, and social work and from clinical directors in managed health organizations. These individuals, selected because of the significant influence they wield upon the current and future patterns of the practice of psychotherapy, were asked to rank order the effectiveness of group therapy for a variety of specific diagnoses, such as anxiety and mood disorders, as well as substance abuse. Not surprisingly, the group treatment of substance abuse was given the highest ranking by both sets of these directors, consistent with the picture from the clinical-theoretical literature.

There is more to this story. The authors of these surveys then calculated correlations among these rankings of perceived effectiveness of group treatment for these discrete disorders and the actual effectiveness of group therapy, as determined from the most recent and comprehensive meta-analysis of group therapy outcome (Burlingame, Fuhriman, and Anderson, 1995). Strikingly, the obtained correlations were almost perfect, in the .8 to .9 range, but in the negative direction! That is, these directors of training and managed care essentially reversed the order of effectiveness compared to the rankings derived from the empirical outcome literature. The perceptions of the effectiveness of group treatment of substance abuse were very positive, consonant with its prominent role in most treatment programs and agencies, but, as we shall review, the scientific basis for these strongly held convictions is lacking.

THE FACTS, OR LACK OF THEM

Review after review of the research literature all draw the same general conclusion about the insubstantiality of the empirical evidence pertaining to the effectiveness of group therapy for the treatment of substance abuse. What follows is a selective report of some of these reviews. We start with an elaboration of the meta-analysis by Burlingame, Fuhriman, and Anderson (1995) cited previously. These researchers conducted an exhaustive literature search spanning the years 1980 through 1992 and found 116 studies that met their stringent methodological criteria for experimental design and definitional criteria for group therapy. In an effort to discern the influence of various moderator variables, they categorized these studies in terms of specific characteristics of the patients, therapists, treatments, and experimental methodologies. Of the ninety-eight studies that could be classified in terms of fourteen various psychodiagnostic categories, only two focused on substance abuse. For each diagnosis, the authors derived an effect size, calculated as the overall pre-post difference averaged first over all the dependent variables within each study and then over the pertinent studies. With respect to substance abuse, the obtained effect size, while in the right direction, was not found to be statistically significant, one of only four categories of diagnoses that failed to demonstrate reliable improvement as a function of treatment.

Complementing this meta-analysis are a spate of qualitative reviews of the experimental literature that span the decades and consistently underscore the lack of definitive findings. More important, they have provided some useful methodological critiques of the flaws and inadequacies in the published research that consequently limit the inferences and conclusions that can be drawn from the findings. On a more positive note, they also suggest a gradual evolution and developing sophistication of the work, at least with regard to methodology. The early reviews (e.g., Brandsma and Pattison, 1985; Parloff and Dies, 1977) revealed, for example, that many of the studies—driven by the then-prevailing theories of substance abuse as a symptom of underlying psychological conflict—only examined changes in psychological status and failed to incorporate variables directly measuring substance abuse. Today, given the increasing pressures on researchers to produce findings of direct clinical relevance (e.g., Piper, 1993), these early projects would neither be funded nor published.

The more recent and current reviews (Carroll and Rounsaville, 1995; Crits-Christoph and Siqueland, 1996; Holder et al., 1991; Stinchfield, Owen, and Winters, 1994) indicate that research efforts are clearly showing increasing methodological refinements, though they still fall short of the gold standard of clinical trials. As we shall posit, this progress in methodology is not accompanied by increasing conceptual rigor; in fact, the literature reviews suggest a gradual decline in the conceptual power of research as investigators attend increasingly to designing and implementing laboratory-tight methodologies.

Stinchfield, Owen, and Winters (1994) offer the most detailed, up-to-date critique of the research literature that focuses specifically on group therapy for substance abuse. Their review covers essentially the same years as the meta-analysis described earlier and uses similar inclusionary and exclusionary criteria. However, by casting a wider net in searching the literature, they find eight outcome studies that they categorize into three design types based on how the group fits into the overall treatment program: those in which group therapy is the primary treatment, those in which group therapy is "added on" to supplement the primary treatment, and those in which group therapy is an "aftercare" or maintenance component following a more intensive, recovery-phase treatment.

Most prominent among the methodological limitations identified by the authors is the lack of internal validity. Although treatment manuals have begun to appear in drug abuse studies using various individual therapies, they have not substantially made their way into research employing group modalities. In the absence of standardized and verified treatments, it is unknown to what degree the therapeutic approach that is purportedly occurring is actually being implemented. Indeed, in one of the studies cited (Ito, Donovan, and Hall, 1988), the authors provide anecdotal evidence indicating that the treatment protocol was not always followed, especially during clinical crises. Further, in most of the reviewed studies, the treatment conditions were confounded by other potentially influential variables, such as treatment goal (i.e., abstinence versus moderation), therapist, treatment "dosage," and concurrent treatments. By having covarying factors across conditions, as occurs in nested rather than crossed designs, it is impossible to conclude what made the difference when significant effects were obtained.

As detailed by Stinchfield, Owen, and Winters (1994), a range of other design weaknesses plague these works; these are not mere niceties, but fundamental deviations from the scientific experimental paradigm that make interpretation of the findings tenuous. To be fair, many of these shortcomings are borne of real-world, insurmountable restrictions imposed by the clinical setting. Unlike outcome studies with other psychodiagnostic categories, research on group therapy for substance abuse has not moved into the academically based laboratory replete with its tight controls over variables. To date, most of the psychosocial substance abuse empirical work is an amalgam of efficacy (i.e., laboratory) and effectiveness (i.e., field) research; it reflects the real obstacles and necessary compromises to carrying out methodologically tight studies in actual clinical settings. Unfortunately, the consequence is a growing number of small scale studies that have sacrificed, in varying degrees, the logic and beauty of the experimental paradigm.

But even more problematic than these methodological considerations is the lack of what we are calling the conceptual power of these studies. Despite the repeated urgings from group psychotherapy critics (Bednar and Kaul, 1978, 1993; Kaul and Bednar, 1986; Parloff and Dies, 1977; Piper, 1993) for careful and detailed observation, there is only minimal description and rarely any systematic assessment of the therapeutic enterprise. Often, the therapy group is dubbed the "traditional" treatment that serves as the background comparison condition for the experimental treatment of interest and allegiance of the researchers, typically behavioral or cognitive-behavioral techniques implemented in a relatively structured and didactic group context. The psychoeducative format of the experimental group is probably more analogous to a classroom or to individual instruction in a group context than to a free-flowing interactive and dynamically oriented therapy group. Several clinical and conceptual problems ensue from this prototypical experimental design. First, as several observers have suggested (Ettin, 1992; Rose, Tolman and Tallant, 1985; Satterfield, 1994), the cognitive-behavioral group approach typically fails to incorporate group therapeutic factors into the work process and thus likely fails to maximize the impact of the experimental condition. Next, given the wide variations in group treatment and the minimal descriptions of the groups in the studies, making generalizations beyond the specific context in which the research was conducted is difficult. That is, external validity, as much as internal validity, is unknown but suspect in these studies. Finally, a reasonable possibility is that the lack of sophisticated and detailed descriptions of the therapy groups may reflect a similar lack of sophistication in the actual group treatment practice, especially for those conditions in which the therapy group is the "treatment as usual."

As Flores warns (1993, p. 430), "What often gets passed off as group psychotherapy . . . is a model that inadequately uses all the curative forces available in a therapy group." The skepticism about the utility of research often voiced by clinicians does, in fact, seem partly justified on the basis of the very real weaknesses in conceptual-clinical rigor of the studies to date.

To illustrate this point, an example described in the Stinchfield, Owen, and Winters (1994) review is cited. Olson et al. (1981) published an outcome study of the "add-on" type in which they compared four groups specially created within an ongoing inpatient setting for alcohol disorders: a behaviorally oriented group involving covert sensitization and relaxation, an insight-oriented group following transactional analytic principles, a group that, inexplicably, combined both of these approaches, and the so-called treatment as usual in the inpatient setting. In terms of methodological considerations, the study, published in a prestigious journal, excelled with its randomized assignment, multiple dependent variables, and several measurement periods. The findings revealed that all four conditions significantly reduced levels of drinking over time, but the insight-oriented group fared worst of all, even inferior to the control condition. In their discussion, the authors emphasize the evidence supportive of the behavioral approach, but they fail to account for the suppressed performance—significantly below baseline—of those patients in the insight-oriented group. Without a clinically meaningful explanation of this lower-than-expected performance in this condition, the authors' conclusions about the purported benefits of behavioral group therapy in this setting may be misleading.

What factors could explain this phenomenon? A closer look at the description of the standard milieu treatment reveals that all the patients already had a "traditional" (i.e., dynamically and analytically oriented) therapy group, in fact, for two hours a day for six days a week. How was the addition of yet another similar group perceived not only by the patients within that condition but also by the patients in the other conditions, all of whom shared the same common setting? It cannot be determined, of course, from the data at hand what contributed to the lowered scores for those in the insight group, but it does seem reasonable to consider that this group was negatively experienced, perhaps as an aspect of envy toward those who received new kinds of groups.

Raising a similar argument, Stinchfield, Owen, and Winters (1994) assert that if group therapy is seen as unimportant or inconsistent with other parts of treatment, patients may resent this inconsistency. The more general issue here is that the potential for causal misattribution is significant in outcome research (e.g., Greene, 2000) and is even more likely when a host of dynamic or motivational factors are not considered as possible covarying and confounding influences.

Before discussing future directions for research, we cite two other recent authoritative reviews of the literature that cogently illustrate the influence of research—or lack of it—for shaping clinical practice, namely the works in progress undertaken by the American Psychiatric Association and the American Psychological Association. The exhaustive review of the clinical and research literature undertaken by the former organization has served in the development of the published practice guidelines for substance abuse disorders (American Psychiatric Association, 1995). This project entailed the codification of 481 references based on the approximation of each to the gold standard of a controlled clinical trial. By far, the majority of studies that were designated with this highest rating were pharmacotherapy investigations. The psychosocial treatment studies that earned this classification were much fewer in number and only three of these pertained to group therapy. As a consequence of this dearth of empirical study, the practice guidelines conclude that although psychosocial treatments in general are an "essential" part of a comprehensive drug treatment program, the specific endorsement of group therapy as a recommended modality attains only a "moderate" level of clinical confidence. The developers of the practice guidelines join the chorus of others in their call for more formal research studies to corroborate the primarily clinical claims about various treatment approaches.

The response of the American Psychological Association to pressures to develop its own practice guidelines has been to construct a list of so-called empirically validated treatments. A developing list of well established and probably efficacious treatments, again based on rigorous experimental criteria, is being continuously updated (Chambless et al., 1998; DeRubeis and Crits-Christoph, 1998). Of the handful of treatments that pass the muster of this highly selective screening process, only one study (Eriksen, Bjornstad and Gotestam, 1986) showed positive evidence for a specific group psychological treatment for alcohol dependence. As is characteristic of most of the group therapy research literature in this area, the experimental group format in this one study was highly structured and psychoeducative, which thus limits the degree to which its findings are generalizable to the larger field. Further, the design and execution of this inpatient study reflected a naiveté with regard to current theories about group therapy, as well as group and organizational dynamics. The covariation of dimensions other than leader technique likely had an influential role in the observed differences between the behaviorally oriented experimental groups and the so-called "discussion" groups. For example, the patients in the experimental condition were placed together in their own specially composed and created homogeneous groups, while the patients in the control condition were dispersed among ongoing discussion groups in the milieu. The differences in group ecology and group development that likely result can have profound effects on process and outcome. For example, the hopefulness engendered in a specially created experimental group compared to the disruption created by adding new "subjects" into an ongoing discussion group may be as much or even more potent a determinant of the obtained effects than the differences in leader techniques.

The point here is not to criticize a single study but rather to highlight the importance of relying upon prevailing clinical wisdom about group process to guide experimental design and thus increase the external validity of efficacy research.

While the databases from these diverse reviews fail to overlap for the most part, the major conclusion drawn from them is consistent. In the words of Stinchfield, Owen, and Winters (1994): "Outcome research has not answered the fundamental question of whether substance abuse group therapy is better than no treatment." Margolis and Zweben (1998) assert—in our view overly optimistically—that "it will likely be near the end of the decade before basic issues of effectiveness are clarified" (p. 134). Whether it is because of the "general popularity and widespread acceptance" of this modality (Stinchfield, Owen, and Winters, 1994) or because of the relatively late entrance of this work into academically based treatment facilities (Margolis and Zweben, 1998) or other factors, the formal study of group psychotherapy for substance abuse lags behind research on group treatments for other disorders and the data are not yet at hand.

The good news in this evaluation is that the opportunity exists for researchers to learn from the weaknesses and improve upon the designs in other areas of group psychotherapy research. What follows is a listing of both recommendations and predictions, based on the patterns reflected in the extant research and foregoing reviews; the future is charted in terms of five experimental designs (see Table 22.1).

THE FUTURE

Outcome Research

Critics of efficacy research notwithstanding, demonstrating outcome in scientifically unassailable terms is the name of the game in this era of bottom-line accountability. Clearly, the pressures are on to execute well-controlled studies of high internal validity and to leave aside—at least for the short term—questions of their applicability to real-world clinical contexts. The next generation of outcome studies likely will further approximate the gold standard by their increasing

TABLE 22.1. Research Designs and Questions for Group Therapy of Substance Abuse Disorders

Experimental Design	Major Question Addressed
Outcome	Is group therapy superior to no treatment on measures of drug abuse and psychological status?
Patient-treatment matching	Do different kinds of groups have differential effects for different kinds of patients?
Group versus individual therapy	Which modality is superior in terms of clinical and cost-effectiveness?
Process-outcome	What processes or patterns within the group affect outcome?
Motivational	Does group therapy affect recruitment and retention of patients for drug abuse treatment?

reliance upon treatment manuals and adherence checks—steps designed to standardize therapeutic approaches—and upon a developing core battery of research instruments, such as the Addiction Severity Index (McLellan et al., 1980), which should facilitate the integration and synthesis of the expanding database.

Unfortunately, the trends also suggest that new studies will continue to be plagued by conceptual and clinical shortcomings. Like most of the extant research, studies in the foreseeable future will likely focus on short-term, cognitive-behaviorally oriented formats that ignore the group qua group, both conceptually and statistically. As suggested elsewhere (Greene, 1998), the schism between cognitive and dynamic perspectives in group psychotherapy research is unnecessarily limiting, not only for the cognitive-behavioral orientation, but also for the dynamic viewpoint that too often is accompanied by a dismissive stance toward quantitative research.

Acknowledging and addressing this schism could facilitate the designing and executing of studies with enhanced clinical meaningfulness. Future research using a cognitive-behavioral orientation might benefit, for example, by including a dynamically oriented group expert to provide input into the design of the study. Expertise regarding group-as-a-whole and individual-in-the-group processes could serve to strengthen the conceptual basis of the study without jeopardizing its methodological rigor. At the same time, Piper's (1993) recent call for group therapy research other than within a cognitive-behavioral framework is to the point. Although manuals may be more readily scripted for cognitive-behavioral treatment, they are beginning to appear in the research literature for dynamically oriented individual therapies, which should lead to their adaption to the group setting. Given the range of dynamically oriented theories regarding the etiology and treatment of substance abuse (Morgenstern and Leeds, 1993), it behooves group therapists within this theoretical framework to acknowledge the need for empirical and systematic verification of the efficacy of these approaches. Continuing to relegate dynamic or interactive group therapies to the "standard" or "treatment as usual" background condition will only further the gap between cognitive-behavioral groups supported by accumulating quantitative evidence and dynamically oriented groups that rely chiefly on anecdotal and impressionistic data.

Patient-Treatment Matching Studies

Some increase in theoretical understanding can be gained by adding to the standard group therapy outcome design clinically or theoretically relevant personality dimensions of the patients in order to assess hypothesized interactions between treatment conditions and patient variables. The research literature reveals that these person by group interactive designs are typically more fruitful than either studies that look only at main effects of groups—those that compare schools of group psychotherapy—or works that investigate only the effects of personality in groups. The research paradigm here follows the common sense and appealing idea of "different strokes for different folks," though, as Finney and Moos (1986) warn, these studies of first-order interactions need to be understood as modestly adding only one level of complexity; they fail to examine higher order interactions as well as nonlinear relationships.

One of the best examples of this design is the recent series by Kadden and colleagues (Cooney et al., 1991; Kadden et al., 1989; Litt et al., 1992; Getter et al., 1992). As a set of comparative analyses, this series examined main and interactive effects of two prominent group approaches for treating substance abuse: cognitive-behavioral and interactional. Among the innovative and methodologically sophisticated procedures of these studies was the development of training manuals for both orientations. Further, as reported by Getter et al. (1992), these researchers conducted a formal assessment of selected group processes thought to discriminate the two kinds of group experience. Supporting the internal validity of their studies, the two group orientations were rated as significantly different on six of their seven process dimensions with greater skill training, problem solving, and role-playing in the cognitive-behavioral groups and greater interpersonal learning, exploration of feelings, and focusing on the here-and-now process in the interactive groups.

As frequently occurs, the main effects of these studies were inconclusive: patients in both kinds of groups improved on measures of alcohol consumption and psychological status over the course of the twenty-six weeks of these aftercare groups, and these pre-post changes generally held in both group conditions over a two-year follow-up period. Without a no- or minimal-treatment condition, however, the determinants of this improvement cannot be identified. Logically, the causative agent might just as likely be some unknown concomitant of the passage of time as a much as specific aspects of the treatment conditions.

More interesting and definitive, however, are the interactions of the two group treatment modalities with clinical features of the patients. As hypothesized, those patients assessed as having comparatively greater sociopathy or global psychopathology improved more in the structured cognitive-behavioral groups, while those assessed as lower in sociopathy or psychopathology did better in the interactional groups. Studies such as these add to a growing empirical database on interactions between characteristics of the individual and the social setting. Although the present findings have practical and prescriptive value, they are limited in terms of adding to theoretical understanding of personality-group interactions primarily because the individual variables that were investigated were of the clinical-descriptive type rather than those derived from a theoretical framework. As Finney and Moos (1986) posit, the latter type of variable is more likely to facilitate the conceptual synthesis of the accumulated findings and to lead to the development of more refined hypotheses. The recent study by McKay et al. (1997), based in a cognitive-behavioral framework, serves as a good illustration of how such theoretically based variables—self-efficacy and commitment to abstain in that study—interact with situational variables to influence clinical outcome.

Just as with straightforward outcome designs, input from a clinical-dynamic perspective could enhance the conceptual power of these patient-matching experiments. Psychological variables extracted from prevailing dynamic theories of substance abuse treatment could be linked interactively with salient aspects of the therapeutic group environment. For example, it would be interesting to study contrasting defensive styles (e.g., internalizing versus externalizing) of patients in group cultures that hold the patients accountable, to lesser or greater degrees, for their addictive behaviors, as might well be found in groups that espouse either disease or psychodynamic viewpoints of substance abuse pathology. Among other benefits accruing from such theoretically informed matching studies is the likelihood that obtained findings might serve to clarify and resolve ongoing controversies in the clinical literature.

Group versus Individual Psychotherapy

The call (e.g., McRoberts, Burlingame, and Hoag, 1998) for more investigations of the differences between individual and group therapy seems based more on economic considerations than on interest in scientific advancement. In the context of managed care, demonstrating the cost-effectiveness of a modality is critical to its viability as a reimbursable practice. McRoberts, Burlingame, and Hoag (1998) recently conducted a comprehensive meta-analysis of twenty-three studies that rigorously compared individual and group therapies across a variety of diagnostic categories. With respect to substance abuse, their findings very tentatively suggest the superiority of group therapy over individual treatment. Of course, strictly in terms of cost-effectiveness, even no differences between the modalities on clinical outcomes is still supportive of the use of the more time-efficient group modality.

Some of the most recent published studies (Graham et al., 1996; McKay et al., 1997; Schmitz et al., 1997) are designed to compare these modalities and are providing corroborating evidence in support of their essential equivalence on both measures of substance abuse and psychological status. These data should serve to strengthen the argument about the general advantages of group therapy over individual therapy for substance abuse, although more refined questions need to be posed to assess conditions under which individual therapy may prove to be superior.

Process-Outcome Studies

Methodology aimed exclusively at demonstrating efficacy has been pejoratively dubbed "black box" and "prescientific" research because it is devoid of essential observation, description, and explanation of the fundamental processes and relationships—the interior of the therapeutic enterprise—by which so-called suboutcomes or "small o" outcomes become ultimate or "big o" outcomes. In an earlier paper (Greene, 2000), we reviewed some of the shortcomings of this approach. In particular, an exclusive outcomes orientation raises the question of generalizability or external validity of findings from the laboratory to treatment as actually practiced in the field. An assessment and elucidation of the therapeutic processes that make a difference would help link laboratory and field and bridge the distinction between efficacy and effectiveness studies. Failure to identify mediating variables can also lead to causal misattribution. Whether the effects of group cognitive-behavioral therapy, for example, are due to specific therapist techniques, as typically concluded, or to pantheoretical dynamic processes occurring at the interpersonal, group, or supragroup contextual level is an open, though empirically addressable, question. Relatedly, without a process orientation, opportunities for theory building are curtailed. Finally, the typical outcome experiment that ignores process variables yields findings of the lowest common denominator; pre-post average change scores from experimental and control groups obscure those dynamic aspects of the situation and person that could maximize therapeutic gain, as well as those processes that impede clinical progress.

As exhaustively documented by Burlingame, Kircher, and Taylor (1994), the failure to study clinical processes within group therapy has been the most frequently raised critique of the group psychotherapy research over the past fifty years, and the criticism certainly applies to the field of substance abuse. Although there are many clinical ideas about therapeutic group processes for substance abuse disorders, very little can be gleaned from the research literature that provides empirical support for these formulations. Rugel (1991) reviews the very few extant works that attempt to examine such eclectic factors as group cohesion and emotional climate on clinical outcome.

The overall development of group psychotherapy research in substance abuse suggests inverse relationships between process and outcome and between conceptual and methodological rigor. As the pressures to demonstrate outcome effects via laboratory-tight experimental designs have increased over the decades, the initial interest seen in studying the more theory-bound psychological change processes has waned. However, just as most of the present day outcome studies can be criticized for their failure to incorporate process variables into their designs, many of the earliest studies—driven by the then-prevailing view of substance abuse as a symptom of underlying psychopathology—could be equally faulted for their exclusive focus on examining psychological processes with poorly validated measures and without linking process to outcome.

One such early study by Ends and Page (1957), for example, explored the effects of different kinds of inpatient group psychotherapy on changes in alcoholic patients' sense of self. Using a Q-sort methodology, these researchers developed an intricate and ingenious series of indices designed to assess intrapsychic changes and thus better understand the therapeutic action of different schools of group psychotherapy. Almost as an afterthought, they examined indices of alcohol consumption, but failed to study the relationships between their process and outcome measures. This omission—the study of therapy process in isolation—likely has contributed to the general decline in studying process variables in psychotherapy research.

Today, the study of process in this field is virtually limited to the exploration of the Yalom-inspired questionnaire of therapeutic factors (e.g., Lovett and Lovett, 1991; Mahon and Kempler, 1995). Unfortunately, as noted before (Greene, 2000), these studies have relatively little value for furthering the understanding of therapeutic action in groups, not only because they fail to examine process-outcome relationships, but also because of the unexplored construct validity of the self-report questionnaire. There is no evidence, nor is there any compelling conceptual rationale, that what patients report to be helpful in groups—instillation of hope, catharsis, universality, and the like—are in fact the active ingredients in therapeutic change. A reasonable argument is that patients' perceptions of therapeutic factors may be as much or more related to resistance and defense than to therapeutic work.

Despite this generally negative assessment, some encouraging signs suggest a current renewal of interest in the study of process in group psychotherapy. In the general group psychotherapy research literature, there is an impressive array of developing systems for the analysis of group process (Beck and Lewis, 2000). Also, there is a burgeoning of applications of new statistical procedures, such as hierarchical linear modeling (Kivlighan and Lilly, 1997), social relations and social network analyses (Koehly and Shivy, 1998; Marcus and Kashy, 1995), and time series analysis (Sexton, 1993), that permit the exploration of complex relationships between behavioral patterns in the group and outcome in much more sophisticated manner than simple correlational analyses. Specifically with respect to substance abuse therapy, interests are developing in measuring the social environment of treatment programs (Swindle et al., 1995) and in assessing the active ingredients in various treatment approaches (e.g., Finney et al., 1998). Taken together, these developments hold promise of movement toward the renewed study of process within substance abuse therapy groups within the not-distant future.

Motivational Studies

Most of the experimental work to date suffers from comparatively high numbers of patients who drop out or prematurely terminate treatment, events considered to reflect the high degree of ambivalence about stopping drug use. A small but growing body of literature turns what has been a methodological weakness that potentially introduces serious biases into the data in other substance abuse studies into the dependent variable of primary focus. On the arguable assumption that longer durations of therapy are better, the question addressed experimentally in these studies is "What factors help to attract or keep patients in treatment?" Several of these recent studies (e.g., Kofoed and Keys, 1988; Lash and Dillard, 1996; Pfeiffer, Feuerlein, and Brenk-Schulte, 1991) rely upon various group psychological formulations in the development of hypotheses about the "holding" capacity of small groups. Kofoed and Keys (1988), for example, analyze retrospective data from two comparable psychiatric wards, one instituting a "persuasion" group for dual diagnosis patients to encourage them to face their drug abuse issues and the other without any special intervention for drug abuse. The researchers found that significantly more patients discharged from the innovative ward went into drug abuse follow-up treatment. These kinds of studies, although too few in number and too preliminary to draw conclusions, has the potential for providing unique evidence about the value of group therapy for the treatment of substance abuse.

CONCLUDING REMARKS

Although neither mutually exclusive nor comprehensive, these five kinds of design paradigms, if implemented in sufficient numbers and with sufficient methodological and conceptual rigor, would provide the kinds of data that would make a difference. They would serve in answering not only the fundamental question of whether group treatment for substance abuse really does work, but could enhance, through the development of ever more refined hypotheses, our current understandings of how, when, why, and for whom group treatment works.

REFERENCES

American Psychiatric Association. Practice guidelines for the treatment of patients with substance use disorders: Alcohol, cocaine, opioids. *American Journal of Psychiatry* 152 (suppl), 1995.

Beck P, Lewis M (eds.). Process in Therapeutic Groups: Systems for Analyzing Change. Washington, DC: American Psychological Association, 2000.

Bednar RL, Kaul TJ. Experiential group research: Current perspectives. In *Handbook of Psychotherapy and Behavior Change: An Empirical Analysis,* Second Edition, edited by Garfield SL, Bergin AE. New York: Wiley, 1978, pp. 769-815.

Bednar RL, Kaul TJ. Experiential group research: Can the canon fire? In *Handbook of Psychotherapy and Behavior Change: An Empirical Analysis,* Fourth Edition, edited by Garfield SL, Bergin AE. New York: Wiley, 1993, pp. 631-663.

Brandsma J, Pattison E. The outcome of group psychotherapy in alcoholics: An empirical review. *American Journal of Drug and Alcohol Abuse* 11:151-162, 1985.

Burlingame G, Fuhriman A, Anderson E. *Group psychotherapy efficacy: A meta-analytic perspective.* Paper presented at the annual convention of the American Psychological Association, New York, NY, August 1995.

Burlingame G, Fuhriman A, Taylor N. *Group psychotherapy training and effectiveness: The eye of the beholder.* Paper presented at the annual conference of the American Group Psychotherapy Association, New York, NY, February 1997.

Burlingame GM, Kircher JC, Taylor S. Methodological considerations in group psychotherapy research: Past, present, and future practices. In *Handbook of Group Psychotherapy: An Empirical and Clinical Synthesis,* edited by Fuhriman A, Burlingame GM. New York: John Wiley, 1994, pp. 41-80.

Burlingame G, Taylor N. *A survey of mental health provider and managed care organization attitudes toward, familiarity with and use of group psychotherapy.* Paper presented at the annual conference of the American Group Psychotherapy Association, Chicago, IL, February 1998.

Carroll K, Rounsaville B. Psychosocial treatments. In *American Psychiatric Press Review of Psychiatry* Volume 14, edited by Oldham J, Riba M. Washington, DC: American Psychiatric Press, 1995, pp. 127-149.

Chambless D, Baker M, Baucom D, Beutler LE, Calhoun KB, Crits-Christolph P, Daiuto A, DeRubeis R, Detweiler J, Haaga DAF, et al. Update on empirically validated therapies, II. *The Clinical Psychologist* 51:3-16, 1998.

Cooney N, Kadden R, Litt M, Getter H. Matching alcoholics to coping skills or interactional therapies: Two year follow-up results. *Journal of Consulting and Clinical Psychology* 59:598-601, 1991.

Crits-Christoph P, Siqueland L. Psychosocial treatment for drug abuse: Selected review and recommendations for national health care. *Archives of General Psychiatry* 53:749-756, 1996.

DeRubeis R, Crits-Christoph P. Empirically supported individual and group psychological treatments for adult mental disorders. *Journal of Consulting and Clinical Psychology* 66:37-52, 1998.

Ends E, Page C. A study of three types of group psychotherapy with hospitalized male inebriates. *Quarterly Journal of Studies on Alcohol* 18:263-277, 1957.

Eriksen L., Bjornstad S, Gotestam K. Social skills training in groups for alcoholics: One-year treatment outcome of groups and individuals. *Addictive Behaviors* 11: 309-329, 1986.

Ettin M. *Group Psychotherapy. A Sphere of Influence.* Boston: Allyn and Bacon, 1992.

Finney J, Moos R. Matching patients with treatments: Conceptual and methodological issues. *Journal of Studies on Alcohol* 47:122-134, 1986.

Finney J, Noyes C, Coutts A, Moos R. Evaluating substance abuse treatment process models: I. Changes on proximal outcome variables during 12-step and cognitive behavioral treatment. *Journal of Studies on Alcohol* 59:371-380, 1998.

Flores P: Group psychotherapy with alcoholics, substance abusers, and adult children of alcoholics. In *Comprehensive Group Psychotherapy,* Third Edition, edited by Kaplan H, Sadock B. Baltimore: Williams and Wilkins, 1993, pp. 429-443.

Flores P, Mahon L. The treatment of addiction in group psychotherapy. *International Journal of Group Psychotherapy* 43:143-156, 1993.

Getter H, Litt M, Kadden R, Cooney N. Measuring treatment process in coping skills and interactional group therapies for alcoholism. *International Journal of Group Psychotherapy* 42:419-430, 1992.

Graham K, Annis H, Brett P, Venesoen P. A controlled field trial of group versus individual cognitive-behavioural training for relapse prevention. *Addiction* 91: 1127-1140, 1996.

Greene LR. Group therapy for medically ill patients (review). *Group Dynamics: Theory, Research, and Practice* 2:57-59,1998.

Greene LR. Introduction to process analysis of group interaction in therapeutic groups. In *Process of Group Psychotherapy: Systems for Analyzing Change,* edited by Beck AP, Lewis CM. Washington, DC: American Psychological Association, 2000, pp. 23-47.

Holder H, Longabaugh R, Miller W, Rubonis A. The cost effectiveness of treatment for alcoholism: A first approximation. *Journal of Studies on Alcohol* 52:517-540, 1991.

Ito J, Donovan D, Hall J. Relapse prevention in alcohol aftercare: Effects on drinking outcome, change process, and aftercare attendance. *British Journal of Addiction* 83:171-181, 1988.

Kadden R, Cooney N, Getter H, Litt M. Matching alcoholics to coping skills or interactional therapies: Posttreatment results. *Journal of Consulting and Clinical Psychology* 57:698-704, 1989.

Kaul TJ, Bednar RL. Experiential group research: Results, questions, and suggestions. In *Handbook of Psychotherapy and Behavior Change: An Empirical Analysis,* Third Edition, edited by Garfield SL, Bergin AE. New York: Wiley, 1986, pp. 671-714.

Kivlighan D, Lilly R. Developmental changes in group climate as they relate to therapeutic gain. *Group Dynamics: Theory, Research, and Practice* 1:208-222, 1997.

Koehly L, Shivy V. Social network analysis: A new methodology for counseling research. *Journal of Counseling Psychology* 45:3-17, 1998.

Kofoed L, Keys A. Using group therapy to persuade dual-diagnosis patients to seek substance abuse treatment. *Hospital and Community Psychiatry* 39:1209-1211, 1988.

Lash S, Dillard W. Encouraging participation in aftercare group therapy among substance-dependent men. *Psychological Reports* 79:585-586, 1996.

Litt M, Babor T, DelBoca F, Kadden R, Cooney N. Types of alcoholics. II. Application of an empirically derived typology to treatment matching. *Archives of General Psychiatry* 49:609-614, 1992.

Lovett L, Lovett J. Group therapeutic factors on an alcohol in-patient unit. *British Journal of Psychiatry* 159:365-370, 1991.

Mahon L, Kempler B. Perceived effectiveness of therapeutic factors for ACOAs and non-ACOAs in heterogeneous psychotherapy groups. *Alcoholism Treatment Quarterly* 13:1-11, 1995.

Marcus D, Kashy D. The social relations model: A tool for group psychotherapy research. *Journal of Counseling Psychology* 42:383-389, 1995.

Margolis R, Zweben J. *Treating Patients with Alcohol and Other Drug Problems: An Integrated Approach.* Washington, DC: American Psychological Association, 1998.

McKay J, Alterman A, Cacciola J, Rutherford MJ, O'Brien CP, Koppenhaver J. Group counseling versus individualized relapse prevention aftercare following intensive outpatient treatment for cocaine dependence: Initial results. *Journal of Consulting and Clinical Psychology* 65:778-788, 1997.

McLellan A, Luborsky L, Woody G, O'Brien C. An improved diagnostic evaluation instrument for substance abuse patients. *Journal of Nervous and Mental Disease* 168:26-33, 1980.

McRoberts C, Burlingame G, Hoag M. Comparative efficacy of individual and group psychotherapy: A meta-analytic perspective. *Group Dynamics: Theory, Research, and Practice* 2:101-117, 1998.

Morgenstern J, Leeds J. Contemporary psychoanalytic theories of substance abuse: A disorder in search of a paradigm. *Psychotherapy* 30:194-206, 1993.

Olson R, Ganley R, Devine V, Dorsey G. Long-term effects of behavioral versus insight-oriented therapy with inpatient alcoholics. *Journal of Consulting and Clinical Psychology* 49:866-877, 1981.

Parloff M, Dies R. Group psychotherapy outcome research 1966-1975. *International Journal of Group Psychotherapy* 27:281-319, 1977.

Pfeiffer W, Feuerlein W, Brenk-Schulte E. The motivation of alcohol dependents to undergo treatment. *Drug and Alcohol Dependence* 29:87-95, 1991.

Piper W. Group psychotherapy research. In *Comprehensive Group Psychotherapy, Third Edition,* edited by Kaplan H, Sadock B. Baltimore, MD: Williams and Wilkins, 1993, pp. 673-682.

Price R, Burke A, D'Aunno T, Klingel DM, McCaughrin WC, Rafferty JA, Vaughn TE. Outpatient drug abuse treatment services, 1988: Results of a national survey. In *Improving Drug Abuse Treatment* (NIDA Research Monograph 106), edited by Pickens R, Leukefeld C, and Schuster C. Rockville, MD: National Institute on Drug Abuse, 1991, pp. 63-92.

Rose S, Tolman R, and Tallant S. Group process in cognitive-behavioral therapy. *Behavior Therapist* 8:71-75, 1985.

Rugel R. Addictions treatment in groups: A review of therapeutic factors. *Small Group Research* 22:475-491, 1991.

Satterfield J. Integrating group dynamics and cognitive-behavioral groups: A hybrid model. *Clinical Psychology: Science and Practice* 1:185-196, 1994.

Schmitz J, Oswald L, Jacks S, Rustin T, Rhoades HM, Grabowski J. Relapse prevention treatment for cocaine dependence: Group vs. individual format. *Addictive Behaviors* 22:405-418, 1997.

Sexton H. Exploring a psychotherapeutic change sequence: Relating process to intersessional and posttreatment outcome. *Journal of Consulting and Clinical Psychology* 61:128-136, 1993.

Stinchfield R, Owen P, Winters K. Group therapy for substance abuse: A review of the empirical research. In *Handbook of Group Psychotherapy,* edited by Fuhriman A, Burlingame G. New York: Wiley, 1994, pp. 458-488.

Swindle R, Peterson K, Paradise M, Moos R. Measuring substance abuse program treatment orientations: The drug and alcohol program treatment inventory. *Journal of Substance Abuse* 7:61-78, 1995.

Chapter 23

Group Psychotherapy in the Treatment of Addictive Disorders: Past, Present, and Future

Sheila B. Blume

INTRODUCTION: A PERSONAL NOTE

The use of group therapy in alcohol dependence treatment was the original impetus to my thirty-five-year career of specialization in addiction psychiatry. As a first-year psychiatric resident on the women's admission service of a large state hospital, I became interested in helping an alcoholic patient (Blume 1985). I discovered rapidly that although the hospital was structured for the care of my psychotic patients whose needs were well served, the hospital had little to offer this unhappy, desperate woman. I was furthermore appalled by a remarkable lack of interest in alcoholic patients on the part of my colleagues and supervisors, a point of view that they often combined with an attitude of distaste. In my efforts to help this patient, I read all I could find on the subject. I recall reading a recommendation for group therapy, perhaps in Marty Mann's *New Primer on Alcoholism* (Mann 1958). With the consent of my supervisors, I proceeded to establish a therapy group for alcoholic women on the inpatient service. Thus, by the time I was two or three months into my psychiatric training I had begun to specialize. Since I always needed patients for my group, female alcoholic admissions would be assigned to my care. I also traded patients with fellow residents who were glad to "unload" their alcoholics. I led the therapy group for about a year, and from those women I learned about both alcohol dependence and the therapeutic value of groups. Later, I became medical director of the first alcohol dependence treatment unit in New York's state hospital system (for men) and helped open the first unit for women. Group therapies, including psychodrama, interactive groups, and lecture/discussion sessions were an integral part of the state hospital units and of every other program with which I have been associated (Blume 1978; 1986; 1989).

Within the space of my own career in addiction medicine, I have witnessed many changes in the increased effectiveness and accessibility of treatment for addictive disorders accompanied by a progressive improvement in societal attitude. Acceptance of addictive disorders as diseases, by both the public and the medical profession, has increased. For example, the AMA first referred to alcohol dependence as an illness in 1956, then reaffirmed that alcohol dependence is a disease in 1966 and, in a 1987 policy statement, declared that both alcohol dependence and other drug dependencies are diseases and a legitimate part of medical practice (AMA 1992; APA 1995).

The addiction field underwent a remarkable proliferation of treatment programs and facilities, followed by a more recent contraction and limitation of addiction services. There have been advances in securing rights for addicted people, such as the federal confidentiality regulations that cover alcohol- and drug-related medical records and the inclusion of addicted people in the Americans with Disabilities Act. More recently, the public policy pendulum has swung away from guaranteeing such rights. An example is the exclusion of alcoholics and other addicts, as of January 1, 1997, from eligibility for federally funded Supplemental Security Income (SSI) and Social Security Disability Income (SSDI) benefits. History teaches us we can never assume that hard-fought victories on the public policy front are destined to be permanent parts of our society. We Americans tend to swing from pole to pole in our attitudes toward alcohol/drug use and addiction. One outstanding example is the policy debate over legalization versus prohibition of various psychoactive substances, a debate that has waxed and waned for the past 150 years.

Trying to foresee the future of addiction treatment is difficult. Almost the only trend we can predict with certainty is that the addictions, their treatment, their prevention, and the way addicted people and their families are accepted by society will continue to be subjects of heated public controversy.

GROUP THERAPY IN THE PAST

Origins

A collection of twenty-nine lectures presented at the second Yale Summer School of Alcohol Studies in 1944 makes no mention of group psychotherapy in alcohol dependence treatment (Yale 1945). In a 1959 textbook of psychiatry with substantial coverage of drug addictions (Nyswander 1959) and alcohol dependence (Zwerling and Rosenbaum 1959), neither of these chapters mentions group therapy. Dr. Marvin Block, chairman of the AMA's first committee on alcohol dependence, wrote a textbook on alcohol dependence treatment in 1962. This book mentions "psychotherapy" but only in an individual, doctor-patient setting (Block 1962). However, by 1967 a nationwide study of alcohol dependence treatment found, "group therapy is widely used in work with alcoholics—far more so, it appears, than with the general run of psychiatric patients. Furthermore, it seems to be widely used as a treatment of choice rather than as a substitute for individual therapy" (Glasscote et al. 1967, p. 15). In 1977, Doroff wrote in the series *The Biology of Alcoholism,* "In recent years there appears to have emerged a consensus among the scientific and professional community to the effect that among the various psychotherapies a group approach seems to offer the brightest prospect" (Doroff 1977, p. 236). In addition, as part of a transcription of a 1973 conference on drug abuse, Dr. Henry Brill wrote that inpatient drug treatment programs make heavy use of group therapy (Brill 1973).

Somehow, during this relatively short period of roughly ten years, group therapy became an accepted, and even a preferred, modality of addictive disorder treatment. It became so accepted that in many states group therapy is required by regulation for program licensure. How did this come to pass?

Most authors trace the origins of group therapy in the United States to the beginning of the twentieth century, when Dr. Joseph Pratt began to conduct health classes for tubercular patients in Boston. These classes employed lectures as well as self-presentations by recovering patients and supportive group interaction. During roughly the same period, Dr. Elwood Worcester, rector of Emmanuel Church in Boston, established the "Emmanuel Church health classes" or "Emmanuel Movement," using group methods. Worcester and his associate, Samuel McComb, worked with a physician, Dr. Isador H. Coriat, combining medical and spiritual principles. They took an interest in treating alcohol dependence and wrote on the subject as early as 1908. Another member of Emmanuel Movement was Courtney Baylor, who joined the group in 1912. Baylor, a recovered alcoholic, specialized in helping patients with drinking problems and further developed ideas about the interaction of physical and psychological factors in alcohol dependence. The treatment he and the Emmanuel group developed was taught to a line of other recovering alcoholics who became lay therapists, including Richard Peabody and his student, Francis Chambers. Chambers describes the treatment in 1939, however, as depending primarily on individual therapy and training in deep relaxation (Strecker and Chambers 1939). Group methods are not mentioned in his volume. It is interesting, however, that the origins of group therapy and alcohol dependence treatment were so closely linked (Blume 1977).

In Europe, Dr. J. L. Moreno experimented with group methods in his psychiatric practice in Vienna as early as 1910. Moreno coined both the terms "group therapy" and "group psychotherapy" in 1914 (Moreno 1975). During the early 1920s, Moreno began to develop the technique of psychodrama, a method that has been applied successfully to addictive disorders. In the 1967 textbook on alcohol dependence edited by Dr. Ruth Fox, a psychiatrist and first medical director of the National Council on Alcoholism, Hannah Weiner describes her four years of experience with the "Weiner-Fox group." This outpatient private practice model of alcohol dependence treatment combined or alternated formal group therapy sessions with psychodrama sessions (Weiner 1967). Weiner was a psychodrama student of J. L. Moreno and, in turn, trained other psychodramatists to work with alcoholics and addicts. Thus, the history of alcohol dependence treatment and that of the group therapies are further connected.

One of the most important movements to stimulate the use of group therapy in addiction treatment was the so-called "self-help" movement (perhaps better described as a mutual help movement) exemplified by Alcoholics Anonymous (AA), founded in 1935 (Wilson 1945). AA also had its historical analogs. The earliest of these was the Washington Temperance Society (also known as the Washingtonians) established by six drinkers in a Baltimore tavern in 1840 (Leonard 1997). This society specialized in helping inebriates to attain abstinence on a person-to-person basis. Its meetings featured recovering alcoholics sharing their experiences. There was a religious/spiritual component to the efforts of the Washingtonians, as well as help for the families of the "drunkards" they worked to "reform." The Washingtonians also established several hospitals for alcohol dependence treatment (Leonard 1997). The nature of their work sets the Washingtonians securely into the history of recovering alcoholics acting as "lay therapists" in alcohol dependence treatment.

Some writers have considered AA a type of therapy. For example, when Dr. Jerome Frank and Florence B. Powdermaker wrote their chapter on group therapy for Arieti's 1959 textbook of psychiatry they divided the current array of psychotherapeutic groups into five categories: didactic groups, therapeutic social clubs, repressive-inspirational groups, psychodrama, and free interaction groups. Alcoholics Anonymous was cited as a type of repressive-inspirational group. However, Frank and Powdermaker (1959) also wrote that the field of group psychotherapy was new and reflected many different methods and opinions, without a defining format.

The success of AA helped fuel a renewed interest in alcohol dependence treatment in the 1940s (APA 1995). One outgrowth was the development of the so-called "Minnesota Model" of treatment, which combined professional, medical, and psychologically based treatment with the twelve-step approach developed by AA. Minnesota model programs employed and trained recovering alcoholics as counselors (Spicer 1993). The three original Minnesota programs, Pioneer House founded in 1948, Hazelden founded in 1949 (McElrath 1987), and Wilmar State Hospital alcohol dependence program founded in 1950, all utilized lecture-discussion sessions (what Frank and Powdermaker called "didactic groups") to complement meetings of AA held on site. The Wilmar program also developed a "peer group" model, while Hazelden developed "repeaters' groups" for patients readmitted after a relapse (McElrath 1987).

The first therapeutic community (TC) for narcotic addicts, Synanon, was founded in 1958 by Charles Dederich, a recovered alcoholic. Dederich drew from his experience in AA but aimed, in Synanon, to develop a separate, self-sufficient, drug-free community of ex-addicts (APA 1995; Yablonsky 1965). Synanon was followed in the 1960s by other TCs such as Daytop that incorporated mental health therapeutic community principles and, unlike Synanon, emphasized rehabilitation and reintegration of the recovered addict into society (APA 1995). All of the early TCs relied heavily on group methods.

Early Models

Several authors have commented that early writings on group therapy were long on description of techniques but short on theory (Doroff 1977; Frank and Powdermaker 1959; Vannicelli 1992). Group therapies were often developed in a trial-and-error manner, much like my own experience (Blume 1978), and based on general principles of psychodynamics, the principles of group interaction, and the specific dynamics of the addictive disorders.

Doroff's 1977 review of group methods in alcohol dependence treatment cites nine papers from the 1940s and 1950s that describe a range of groups, including a group made up of alcoholic merchant seamen who were judged unsuitable for AA or refused to attend, selected alcoholic outpatients, a private practice alcohol dependence model, and group therapies in specialized inpatient treatment units.

Several authors made an attempt to apply psychoanalytic principles and/or techniques to the group. Others had unusual methods of encouraging support and minimizing hostile transference, one serving tea and cakes at the halfway point of the two-hour session. Another format was the outpatient lecture-discussion group format used by the "Yale Plan" Clinics developed by the Yale Center of Alcohol Studies in the early 1940s.

As mentioned earlier, Weiner and Fox alternated group therapy and psychodrama outpatient sessions (Weiner 1967), while the three original "Minnesota Model" programs combined the use of recovering alcoholics as group leaders, peer-led groups, and lecture-discussions of the principles of AA in residential settings (McElrath 1987; Spicer 1993).

Groups were also the basic therapeutic vehicle at Bridge House, a residential rehabilitation program for alcoholics established by the New York City Department of Welfare in 1945. This program was based on an educational model of recovery developed by a New York attorney, Edward McGoldrick Jr. McGoldrick, a recovering alcoholic himself, rejected the AA twelve-step model, stating that alcoholics need "information rather than reformation." His groups featured both didactic presentations and group interaction.

Group hypnotherapy was one of three methods tested in 1950-1952 at Winter Veterans Administration Hospital in Topeka, Kansas (Wallerstein 1957). In this study, one of the earliest to compare the efficacy of competing models of alcohol dependence treatment, 178 male patients were semirandomly assigned to receive antabuse, conditioned reflex therapy, group hypnotherapy, or milieu therapy. The patients assigned to "milieu therapy" were treated in small psychotherapy groups twice weekly, along with some individual counseling. After a follow-up period of two years, the antabuse-treated patients did best, although all groups improved significantly. The authors believed their results would have been improved by careful patient-treatment matching, which was prevented by their study methodology.

A 1965 survey of U.S. alcohol dependence treatment programs was cosponsored by the American Psychiatric Association and the National Association for Mental Health, and funded by the National Institute of Mental Health (Glasscote et al. 1967). Fifty-six inpatient and outpatient alcohol dependence facilities were contacted and the authors conducted site visits to eleven of the forty-two that returned the survey instrument. The four state inpatient rehabilitation programs described (in Georgia, West Virginia, Florida, and Connecticut), all relied heavily on group methods, while the two general hospital detoxification programs did not.

The outpatient clinics visited varied in their use of groups. For example, the Massachusetts General Hospital clinic favored individual over group therapy. The Santa Clara clinic in California offered "either individual or group psychotherapy," including a couples' group and a group for wives of male alcoholic patients. One community mental health center was visited (San Mateo County). Its outpatient service offered both individual and group therapy to alcoholics.

"Encounter" group sessions, based on the analysis of interaction in the "here and now," became a basic ingredient of therapeutic community drug treatment as TCs developed during the 1960s. These methods were undoubtedly influenced by the human potential movement of the 1960s and 1970s. One technique to emerge from this movement, Transactional Analysis, also had some application to alcohol dependence treatment.

Although therapeutic communities grew in popularity in the public sector for the residential treatment of so-called "hard-core drug addicts," the private (and to a lesser extent public) sector developed and expanded the residential Minnesota Model in many parts of the country. Originally developed for AA-based alcohol dependence treatment, the facilities expanded to include chemical dependence, treating other drug addictions as well (Spicer 1993). This expansion was originally a result of treating a growing number of alcoholics who were dependent on other drugs in addition to alcohol. However, by incorporating on-site meetings of Narcotics Anonymous (NA), the model could be applied to drug addicts who were not also alcoholics. NA, which began in California in 1953, adapted the twelve steps of AA to drug dependence (Narcotics Anonymous 1982). Cocaine Anonymous (CA), a twelve-step group specifically for cocaine addicts, is also incorporated into Minnesota Model programs.

GROUP THERAPY IN THE PRESENT

This book and others (e.g., Vannicelli 1992) attest to the current popularity of group psychotherapy in the treatment of addicted patients and their "significant others." Group therapies are routinely discussed in textbooks on addictive disorders published in the 1980s and 1990s (e.g., Bratter and Forrest 1985; Frances and Miller 1991; Galanter and Kleber 1994; Lowinson, Ruiz and Millman 1992; Miller 1991; 1994; 1997; Washton and Gold 1987).

According to the results of the last National Drug and Alcoholism Treatment Unit Survey (NDATUS), 944,000 Americans were in treatment in specialty addiction treatment facilities on a single day (October 1) in 1994 (SAMHSA 1996). The vast majority (87 percent or 823,000 clients) were in outpatient rehabilitation. Seventy-five percent of clients were in outpatient drug-free programs and 12 percent in methadone maintenance. An additional 11 percent of the total clients (107,000) were in inpatient or residential rehabilitation programs. It is safe to guess that the vast majority of these 944,000 clients were receiving some form of group therapy specifically geared to addiction treatment.

However, the NDATUS figures do not tell the whole story. NDATUS only supplies data from the 11,716 specialty alcohol dependence/drug addiction programs reporting. Several studies have shown that far more adults with addictive disorders are treated in settings outside of the specialty addiction treatment system than within it (APA 1995). A greater proportion are seen by mental health professionals in private practice, mental health clinics, health plan settings, and in general medical settings. In fact, only 11 percent of individuals with substance use disorders identified in the Epidemiologic Catchment Area (ECA) study who received any help during the previous year were treated in the specialty addiction treatment system (Narrow et al. 1993).

A more recent study, the National Comorbidity Survey, focused specifically on persons aged fifteen to fifty-four in the general population (Kessler et al. 1996). Between 8 and 41 percent of subjects with an active addictive disorder received some kind of treatment in the previous year, depending on whether there was comorbidity with an affective or anxiety disorder. Persons with comorbid disorders were more likely to receive treatment. As in the ECA study, more patients were treated in the mental health treatment system than in specialty addiction programs. Remarkably, this disproportion was evident for subjects who suffered from alcohol or drug abuse or dependence without comorbid psychiatric disorder, as well as for those with affective and/or anxiety disorders. It is difficult to estimate what proportion of the alcoholics and addicts treated outside of the specialty addiction treatment system are likely to be receiving addiction-focused group therapies. In fact, it is possible that many are not receiving addiction treatment at all. We cannot estimate how many addicted persons have been shunted into non-addiction-specific treatment because of a shortage or maldistribution of addiction programs, the lack of appropriate insurance, or patient preference based on societal stigma. Clearly, a large unmet need exists for addiction treatment in general, and for addiction-specific group therapy in particular.

In spite of this unmet need, American society in the late 1990s has witnessed the closing or downsizing of many addiction treatment programs, particularly in the private sector. For instance, the National Association of Addiction Treatment Providers, the trade association for most of the freestanding private inpatient addiction programs, reported that its membership had dropped from 400 in the early 1990s to 250 by 1997 (Alcoholism and Drug Abuse Weekly 1997). Managed care, changes in health insurance, and the demand for cost control have been blamed for this downsizing.

The influences of managed care and other changes in the rapidly shifting American health care system are discussed in Chapter 1.

These changes, along with decreases in entitlement benefits for individuals suffering from addictive disorders and the failure of public funding to meet the addiction treatment needs of the uninsured and underinsured, threaten to widen the gap between the treatment requirements of this population and society's ability to provide specific services. However, even in this climate of inadequate support, group therapies continue to thrive.

ETHICAL CONSIDERATIONS

The current popularity of the group psychotherapies in addiction treatment raises important ethical questions that bear consideration before policy recommendations for the further adoption of group methods are made. The most important ethical problem in all group psychotherapies is confidentiality. The only patient for whom group therapy is absolutely contraindicated is a blackmailer. The risk of such a patient taking advantage of sensitive personal information revealed in the group setting to extort money or favors from another group member is a real hazard, yet most programs assign addicted patients to groups without giving much thought to their antisocial histories. Although patients may be cautioned before beginning group treatment that certain sensitive issues or experiences should be reserved for individual sessions, the level of trust generated in a well-functioning group will encourage self-revelation. "Getting rid of one's secrets" is a highly valued behavior in most therapy groups, while "holding back" is considered an affront to the other members. For some alcoholics and addicts, the very fact of their membership in the group (that is, their participation in addiction treatment) could be used against them in damaging ways.

Recognizing the special sensitivity of alcohol and drug treatment, the U.S. Congress passed legislation in the mid 1970s to establish special confidentiality protection for alcohol- and drug-related patient records. Although these regulations and the penalties for disclosure apply to the group leader, the treatment facility, and the medical record, they do not bind fellow patients to secrecy. Group members are generally told the confidentiality rules of the therapy group before and during their treatment. However, the only constraints on their behavior are their desire to be accepted by the group and, perhaps, revealed secrets of their own that they wish to keep private. These confidentiality problems are experienced most urgently by group members in sensitive occupations such as airplane pilots, practicing lawyers, law enforcement personnel, and health professionals. For such patients, a license and, therefore, a livelihood may be jeopardized by an unauthorized disclosure.

Physicians in treatment have a particularly difficult situation, since some state laws require physicians to report colleagues whom they know or suspect to be impaired to the state licensing board. Although federal confidentiality regulations protect the patient from professional group leader disclosure without consent, these regulations do not cover their fellow physicians who are group members. In many cases, federal and state laws are in conflict. These problems are not merely theoretical. A survey of forty-five state impaired physician programs and the group therapists who work with addicted physicians in these programs revealed many difficult dilemmas (Roback et al. 1996). Although nearly all group leaders discussed confidentiality rules in the group, the fifty-one respondents reported over 300 incidents of breaches of confidentiality by other group members. Most of these involved identifying a member of the group to an outsider, although revelation of illegal activities, sexual behavior, and substance-related behavior were also reported. Twenty-seven percent of the group leaders had been subpoenaed to testify about one or more group members. However, none reported any instances of one group member being subpoenaed to testify about another. All group leaders reported that their physician-patients were intensely concerned about confidentiality. It is reasonable to assume that nonphysician patients have the same concern.

What can be done about this problem? First of all, group therapy should not be the only form of treatment offered to addicted patients. Individual therapy may be more appropriate for some who are either at risk for victimizing fellow group members or have special personal concerns. With those patients to whom group treatment is recommended, the therapist should make clear what kinds of revelations might be better handled in an individual consultation. Individual sessions should be available to all group members as needed. Reluctance to be treated in a group should not always be interpreted as resistance. Second, federal and state law can be changed to protect group members from damaging disclosures by others in the therapy group, and to protect group members from legal compulsion to testify about the contents of group therapy sessions.

GROUP THERAPY IN THE FUTURE

Difficult as it is to predict the final outcome of the many drastic changes taking place in the provision of health care, it is safe to prophesy that the need and demand for addiction treatment will not go away. If for no other reason than the burden placed on the health care system by the serious physical consequences of alcohol dependence and other addictions (APA 1995), and the comorbidity with other psychiatric disorders (Kessler et al. 1996), addiction treatment will survive. Shrinking resources allocated to addiction treatment will require that such treatment be provided in the most cost-effective manner possible. This need makes the group therapies seem even more attractive. However, several important factors must be considered.

The first is if self-help, either in the form of twelve-step programs or other alternatives, can be substituted for professional treatment. Asked another way, is AA a group therapy? If the answer is yes, can a self-help group referral, at no cost to the insurer, be considered adequate treatment? While I was New York State Commissioner for Alcoholism (1979-1983), a business group had issued an "alternative" state budget proposal which, among other things, removed all state funding for alcohol dependence treatment. The report stated that since AA was the best "treatment" for alcohol dependence and AA was free, the millions of dollars allocated for treatment could and should be discontinued. Similar arguments are still being made (e.g., Bower 1997).

Self-help should not be considered group therapy. An adequate definition of group therapy is the one offered by Sadock (1975, p. 1850): "Group psychotherapy is a form of treatment in which carefully selected emotionally ill persons are placed into a group, guided by a trained therapist, for the purpose of helping one another effect personality change." Any such definition contains at least four elements:

1. professional leadership,
2. evaluation (including diagnosis and assessment of severity),

3. a clinical decision based on this evaluation that group therapy is indicated for this individual patient, and
4. professional responsibility/accountability for the individual's care.

Added to these elements is a professional, ethical responsibility for providing or referring for such other care as is needed by the group member and for maintaining confidentiality. None of these elements is present in a self-help group.

Self-help fellowships are an important adjunct to professional treatment. Voluntary AA participation has been shown to reduce health care costs for alcoholic patients (Humphreys and Moos 1996), so that the combination of treatment and self-help makes good sense. However, we should be clear in our own thinking that although they function through group meetings, self-help fellowships are not group therapies, and should not be substituted for professional treatment.

Second, we should reexamine the use of mandates or requirements for group participation in treatment. A review of the confidentiality considerations discussed in the previous section should remind us that groups cannot be looked upon as a "one size fits all" treatment for addictive disorders. The U.S. Supreme Court ruled in 1997 that alcoholics in the criminal justice system cannot be mandated to attend AA or denied privileges if they refuse to attend, based on the religious/spiritual nature of the program (Project MATCH Research Group 1997). No similar ruling has been made concerning the privacy issues involved in AA or in mandated group treatment. However, in 1996 a man was found guilty of homicide based on testimony from fellow AA members that he had confessed to the crime at meetings. The defendant's claim of privilege for material discussed at AA meetings was not accepted by the court.

The final consideration needed to predict the future of group therapy in addiction treatment is the urgent need for research. Considering the popularity of group therapy in treating addicts, surprisingly little outcome research has examined specific group methods. For example, the first results of Project MATCH were reported in 1997 (Project MATCH Research Group 1997). This eight-year, $27 million research study was funded by the National Institute on Alcohol Abuse and Alcoholism. More than 1,700 adult alcoholic outpatients were randomly assigned to one of three outpatient treatment modalities, and treatment outcome at one year was assessed in relation to several patient variables expected to predict response to each specific treatment (i.e., patient-treatment matching). The project found little evidence for the value of such matching, although all of the treatments were effective. All of the modalities studied were individual treatments, and no group methods were evaluated. Unless researchers and those who award grants are convinced of the necessity to study group therapies, the future choice of treatment for the addictive disorders may well be based on considerations of cost alone, rather than sound knowledge of patient needs and treatment effectiveness. Thus, the outlook for group therapy in the future will be to a great degree dependent on the outlook for addiction research today.

In addition to research, training in the group therapies for addiction treatment will be needed to ensure the future of this method. As training funds become more and more restricted, training in group methods will have to compete with other training needs. Let us hope that our national policies support both research and training in this area, in order to ensure continued improvement in our treatment capability.

REFERENCES

Alcoholism and Drug Abuse Weekly. New executive director expects to increase NAATP's profile. *Alcoholism and Drug Abuse Weekly* 9(2):1,4, January 13, 1997.

American Medical Association. Policy 95.983—*Drug Dependencies As Diseases: Policy Compendium.* Chicago, IL: American Medical Association, 1992.

American Psychiatric Association. *Psychiatric Services for Addicted Patients: A Task Force Report of the American Psychiatric Association.* Washington, DC: American Psychiatric Association, 1995.

Block MA. *Alcoholism: Its Facets and Phases.* New York: The John Day Company, 1962.

Blume SB. Role of the recovered alcoholic in the treatment of alcoholism. In *The Biology of Alcoholism: Treatment and Rehabilitation of the Chronic Alcoholic,* Volume 5, edited by Kissin B, Begleiter H. New York: Plenum Press, 1977, pp. 545-565.

Blume SB. Group psychotherapy in the treatment of alcoholism. In *Practical Approaches to Alcoholism Psychotherapy,* edited by Zimberg S, Wallace J, Blume SB. New York: Plenum Press, 1978, pp. 63-76.

Blume SB. Alcoholism rehabilitation: Getting involved—A memoir of the 60's. In *Alcoholism Interventions: A Historical and Socio-Cultural Approach,* edited by

Strug D, Priyadarsimi S, Hyman M. Binghamton, NY: The Haworth Press, 1985, pp. 75-80.

Blume SB. Treatment for the addictions: Alcoholism, drug dependence and compulsive gambling in a psychiatric setting. *Journal of Substance Abuse Treatment* 3:131-133, 1986.

Blume SB. Treatment for the addictions in a psychiatric setting. *British Journal of Addiction* 84:727-729, 1989.

Bower B. Alcoholics synonymous: Heavy drinkers of all stripes may get comparable help from a variety of therapies. *Science News* 151:62-63, January 25, 1997.

Bratter TE, Forrest GG (eds.). *Alcoholism and Substance Abuse: Strategies for Clinical Intervention.* New York: Free Press, 1985.

Brill H. Treatment of drug addiction and abuse. In *Drug Abuse in Industry,* edited by Carone PA, Krinsky LW. Springfield, IL: Charles C Thomas, 1973, pp. 136-141.

Doroff DR. Group psychotherapy in alcoholism. In *The Biology of Alcoholism: Treatment and Rehabilitation of the Chronic Alcoholic,* Volume 5, edited by Kissin B, Begleiter H. New York: Plenum Press, 1977, pp. 235-258.

Frances RJ, Miller SI (eds.). *Clinical Textbook of Addictive Disorders.* New York: Guilford Press, 1991.

Frank JD, Powdermaker FB. Group psychotherapy. In *American Handbook of Psychiatry,* Volume 2, edited by Arieti S. New York: Basic Books, Inc., 1959, pp. 1362-1374.

Galanter M, Kleber HD (eds.). *Textbook of Substance Abuse Treatment.* Washington, DC: American Psychiatric Press, Inc., 1994.

Glasscote RM, Plaut TF, Hammersley DW, O'Neill FJ, Chafetz ME, Cumming E. *The Treatment of Alcoholism: A Study of Programs and Problems.* Washington, DC: American Psychiatric Association, 1967.

Humphreys K, Moos RH. Reduced substance-abuse-related health care costs among voluntary participants in alcoholics anonymous. *Psychiatric Services* 47(7):709-713, July 1996.

Kessler RC, Nelson CB, McGonagle KA, Liu J, Swartz M, Blazer DG. The epidemiology of co-occurring addictive and mental disorders: Implications for prevention and service utilization. *American Journal of Orthopsychiatry* 66:17-31, 1996.

Leonard EC. The treatment of Philadelphia inebriates: From temperance reform to "secret cure." *American Journal on Addictions* 6:1-10, 1997.

Lowinson JH, Ruiz P, Millman RB (eds.). *Substance Abuse: A Comprehensive Textbook,* Second Edition. Baltimore, MD: Williams and Wilkins, 1992.

Mann M. *New Primer on Alcoholism.* New York: Holt, Rinehart and Winston, 1958.

McElrath D. *Hazelden. A Spiritual Odyssey.* Center City, MN: Hazelden-Pittman Archives Press, 1987.

Miller NS (ed.). *Comprehensive Handbook of Drug and Alcohol Addiction.* New York: Marcel Dekker, Inc., 1991.

Miller NS (ed.). *Principles of Addiction Medicine.* Chevy Chase, MD: American Society of Addiction Medicine, Inc., 1994.

Miller NS (ed.). *The Principles and Practices of Addictions in Psychiatry.* Philadelphia: W.B. Saunders Company, 1997.

Moreno JL. Psychodrama. In *Comprehensive Textbook of Psychiatry II,* edited by Freedman AM, Kaplan HI, Sadock BJ. Baltimore, MD: Williams and Wilkins Company, 1975, pp. 1891-1909.

Narcotics Anonymous. *Narcotics Anonymous.* Van Nuys, CA: World Service Office, Inc., 1982.

Narrow WE, Regier DA, Rae DS, Manderscheid RW, Locke BS. Use of services by persons with mental and addictive disorders: Findings from the National Institute of Mental Health Epidemiologic Catchment Area program. *Archives of General Psychiatry* 50:95-107, 1993.

Nyswander M. Drug addictions. In *American Handbook of Psychiatry,* Volume 1, edited by Arieti S. New York: Basic Books, Inc., 1959, pp. 614-622.

Project MATCH Research Group: Matching alcoholism treatments to client heterogeneity: Project MATCH posttreatment drinking outcomes. *Journal of Studies on Alcohol* 58:7-29, 1997.

Roback HB, Moore RF, Waterhouse GJ, Martin PR. Confidentiality dilemmas in group psychotherapy with substance-dependent physicians. *American Journal of Psychiatry* 153:1250-1260, 1996.

Sadock BJ. Group psychotherapy. In *Comprehensive Textbook of Psychiatry,* edited by Freedman AM, Kaplan HI, Sadock BJ. Baltimore, MD: Williams and Wilkins, 1975, pp. 1850-1876.

SAMHSA. *National Drug and Alcoholism Treatment Unit Survey (NDATUS): Data for 1994 and 1980-1994.* Advance Report Number 13. Rockville, MD: Department of Health and Human Services, June 1996.

Spicer J. *The Minnesota Model: The Evolution of the Multidisciplinary Approach to Addiction Recovery.* Center City, MN: Hazelden Foundation, 1993.

Strecker EA, Chambers FT. *Alcohol: One Man's Meat.* New York: Macmillan, 1939.

Supreme Court rejects appeal in coerced AA attendance case. *Substance Abuse Letter* 3(14):3, January 17, 1997.

Vannicelli M. *Removing the Roadblocks: Group Psychotherapy with Substance Abusers and Family Members.* New York: Guilford Press, 1992.

Wallerstein RS (ed.). *Hospital Treatment of Alcoholism.* Basic Books, Inc., 1957.

Washton AM, Gold MS (eds.). *Cocaine: A Clinician's Handbook.* New York: Guilford Press, 1987.

Weiner HB. Psychodramatic treatment for the alcoholic. In *Alcoholism: Behavioral Research Therapeutic Approaches,* edited by Fox R. New York: Springer Publishing Company, Inc., 1967, pp. 218-233.

Wilson W. The fellowship of Alcoholics Anonymous, in Yale University Center of Alcohol Studies: Alcohol, Science and Society. New Haven, CT: *Quarterly Journal of Studies on Alcohol,* 1945, reprinted Westport, Greenwood Press, 1945, pp. 461-473.

Yablonsky L. *Synanon: The Tunnel Back.* Baltimore, MD: Penguin, 1965.

Yale University Center of Alcohol Studies. Alcohol, Science and Society. New Haven: *Quarterly Journal of Studies on Alcohol,* 1945, reprinted Westport, Greenwood Press, 1945.

Zwerling I, Rosenbaum M. Alcoholic addiction and personality (nonpsychotic conditions). In *American Handbook of Psychiatry,* Volume 1, edited by Arieti S. New York: Basic Books, Inc., 1959, pp. 623-644.

Index

Page numbers followed by the letter "b" indicate boxed material; those followed by the letter "i" indicate illustrations; and those followed by the letter "t" indicate tables.

Order a copy of this book with this form or online at:
http://www.haworthpressinc.com/store/product.asp?sku=4717

THE GROUP THERAPY OF SUBSTANCE ABUSE

_____in hardbound at $79.95 (ISBN: 0-7890-1781-4)

_____in softbound at $49.95 (ISBN: 0-7890-1782-2)

COST OF BOOKS_____

OUTSIDE USA/CANADA/
MEXICO: ADD 20%____

POSTAGE & HANDLING_____
(US: $4.00 for first book & $1.50
for each additional book)
Outside US: $5.00 for first book
& $2.00 for each additional book)

SUBTOTAL_____

in Canada: add 7% GST____

STATE TAX____
(NY, OH & MIN residents, please
add appropriate local sales tax)

FINAL TOTAL____
(If paying in Canadian funds,
convert using the current
exchange rate, UNESCO
coupons welcome.)

☐ **BILL ME LATER:** ($5 service charge will be added)
(Bill-me option is good on US/Canada/Mexico orders only;
not good to jobbers, wholesalers, or subscription agencies.)

☐ Check here if billing address is different from
shipping address and attach purchase order and
billing address information.

Signature_____

☐ **PAYMENT ENCLOSED: $**_____

☐ **PLEASE CHARGE TO MY CREDIT CARD.**

☐ Visa ☐ MasterCard ☐ AmEx ☐ Discover
☐ Diner's Club ☐ Eurocard ☐ JCB

Account #_____

Exp. Date_____

Signature_____

Prices in US dollars and subject to change without notice.

NAME_____

INSTITUTION_____

ADDRESS_____

CITY_____

STATE/ZIP_____

COUNTRY_____ COUNTY (NY residents only)_____

TEL_____ FAX_____

E-MAIL_____

May we use your e-mail address for confirmations and other types of information? ☐ Yes ☐ No
We appreciate receiving your e-mail address and fax number. Haworth would like to e-mail or fax special
discount offers to you, as a preferred customer. **We will never share, rent, or exchange your e-mail address
or fax number.** We regard such actions as an invasion of your privacy.

Order From Your Local Bookstore or Directly From
The Haworth Press, Inc.
10 Alice Street, Binghamton, New York 13904-1580 • USA
TELEPHONE: 1-800-HAWORTH (1-800-429-6784) / Outside US/Canada: (607) 722-5857
FAX: 1-800-895-0582 / Outside US/Canada: (607) 722-6362
E-mail: getinfo@haworthpressinc.com
PLEASE PHOTOCOPY THIS FORM FOR YOUR PERSONAL USE.
www.HaworthPress.com

BOF02